5

Name **Figen Yildiz**

Nurse Practitioner Certification Exam Review & Advanced Practice Update

FAMILY & ADULT-GERONTOLOGY PROGRAM

Developed by:
Margaret A. Fitzgerald, DNP, FNP-BC, NP-C, FAANP, CSP, FAAN, DCC, FNAP
President, Fitzgerald Health Education Associates, North Andover, MA
Family Nurse Practitioner, Greater Lawrence (MA) Family Health Center
Editorial Board Member, *The Nurse Practitioner*, *Prescriber's Letter*,
   American Nurse Today
Member, Pharmacy and Therapeutics Committee, Neighborhood Health Plan,
   Boston, MA

Presented by:
Margaret A. Fitzgerald, DNP, FNP-BC, NP-C, FAANP, CSP, FAAN, DCC, FNAP
Susan Feeney, DNP, NP-C, FNP-BC
Louise McDevitt, MS, ACNP-BC, ANP-BC, FNP-BC, FAANP
Sally K. Miller, PhD, AGACNP, AGPCNP, FNP-BC, FAANP
Brett Badgley Snodgrass, MS, FNP-C, CPE, FAANP
Monica Tombasco, MS, MSNA, FNP-BC, CRNA
Wendy L. Wright, MS, ANP-BC, FNP-BC, FAANP, FAAN

Fitzgerald Health Education Associates
Website: fhea.com • Email: review@fhea.com
85 Flagship Drive, North Andover, MA 01845-6154
Phone: 1.800.927.5380 • Fax: 978.794.2455

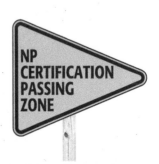

STATEMENT OF LIABILITY

The information contained in this workbook has been thoroughly researched and checked for accuracy. However, clinical practice is a dynamic process and new information becomes available daily. Prudent practice dictates that the clinician consult further sources prior to applying information, whether in printed or verbal form, obtained from this program. Fitzgerald Health Education Associates disclaims any liability, loss, injury, or damage incurred as a consequence, directly or indirectly, of the use and application of any of the contents of this volume or information given in the presentation.

While taking a preparation course such as *NP Certification Exam Review and Advanced Practice Update Course* is useful and will help the candidate prepare for the certification exam, many factors influence successful completion of the certification process. Fitzgerald Health Education Associates disclaims any liability, loss, injury, or damage incurred as a consequence, directly or indirectly, of the use and application of any of the contents of this volume or information given in the presentation with respect to the results the candidate achieves on the certification exam(s).

Taking, completing, and passing a Fitzgerald practice examination does not in any way result in or guarantee passing actual nurse practitioner certification exams offered by various certification organizations. Fitzgerald practice examinations are designed to be an assessment tool of one's strengths and weaknesses requiring further study. They are not designed to be used as a study guide. Fitzgerald offers several products for study and examination preparation, including printed study guides, live, online, and recorded review seminars that provide help in preparing for the certification exams.

All website addresses cited in this document were active when published. Many are sources created and maintained by organizations other than FHEA; in these instances, the websites are subject to change over time and out of our control.

Acknowledgements:
Content contributors: Susan Feeney, DNP, NP-C, FNP-BC; Teresa (Tess) Judge-Ellis, DNP, FNP-BC, PMHNP-BC, FAANP; Sally K. Miller, PhD, AGACNP, AGPCNP, FNP-BC, FAANP

ISBN 978-1-57942583-8

Last digit indicates print number: 10 9 8 7 6 5 4

Editor: June Kuznicki, MBA

Fitzgerald Health Education Associates
85 Flagship Drive
North Andover, MA 01845-6154

VM (978) 794-8366 • FAX (978) 794-2455
email: review@fhea.com
Website: fhea.com

Developing a Study Plan for the NP Certification Exam

Margaret A. Fitzgerald, DNP, FNP-BC, NP-C, FAANP, CSP, FAAN, DCC, FNAP

As a newly prepared nurse practitioner, you are to be congratulated on your success to date. After completing a rigorous graduate program, your days of study are not yet over but continue with a new focus. You need to continue to develop, expand, and refine your NP knowledge base to assure success with certification. But how do you do this? Here is advice I provide in response to commonly asked questions about preparing for the certification exam.

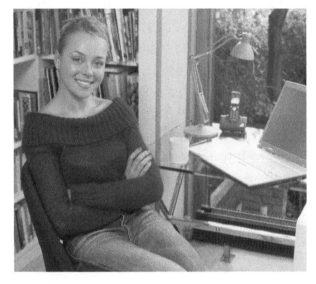

In preparing for the NP certification exam, where should I start?

Start with reviewing the information on the exam content outline, available at your certification agency's website. Make a list of the areas where you feel your knowledge base is secure and where just reviewing material to refresh your memory will likely suffice. Make a second list where you identify areas of weakness and topics where you need to concentrate your review. Since you have taken the Fitzgerald NP review course, you are likely aware that the content of certain parts of the program was truly review, whereas other sections revealed areas where you need to expand your knowledge base. Knowing what areas you need to focus on helps you decide how to allocate your study time.

As you study, please keep in mind that the NP certification examination is a test to see if you possess and can utilize the knowledge base to be a safe entry-level nurse practitioner. As a result, consider that certification tests your knowledge of the following:

- *Why* a patient is at risk for a problem.
- *How* a clinical problem has developed.
- *What* is the most likely clinical presentation of the condition?
- *Why* a given intervention is effective.
- *How* that intervention works.
- *What* is the most likely clinical outcome?
- *Why* this clinical problem is of significance to the overall healthcare system.

Therefore, a poor approach to preparing for the exam and practice is to memorize information, so you know what to do but not why you are doing it. For both the exam room and as part of the larger healthcare system, a better approach to knowledge building is to understand concepts and apply knowledge so you know what to do and why you are doing it. The Fitzgerald *Nurse Practitioner Certification Examination Review and Advanced Practice Update*, with hundreds of practice questions, prepares you in the why, how, and what of NP practice, while helping you to build your knowledge base and prepare you for success on the NP boards.

Another pitfall is not taking the time to complete the entire online portion of the Fitzgerald Health review course. The online presentations are an integral part of the Fitzgerald *Nurse Practitioner Certification Examination Review and Advanced Practice Update* course. Be sure to utilize the resources available through your NPXpert learning portal:

- Review the important additional study resources mentioned at the end of review course chapters.
- Review the questions from the review course, bonus questions, and images from the Fitzgerald Health certification course to help reinforce your learning.
- Wrap up your study with the 150-question practice exam. Complete your course evaluation and print your CE certificate.

How much time should I allow to prepare for my examination?

This issue of time needed for certification preparation is unique to each exam candidate. That said, one of the major pitfalls in study is the failure to put aside the time to prepare. Map out the demands on your time in the first months after completing your NP program, including work hours, family, personal, and professional commitments, as well as time you have perhaps set aside for a well-deserved vacation. After doing this, set up a schedule of study time, allotting a greater amount of time to areas where you have a knowledge deficit and less to areas where you only need to refresh your knowledge base. Make sure you cover all areas listed as possible exam content. Set your exam date only after a period of well-planned, systematic certification-focused study that is focused on increasing your knowledge base and honing your clinical decision-making skills.

How should I organize my study time?

You've taken the first step by selecting the Fitzgerald Health Education NP review course as part of your study for the NP boards. The Fitzgerald Method of NP review begins with a summary of the vast body of knowledge needed for evidence-based NP practice and for successfully passing the NP boards. This summary is followed by sample practice questions to help you hone your clinical decision-making and test-taking skills.

Allow a minimum of 4 to 6 weeks of planned study *after* you complete the review course to maximize your likelihood of success on this important high-stakes exam. Sit down with your calendar and develop a study schedule, in 2- to 3-hour blocks, 6 days per week, giving yourself one day off a week so you do not feel trapped or overwhelmed. Then analyze what you have already reviewed, noting your stronger and weaker points. For example, if you really understand all the cardiac information and can apply this knowledge, and the NP review course was truly review, then you are likely set in this portion of your study. If you are still struggling with thyroid issues, then you know you need additional study in that area. While this seems obvious, often people who are studying for a high-stakes exam gravitate back to the familiar as it is comforting to review what you know. Mark the topics you will review in your schedule; for example:

Monday night, 7–9 PM, study thyroid disease using the book *Nurse Practitioner Certification Examination and Practice Preparation* (5th edition) by Dr. Margaret Fitzgerald and my course materials from the *Fitzgerald Health NP Certification Examination Review and Advanced Practice Update.*

Tuesday, 4–7 PM, review health promotion using my class notes from my NP program, as well as the Fitzgerald Health workbook and online resources.

How do I approach my study for the NP boards?

Setting up a system of study can further enhance the success of a review or study session. One method is the *SQ4R* system:

- The study information is **S**urveyed to establish goals.
- **Q**uestions about the information are formulated. What do you need to learn about this topic so that you have

a firm grasp on the concepts? Are you able to consider the pathophysiology of a condition, how this manifests in the clinical presentation, and how a given intervention modifies or corrects the disease process?

- **R**ead to answer these questions. Study background information so you can correctly answer the questions above.
- **R**ecite the responses to the original questions. Consider w**R**iting up a short summary of what you have learned from your study.
- **R**eview to see if the original goals were met.

At the end of each session, after securing your knowledge base, use the practice questions from Fitzgerald Health to test where you are in your learning. Practice exam questions are a great way to wrap up your study on a topic and demonstrate your mastery of the information. Post-study, you should be scoring in the 85%+ range on practice questions. *Use practice questions to wrap up, not start, your NP certification review.* If you are not scoring well on practice questions, you need additional study of the content area associated with those questions.

What about forming a study group?

Study groups can be helpful and are a terrific vehicle for sharing information and resources. Alternatively, study groups can yield a poor return on time invested if all members are not similarly committed. I hear about study groups that meet in person as well as groups who use Skype or some other service to get together online. Here are some guidelines for forming a successful study group.

- All group members must treat attendance and participation as they would any other professional commitment, such as work or school.
- Well in advance, set a schedule, a place and time to meet, as well as a topic for the meeting.
- Plan a start and end time, with a clear objective for the session.
- Study groups usually work best when a group member volunteers to research and present information on a subject according to a predetermined schedule. The presentation is typically followed with a discussion of the issue and review of sample exam questions and rationales for the correct response.
- The leader of a given session should also assume responsibility for keeping the discussion on track, facilitating the efficient use of time and resources.
- In order to help avoid having the group deteriorate into a chat session, plan for a short period of socialization following high-yield study sessions.

Here is an example of a session planned by a highly successful study group with three members, Sarah, Ben, and Helena:

"The session will start at 7 PM and end at 9 PM with the objective of identifying the clinical presentation, assessment, and intervention in community acquired pneumonia. Sarah is the presenter and also group leader for the evening and is responsible for keeping us on track. A social period from 9– 9:30 PM will follow. We will meet at Helena 's apartment. Ben is responsible for refreshments."

Should I take additional preparation examinations?

I am often asked this question, and taking a prep test prior to study may help you identify areas of weakness that require further study. Attempting to build your knowledge base by taking practice tests does not work and is often cited as the main study method by NPs who fail boards. Taking additional prep tests once you have completed your study can both confirm your knowledge and bolster your confidence. The Fitzgerald Test Bank online prep tests cover the topics found on the certification exam and are available at **https://fhea.com?l=1c6c.**

Conclusion

Successfully passing your certification exam not only marks a critical rite of passage, but is also tangible evidence of your considerable achievement. Make sure you do all that is possible to maximize your likelihood of success.

A list of additional study resources for preparing for the NP certification exam is provided on the following page. Additional courses and resources are available at: **fhea.com**

Resources for NP Certification Examination Preparation

All resources listed are available at: **fhea.com**

Fitzgerald Knowledge Building Courses & Resources

Fitzgerald Comprehensive Pharmacology Courses help NPs gain the broad-based pharmacology knowledge needed for clinical practice:

- **Family Pharmacology Package** (available at: **https://fhea.com?l=76f5**)
- **Adult-Gerontology Pharmacology Package** (available at: **https://fhea.com?l=8c0c**)

Improve your cardiology knowledge through the following Fitzgerald courses:

- **12-Lead ECG Interpretation: A Primary Care Perspective**. Gain critical skills such as how to identify and recognize common ECG alterations.
- **Cardiac Rhythms**. Master the skills needed to interpret cardiac rhythms using this 5-step approach.
- **Honing Your Cardiac Exam**. Learn how to differentiate normal and abnormal heart sounds, identify common murmurs, and obtain a symptom-focused cardiac health history.

This practical case-based course is designed to help you learn when and what to order and how to analyze the results of lab tests:

- **Laboratory Data**

The Fitzgerald **Cue Cards** are step-by-step guides designed to help you provide a thorough and accurate physical exam. Available **Cue Cards**:

- *Adult Physical Assessment*
- *Pediatric Physical Assessment*
- *Orthopedic Physical Assessment*

NP Review & Practice Prep

Dr. Fitzgerald's comprehensive study guide for NP certification prep featuring more than 2,300 sample questions and 177 quick-look tables:

- Fitzgerald, Margaret A. (2017) *Nurse Practitioner Certification Examination and Practice Preparation*, 5th edition. Philadelphia: F.A. Davis. This book is the most comprehensive NP review text on the market. Make sure you study the entire text, and not simply focus on the practice questions. This will help expand your knowledge and clinical decision-making skills.

Test Taking Skills

A resource that will be helpful in developing test-taking skills:

- Sefcik, Donald, Gillian Bice, Frank Prerost. (2012) *How to Study for*

Standardized Tests. Sudbury, MA: Jones & Bartlett Publishers.

Certification Exam Practice Questions

Excellent sources of practice questions for the family and adult-gerontology NP certification examinations:

- **Fitzgerald Test Bank**. (Available at **https://fhea.com?l=1c6c**) Online tests provide detailed rationales for every question and analysis of knowledge gaps help you focus your study.
- Winland-Brown, Jill E., Lynne M. Dunphy. (2013) *Family and Adult-Gerontological Nurse Practitioner Certification Examination: Review Questions and Strategies*, 4th edition. Philadelphia: F.A. Davis.
- Kennedy-Malone, Laurie, Kathleen Ryan Fletcher, Lori Martin Plank. (2014) *Advanced Practice Nursing in the Care of Older Adults*. Philadelphia: F.A. Davis.

Clinical Resources

A helpful resource for honing high-level assessment and differential diagnosis skills:

- Goolsby, Mary Jo, Laurie Grubbs.

(2014) *Advanced Assessment: Interpreting Findings and Formulating Differential Diagnoses*, 3rd edition. Philadelphia: F.A. Davis.

A helpful overall guide to primary care NP practice:

- Cash, Jill C., Cheryl A. Glass. (2014) *Family Practice Guidelines*, 3rd edition. New York, Springer Publishing.

A comprehensive guide to diagnostic imaging and laboratory diagnosis that uses an algorithmic approach to choosing the best study:

- Ferri, Fred. (2014) *Ferri's Best Test: A Practical Guide to Clinical Laboratory Medicine and Diagnostic Imaging*, 3rd edition. St. Louis: Elsevier Health Sciences.

Fully illustrated in a unique format, this is one of the clinical resources I find most helpful in my practice:

- Habif, Thomas. (2012) *Dermatology DDxDeck*, 2nd edition. St. Louis: Elsevier Health Sciences.

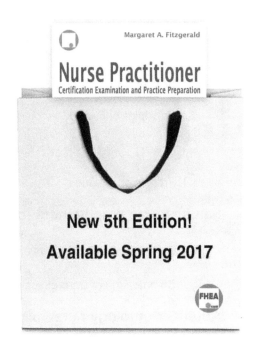

Online Course Resources

See Table of Contents for
Online Course Resources: Instructions and detailed listing

These resources are <u>integral parts of the course</u> and <u>important to your</u> <u>success on the exam</u>. No part of this program is optional. Be sure to complete all of the online portions of this course in order to maximize your results on the exam and preparation for practice. Printable handouts are available through your online learning portal for these programs.

Use this as your checklist for success!

☐ Completed workbook chapters

Family and Adult-Gerontology nurse practitioners

☐ AANPCP vs. ANCC: A Comparison of the Examinations

☐ Disorders Revealed by the Cardiac Exam: A Focus on Heart Sounds and Murmurs

☐ Common Musculoskeletal Problems

☐ Principles of Family Planning

☐ Special Considerations in Geriatric Prescribing Issues of Safety and Efficacy

☐ Professional Issues

Family nurse practitioners (only)

☐ Primary Care of the Woman during Pregnancy

☐ Common Infant Dermatological Conditions

Adult-Gerontology nurse practitioners (only)

☐ Foundations of Gerontology: Theories of Aging, Care of the Frail Elder

☐ Primary Care of the Adolescent

Final resources for all

☐ Final review of the hundreds of course questions **PLUS** 87 bonus questions

☐ 150-question practice test

☐ Supplemental exam preparation materials to enhance your learning experience listed at the end of workbook chapters

☐ Color illustrations referred to in the live and recorded programs.

Table of Contents for Workbook

*Color illustrations referred to during this program and all additional resources
listed throughout this workbook are available through your Fitzgerald Health
online learning portal at fhea.com/npexpert.*

Live Seminar Faculty

Family and adult-gerontology seminars are taught by one of these associates, who have extensive experience as both clinicians in active practice and as professional speakers.

Margaret A. Fitzgerald, DNP, FNP-BC, NP-C, FAANP, CSP, FAAN, DCC, FNAP

Susan Feeney, DNP, NP-C, FNP-BC

Louise McDevitt, MS, ACNP-BC, ANP-BC, FNP-BC, FAANP

Sally K. Miller, PhD, AGACNP, AGPCNP, FNP-BC, FAANP

Brett Badgley Snodgrass, MS, FNP-C, CPE, FAANP

Monica Tombasco, MS, MSNA, FNP-BC, CRNA

Wendy L. Wright, MS, ANP-BC, FNP-BC, FAANP, FAAN

The online and MP3 versions of this program are taught by Dr. Margaret A. Fitzgerald. Available at fhea.com

Additional courses available

Adult-Gerontology Acute Care Nurse Practitioner Certification Exam Review and Advanced Practice Update by Anthony Angelow, PhD(c), ACNPC, AGACNP-BC, CEN, *available live, online, and MP3*

Psychiatric-Mental Health Nurse Practitioner Certification Exam Review and Advanced Practice Update by Teresa Judge-Ellis, DNP, FNP-BC, PMHNP-BC, FAANP, *available live, online, and MP3*

Women's Health Nurse Practitioner Certification Exam Review and Advanced Practice Update by Ursula A. Pritham, PhD, FNP-BC, WHNP-BC, SANE and Margaret A. Fitzgerald, DNP, FNP-BC, NP-C, FAANP, CSP, FAAN, DCC, FNAP, *available online*

Pediatric Nurse Practitioner Certification Exam Review and Advanced Practice Update by Karen B. Farnum, DNP, PPCNP-BC, *available online*

Continuing Education Approved Provider

Fitzgerald Health Education Associates, LLC is approved as a provider of nurse practitioner continuing education by the American Association of Nurse Practitioners. Provider number: 070201

Provider approved by the California Board of Registered Nursing. Provider #CEP 13785.

Additional Continuing Education Available (see fhea.com)

- ❖ Pharmacology Updates *available live and online*
- ❖ Clinical Skills Workshops *available live and online*
- ❖ Advanced Pathophysiology for Nurse Practitioners and Advanced Practice Clinicians *available online*
- ❖ Clinical Pharmacology for Nurse Practitioners and Advanced Practice Clinicians *available online*
- ❖ Clinical Updates *available live and online*

Table 1-1: When Preparing for All NP Certification Examinations

Passing the NP certification examination implies that you have demonstrated mastery of the broad knowledge base and its application needed for entry-level NP practice.

NP certification examination is based on national, not regional or local, practice.	Anticipate being tested on nationally and internationally recognized standards of care and clinical guidelines, evidence-based practice (EBP).	Evidence-based practice (EBP) defined: The delivery of **individualized healthcare** on the basis of an awareness of the impact and strength of **related scientific evidence***. ***This course's content reflects current evidence-based practice.**
The broad stroke of practice, not the mix you see in a typical clinical day	**Location of practice cited in questions on above-mentioned exams will be largely in a primary care-oriented practice in the outpatient setting.**	For FNP, AGNP • As much thyroid as DM • As much male GU as female GYN For AGNP • Scope of practice starts with the teenager • Family planning is part of these examinations but there are no childbearing questions on the AGNP exam.
These tests are developed to rigorous standards and have been deemed to be psychometrically sound.	Assume the content and, therefore, questions on the NP examinations provide a valid evaluation of your ability to practice as a safe, entry-level NP.	According to the NCSBN, the NP certification programs provide a **legally defensible examination** suitable for the **regulation of advanced practice registered nurses.**
Common diseases occur commonly.	Not an examination of the esoteric	Most nursing practice at the RN level is one of exceptions rather than rules. Often, specialty RN experience does not translate well to the broad-based content of the NP board examination.

*www.encyclopedia.com/doc/1O62-evidencebasedpractice.html

Table 1-2: Pass Rate for the FNP, AGNP NP Boards

American Academy of Nurse Practitioners (AANP)	American Nurses Credentialing Center (ANCC)
~ 79% for all candidates	~75% for all candidates

Source:
https://www.aanpcert.org/resource/documents/AANPCP%202015%20Annual%20Report%20Final%205.28.2016.pdf
http://www.nursecredentialing.org/Certification/FacultyEducators/FacultyCategory/Statistics/2015-CertificationStatistics.pdf

Test-taking tip:

The purpose of NP certification examination questions is the measurement of your knowledge, reasoning, and clinical decision-making skills in assessment, diagnosis, plan/intervention, and evaluation.

Test-taking tip:
The NP certification examination tests your ability to know...

- *Why* a patient is at risk for a problem.
  - Epidemiology of disease
- *How* a clinical problem has developed.
  - Pathophysiology
- *What* is the most likely clinical presentation of the condition.
  - Assessment (gathering subjective, objective information)
- *Why* a given intervention is effective.
  - Evidence-based practice
- *How* that intervention works.
  - Modification of disease process via lifestyle or pharmacologic intervention
- *What* is the most likely clinical outcome.
  - Evaluation, gauging response to therapy
- *Why* this clinical problem is of significance to the overall healthcare system.
  - Mortality, morbidity, healthcare finances
- *How* this problem can be approached from both a macro and micro healthcare viewpoint.
  - Primary, secondary, tertiary prevention
- *What* is the role of the NP on the overall health of the nation and beyond.
  - NP as a healthcare leader

Test-taking tip: The best approach in preparing for the exam and practice is to have a firm grasp of knowledge critical to safe practice as your foundation so that you are able to analyze and synthesize the data presented so you know what to do and why you are doing it at both the micro (exam room) and macro (public) healthcare level.

- *Analyze* defined: To examine methodically by separating into parts and studying their interrelations
- *Synthesize* defined: To combine so as to form a new, complex product
- *Critical thinking:* The mental process of actively and skillfully conceptualizing, applying, analyzing, synthesizing, and evaluating information to reach an answer or conclusion.
- *Practice includes application.*

There are no shortcuts to success on the NP boards!

Source: National Council of State Boards of Nursing, available at
www.ncsbn.org/boards.htm, http://dictionary.reference.com/browse/critical+thinking

Table 1-3: What is the question asking? The clinical decision-making process has 5 major components, usually performed sequentially: *ADPIE*	
Assessment	Collect subjective (health history including HPI) and objective (physical examination, available diagnostic results) data.
Diagnosis	Analyze assessment data to determine a (working) diagnosis, keeping in mind common health problems seen in primary care.
Plan	Develop a plan of care and prescribe intervention to attain expected outcome. ***Assume the resources needed to provide cost-effective diagnosis and treatment based on the evidence are available.***
Implementation	Actualizing the plan of care, the application portion of the above-mentioned process.
Evaluate	Performed post diagnosis, plan and intervention. Evaluate patient's attainment of treatment goals, keeping in mind the ongoing need to adjust the plan of care based on patient response.

Test-taking tip: When unsure about the answer to a clinical question, apply ADPIE. Often the answer becomes easily apparent.

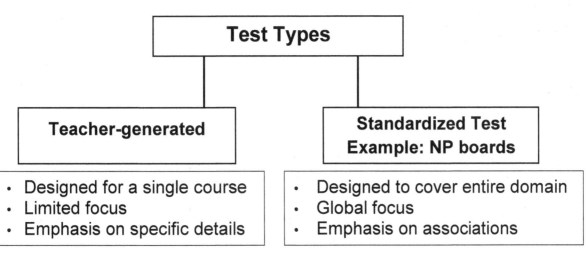

Source: Sefcik, D. (2012) <u>How to Study for Standardized Tests</u>, Sudbury, MA: Jones & Bartlett Publishers.

Figure 1-1

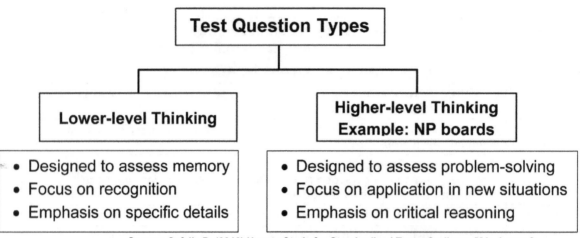

Test Question Types

Lower-level Thinking
- Designed to assess memory
- Focus on recognition
- Emphasis on specific details

Higher-level Thinking
Example: NP boards
- Designed to assess problem-solving
- Focus on application in new situations
- Emphasis on critical reasoning

Source: Sefcik, D. (2012) <u>How to Study for Standardized Tests</u>, Sudbury, MA: Jones & Bartlett Publishers.

Figure 1-2

Table 1-4: Recognition question
Test-taking tip: Relatively few questions on the NP boards are at this level. The simplest exam question. There is no opinion on the correct answer to a fact-oriented question.

The test taker should be able to quickly recognize the correct answer.	These questions are fact-oriented and test generalizations, principles, and theories. Mnemonics can be helpful.

1. Assessment of the optic disc is a component of the evaluation of cranial nerve:
   A. I.
   B. II.
   C. III.
   D. IV.

Table 1-5: Anticipate the information in the question will build in order to test your knowledge base as well as your critical thinking and clinical decision-making skills.

Test-taking tip: Given that questions often have more than one correct answer, every piece of information is important and helps direct you to the BEST answer for that particular question.

Example	Information	Clinical significance
Fact-oriented information	Cardiac anatomy and physiology: Lower pressure right-sided venous system, higher pressure left-sided arterial system **Figure 1-4**	Abnormalities in the cardiac examination are more likely to arise from left-sided heart problems.
Comprehension of the information presented	With mitral regurgitation, incompetent mitral valves fail to close properly, allowing blood to regurgitate to left atrium. End result is decreased cardiac output potential.	Symptoms of low cardiac output can include dyspnea with exertion, chest pain, orthopnea, syncope, and near-syncope.
Assessment, diagnosis, application, evaluation question: Requires the examinee to analyze the condition, then decide what is pertinent to the given situation	The cardiac exam features in mitral regurgitation (MR) include the presence of a holosystolic murmur with a blowing quality that is typically Gr II–III/VI with a predictable pattern of radiation. **Figure 1-6** Holosystolic Murmur S1 S2 S1 S2 Systole Diastole Systole Diastole	Given that with MR, blood is regurgitating in left atrium, instead of being in left ventricle, there is a potential for low cardiac output and resulting patient report of corresponding symptoms. Classic symptoms of low cardiac output include dyspnea with exertion, chest pain, orthopnea, syncope, and near-syncope.

2. You examine a 62-year-old woman with a 20-year history of hypertension. She reports intermittent use of antihypertensive medications, stating, "I feel better without the medications." Today she presents for a "check-up." On physical examination, you note the following: PMI with a downward and lateral shift as well as a Gr II/VI holosystolic murmur with radiation to the axilla.

Table 1-6: Analysis, Synthesis, and Application of the Information Presented	
Long-standing hypertension (HTN) with history of intermittent medication use, therefore increasing risk of HTN target organ damage (TOD). Left ventricular hypertrophy (LVH) is a common form of HTN TOD.	Point of maximum impulse (PMI) shift common in LVH; NL PMI location=5th intercostal space (ICS), midclavicular line (MCL) in most adults • An example of the clinical presentation of a disease's pathophysiology
Holosystolic murmur with a predictable pattern of radiation to the axilla	Mitral regurgitation (MR) common in LVH. Description is consistent with the murmur of mitral regurgitation.
MR=Decreased cardiac output potential	Symptoms of low cardiac output include dyspnea with exertion, chest pain, orthopnea, syncope, and near-syncope.

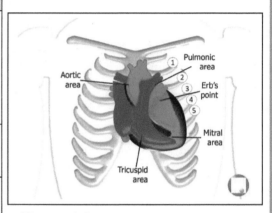

Figure 1-9

This patient's health history is likely to include a report of:

A. Syncopal episodes.

B. Episodes of chest pain at rest.

C. Dyspnea with exertion.

D. Vertigo.

Table 1-7: *Test-taking Tip:*	
Look for key words in stem that set priority in the question.	
First	
Airway, breathing, circulation (ABC) often directs the answer.	Answering a question containing the term "first" allows the test taker to demonstrate skills at assessing clinical priorities.
Initially	
Assess before diagnosis, (working) diagnosis before plan, plan before intervention, intervention prior to evaluating response to care.	Answering a question containing the term "initially" allows the test taker to demonstrate skills at assessing where in the care continuum (ADPIE) the patient is.
Most appropriate	
Evidence-based practice guides the choice of diagnostics, plan/intervention, and follow-up and therefore dictates the correct answer.	Using the "most appropriate" term increases the difficulty of a question and allows the test taker to demonstrate clinical decision-making skills.

3. Of the following, which should be performed first in assessing a 48-year-old woman who has a 25-year history of moderate persistent asthma and who now presents with an acute asthma flare?

  A. Oxygen saturation

  B. Arterial blood gas

  C. FEV_1 (forced expiratory volume at 1 second)

  D. Chest x-ray

Table 1-8: Timing Clinical Findings During an Asthma Flare	
Oxygen saturation	
Arterial blood gas	
FEV_1	
Chest x-ray	

Relationship between SaO_2 and PaO_2

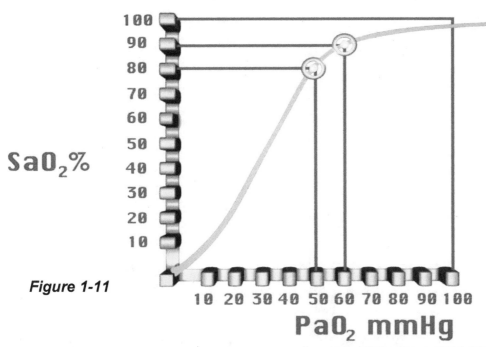

Figure 1-11

Table 1-9: *Test-taking Tip: Look for clues in the question's stem.*	
Word or phrase that leads to correct answer	Match the modifier if possible.
This is a national NP certification examination. ***Think healthcare principles that will impact not only a community or region but the entire nation.***	The NP in the rural Northeast will take the same exam as the NP in urban Southeast who will sit for the same exam as the NP in the suburban Midwest, who will sit for the same exam…

mobile

4. You are setting up a healthcare clinic for *mobile* migrant farm workers. Which of the following sites is most desirable?

    A. Community hall of a local church

    B. Local hospital ambulatory care center —

    (C.) Mobile van — *to bring health care mobile people*

    D. Space in a shopping center

Would your response differ in setting up a healthcare clinic for homeless adults?

5. A 58-year-old woman presents for an initial examination in order to become a patient in your primary care practice. She is a nonsmoker, drinks 1 to 2, 5 oz (0.15 L) glasses of wine per week, and works as an administrative assistant in a law office. She is without complaint and reports that she is generally in good health. Physical exam reveals BMI=34 kg/m^2 and BP=144/98 mm Hg bilaterally. The rest of her examination is unremarkable.

Calzones *Spinach*

Table 1-10: *Test-taking Tip: Analyze, synthesize, and apply the information provided.*	
Given social history	Likely sedentary work Assume alcohol intake is accurate as given and is not a significant contributor to her health issues today.
BMI=34 kg/m^2	Obesity=BMI≥30 kg/m^2 *Obesity*
Age 58 years	Average age at menopause for women in North America=Age 51 years, therefore assume postmenopause. —
Without complaint with elevated BP finding	Hx negative for HTN target organ damage (TOD) symptoms - No visual changes - No chest pain - No shortness of breath - No dizziness
PMI WNL	Usually displaced in LVH
No S$_3$	Noted with systolic dysfunction - Often present in heart failure
No S$_4$	Noted with diastolic dysfunction - Often present in poorly-controlled HTN, recurrent myocardial ischemia
No murmurs	Murmur of mitral regurgitation (MR) common in LVH
No hypertensive retinopathy	Grade 1 and 2 HTN retinopathy is common in poorly-controlled HTN. Patient does not have visual changes with these low-grade findings. ✓
No renal artery bruit	Occasionally noted with renal artery stenosis, a cause of secondary hypertension, usually with markedly elevated BP at presentation

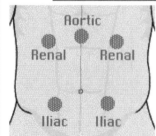

Figure 1-15

Patient is clinically stable with a one-time elevated BP reading.

Your next best action is to:

    A. Prescribe a low-dose thiazide diuretic.

    (B.) Arrange for additional blood pressure measurements within the next four weeks.

    C. Check renal function.

    D. Advise restricting sodium intake and limiting alcohol intake to no more than 1 glass of wine per week.

Table 1-11: Establishing the Diagnosis of HTN	
HTN diagnosis in absence of TOD	≥2 abnormal readings on ≥2 occasions

Table 1-12: *Test-taking Tip: Use your experience from your NP studies and RN role and common sense in answering professional issues questions.*	
Leadership defined	A process by which a person influences a group of individuals to achieve a common goal, regardless of setting.
Look for the leader to direct activities that have the most wide-reaching influence.	

6. The NP demonstrates fulfillment of the advanced practice nursing leadership role by participating in which of the following activities?

 A. Teaching a 56-year-old man with newly-diagnosed type 2 diabetes mellitus about the importance of self-glucose monitoring

 B. Volunteering to teach a class on contraceptive methods to a group of teen mothers

 C. Discussing barriers to achieving blood pressure control with a 65-year-old woman with hypertension who "does not want to take any medicine"

 D. Collaborating with the regional public health department on an initiative to combat obesity through a community-based exercise program

Table 1-13: What is more powerful? Input or output?	
Input	The sum of the NP's academic, clinical, personal, and professional background
Output	The evidence of the impact of NP practice on a patient population health outcomes

Source for additional information on NP practice outcomes:
http://www.aanp.org/images/documents/publications/clinicaloutcomesyardstick.pdf

7. You are asked to speak to a group of healthcare executives on the NP role. Which of the following provides the strongest support for NP practice?

 A. Number of academic credits earned during the NP program

 B. NP practice outcomes

 C. The quantity of clinical hours and type of clinical rotations in the NP program

 D. The professional experience of the person prior to entering the NP program

Notes:

8. Rank the following from highest to lowest level of research design.
   ____Case reports
   ____Randomized controlled trials
   ____Expert opinion

Evidence Hierarchy

Figure 1-16

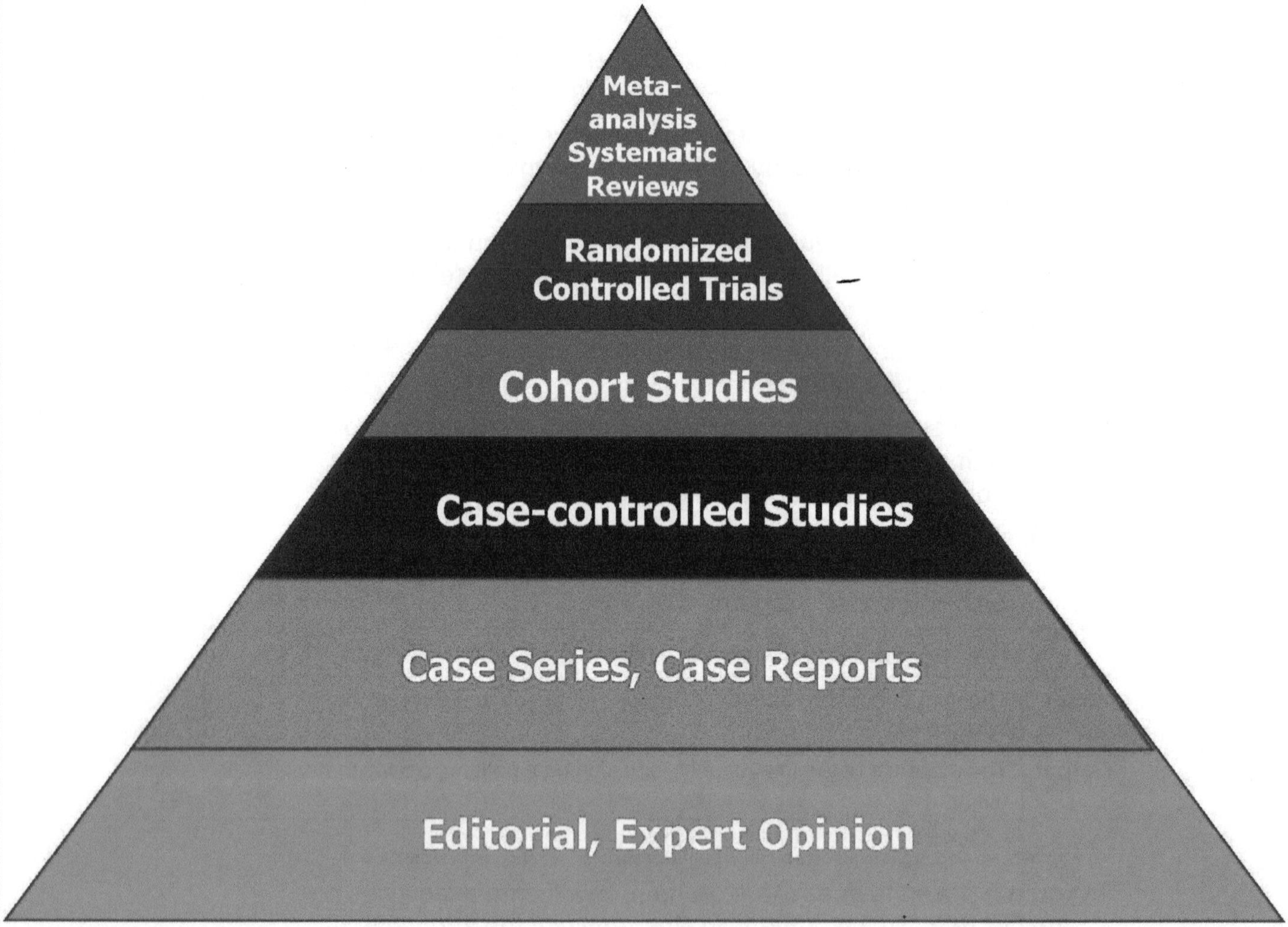

Meta-analysis Systematic Reviews
Randomized Controlled Trials
Cohort Studies
Case-controlled Studies
Case Series, Case Reports
Editorial, Expert Opinion

	**Table 1-14: Evidence Hierarchy** **This component of evidence-based medicine lists the types of medical research in order of weight of authority (from greatest to least)**	
I	Systematic review (meta-analysis)	A review of high-quality published research (i.e., randomized controlled trials meeting stated parameters) that addresses a specific clinical issue in which the reported evidence and resulting conclusions are evaluated and summarized
II	Randomized controlled trial	A study designed to evaluate the effectiveness of a medication or clinical procedure in carefully selected patients. These subjects are divided randomly into groups whose members either receive treatment or serve as controls (i.e., take a placebo instead of the study medication, or undergo a sham procedure). Other possibly confounding factors are minimized as possible. Response to treatment (or to lack of treatment) and development of adverse effects are monitored and reported
III	Cohort study	A study—prospective or retrospective—in which the hypothesized association between a specific variable (such as use of a certain medication) and a specific outcome is tested; subjects in the cohort are either exposed or not exposed to the variable, and all are followed over time for development of the stated outcome
IV	Case-control study	A retrospective study in which *cases* (patients with a particular condition) and *controls* (those unaffected by that condition) who otherwise share specified characteristics (such as age and gender) are compared for the presence of potential risk factors for the condition under study
V	Case series	A retrospective study examining the experience of a group of patients affected by a specific illness or treated with a specific medication or procedure
	Case report	A clinical narrative describing a single patient with a particular condition or illness, including presentation, history and physical findings, diagnostic test results, course of treatment, and the patient's outcome and/or prognosis
VI	Editorial	An essay, authored by a journal editor or a qualified clinician or group of clinicians, that addresses a specific clinical topic; it often accompanies one or more related clinical studies or other research published in the same issue of a publication
	Expert opinion	Essay by a qualified author on a clinical topic of current concern, often citing relevant research and/or personal observation

Source: Ho PM, Peterson PN, Masoudi RA. Evaluating the evidence: Is there a rigid hierarchy? *Circulation.* 2008;118:1675-1684.

Table 1-15: *Test-taking Tip: Give yourself positive, not negative, self-messages as you prepare for the NP boards.*	
Comment	**Response**
"I froze when I saw how hard the questions were."	Anticipate that the first few questions will be challenging, particularly as you get accustomed to the test. ***Recall you can highlight questions and go back to revisit later.***
"I never do well on standardized tests."	SAT? GRE? NCLEX? Other certifications? **For help with test taking, please see Sefcik, D. (2012) <u>How to Study for Standardized Tests</u>, Sudbury, MA: Jones & Bartlett Publishers. A concise guide developed by a team who are experts in high-stakes professional exam-taking skills.**
"I have crippling test anxiety."	You have completed or will soon complete rigorous graduate study. This is the true testimony to your academic success. ***A solid knowledge base is the best action against test anxiety.***
With either certifying body, you will answer approximately 130–140 clinically-based questions encompassing the entire range of NP practice in your area of preparation. ***Therefore, the test is not focused on any particular topic or practice area.***	Regardless of certifying agency, NPs who fail the boards do so because of poor performance in clinical portions of the examinations. Remember, this is a test to measure your ability to possess and apply the knowledge base needed to perform as a safe, entry-level NP. Insufficient clinical knowledge base and/or inability to utilize that knowledge base are the reasons NPs fail the boards. ***Please recall, the NP boards have failure rates of approximately 1 in 4 to 1 in 5 candidates.***

Table 1-16: Frequently Asked Questions, Study Recommendations, and Sample Exam Questions to Aid in Preparing for Certification, Including Archives of Margaret Fitzgerald's Certification Issues Articles Available Free-of-Charge www.fhea.com/certificationcols/certfaqfhea.shtml		
General information	**Tips for successfully passing the test**	**Building your knowledge base**
Frequently Asked Questions about NP Certification Certification: Myths and Realities How do I sign my name? Certification after Years of NP Practice	Test Question Analysis Preparing for the NP Certification Exam Passing on the First Try Tips for Taking a Certification Exam	Levels of Prevention Important in Certification Enhancing your Understanding of Assessment What's the Sign? Evaluating your Broad Knowledge Base Mnemonics and Memory Aids What Nerve! Honing Your Skills in Cranial Nerve Assessment The Certification Exam: Intersection of Skills Required Test Questions about Pregnancy (FNP only) Professional Issues on the Certification Exam

Table 1-17: Focusing Your Study:

Test-taking Tip: Please ensure you are familiar with the content outline of the examination you plan to take. This is available on your NP certification agency website.

Information on exam will be at least 6 months old.

Study with purpose, intent, and goals.	*This is best achieved with a well-developed plan that works on increasing knowledge base and honing clinical decision-making skills. Use practice questions to wrap up, not start, your board study.*
Subjective	History-taking skills • When to use open- and closed-ended questions, interviewing techniques that demonstrate cultural competency Symptom analysis • One of the most helpful tools in clinical practice o OLD CARTS mnemonic for symptom analysis=**O**nset, **L**ocation/radiation, **D**uration, **C**haracter, **A**ggravating factors, **R**elieving factors, **T**iming and **S**everity
Objective	Normal PE findings • Including age-appropriate examination findings in the child (FNP) and elder (FNP, AGNP) Abnormal PE findings • For commonly encountered health problems in primary care, not acute care, setting **For help with conducting the health history and physical examination, please see Feeney, S., Fitzgerald, M.A. <u>Pediatric Physical Assessment Cue Cards;</u> Wright, W. L. <u>Adult Health History and Physical Exam Cue Cards</u>; Tombasco, M., McDevitt, L., <u>Orthopedic Physical Assessment Cue Cards</u>, North Andover, MA: Fitzgerald Health Education Associates, available at fhea.com**
Assessment	Differential diagnosis • Defined: The process of determining which of ≥2 conditions or diseases with similar symptoms is the one which the patient most likely has, by a systematic analysis, comparison, and contrasting of the clinical findings **Source: http://dictionary.webmd.com/terms/differential-diagnosis**

Plan	Broad strokes of intervention
	• Drug classes rather than specific products
	   o ACEI (-pril): Lisinopril vs. trandolapril
	   o Fluoroquinolones (-floxacin): Levofloxacin vs. moxifloxacin
	   o Beta$_2$-adrenergic agonist (-terol): Albuterol vs. salmeterol
	• Across drug classes and lifespan
	   o Pharmacodynamics (PD, what the drug does to the body and/or disease) ***does not*** differ, but pharmacokinetics (PK, what the body does to the drug, including absorption, distribution, biotransformation [metabolism], and elimination) ***does*** differ.
	   o Major drug adverse effects tend to be found consistently across a given drug class and are often consistent with the drug's mechanism of action.

Safety issues in medication use	Who should take a given med (often using EBP standards), who should not (typically safety issues) Consideration in special groups • Elders (FNP, AGNP) • Pregnancy and lactation (FNP only) • Infants and children (FNP only)
Consider all the roles the NP fulfills.	Clinician, coach, teacher, healthcare leader who applies micro and macro healthcare principles. Be familiar with national statements on scope of NP practice. **AANP's Statement on NP Scope of Practice, www.aanp.org/publications/position-statements-papers**

Learning activities are an integral part of the course available through your Fitzgerald Health learning portal at fhea.com/npexpert:

Online program for Family and Adult-Gerontology NPs:

AANPCP vs. ANCC: A comparison of the examinations

and

Professional Issues

Study resources
- Archived FHEA electronic newsletters. This newsletter provides timely information on pharmacology, clinical issues of interest to nurse practitioners, schedules for upcoming seminars, and special offers not generally advertised in other media.
    - www.fhea.com/ezine_archive.shtml
- AANP: Position Papers and Statements
    - www.aanp.org/publications/position-statements-papers
        - Clinical Outcomes: The Yardstick of Educational Effectiveness
        - Doctor of Nursing Practice (DNP) Discussion Paper
        - Nurse Practitioner Cost-effectiveness
        - Nurse Practitioner Curriculum
        - Nurse Practitioners and Team-based Care
        - Nurse Practitioners in Primary Care
        - Nurse Practitioner Prescriptive Privilege
        - Quality of Nurse Practitioner Practice
        - Scope of Practice for Nurse Practitioners
        - Standards for Nurse Practitioner Practice in Retail-based Clinics
        - Standards of Practice for Nurse Practitioners
        - Use of Terms Such as *Mid-level Provider* and *Physician Extender*

Web resources
- Guideline.gov
    - AHRQ's National Guideline Clearinghouse, a public resource for summaries of evidence-based clinical practice guidelines
- www.fda.gov/Safety/MedWatch
    - MedWatch: The FDA Safety Information and Adverse Event Reporting Program, site where you can report as well as learn about recent drug recalls and advisories."
- CDC.gov
    - Centers for Disease Control and Prevention, helpful updates on emerging infectious diseases, immunization and a myriad of other important health issue

Resources for Additional Study

Books:

Feeney, S., Fitzgerald, M.A. (2017) <u>Pediatric Physical Assessment Cue Cards</u>, 10th Edition, North Andover, MA: Fitzgerald Health Education Associates.

Fitzgerald, M.A. (2017) Answers to Your Most Common Test Taking Questions, <u>Nurse Practitioner Certification Examination and Practice Preparation</u>, 5th Edition, Philadelphia, PA: F. A. Davis.

Wright, W. L. (2015) <u>Adult Physical Assessment Cue Cards</u>, 8th Edition, North Andover, MA: Fitzgerald Health Education Associates.

Video program:

Wright, W. L. <u>Expert Exam: Physical Examination of the Adult</u>, North Andover, MA: Fitzgerald Health Education Associates.

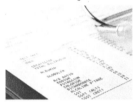
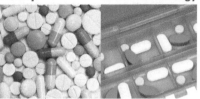

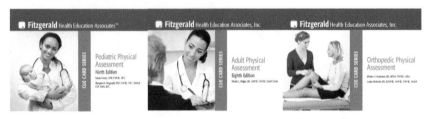
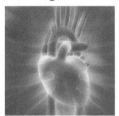
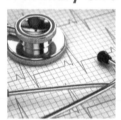
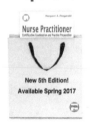
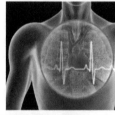

Chapter 2: Primary Prevention: Health Promotion and Immunization

Table 2-1: Healthcare Principle: Intervene at Lowest Level Possible		
Level of prevention	**Goal**	**Example**
Primary	Preventing the health problem, the most cost-effective form of healthcare	Immunizations, counseling about safety, injury, and disease prevention
Secondary	Detecting disease in early, asymptomatic, or preclinical state to minimize its impact	Screening tests, such as BP check, mammography, colonoscopy.
Tertiary	Minimizing negative disease-induced outcomes	In established disease, adjusting therapy to avoid further target organ damage. Potentially viewed as a failure of primary prevention.

Source: Office of Disease Prevention and Health Promotion, available at http://health.gov/

1. In a 46-year-old woman with hypertension and dyslipidemia:

Action	Primary, Secondary, or Tertiary
Counseling about reducing risk for sexually transmitted infection ✓	primary
Skin survey for precancerous lesions ✓	Secondary

2. In a 66-year-old woman with type 2 diabetes mellitus (T2DM):

Action	Primary, Secondary, or Tertiary
Administering influenza vaccine	primary
Adjusting therapy to enhance glycemic control	Tertiary ✓

3. In a 25-year-old well woman with a strong family history of T2DM:

Action	Primary, Secondary, or Tertiary
Checking fasting lipid profile	Secondary
Teaching the benefits of participating in a consistent program of moderate-intensity physical activity	primary

4. In a 76-year-old man with chronic obstructive pulmonary disease (COPD):

Action	Primary, Secondary, or Tertiary
Ensuring adequate illumination at home	*primary*
Screening for physical, emotional, or financial abuse	*secondary*

Table 2-2: Before We had Immunizations Against these Diseases...	
Per-year toll in the United States	
Disease	**Comments**
Polio	10,000 children paralyzed, 3,000 children died
Rubella (German measles)	20,000 newborns with birth defects, including developmental disability, blindness, hearing loss
Measles	4 million children infected, 3,000 died If measles vaccine did not exist, each year _____ measles-related deaths worldwide would be expected.
Influenza	With immunization, up to 9,400 deaths prevented annually (~90% in people 65 years and older)
Pneumococcal disease	Estimated _____ deaths annually, of which 50% could be prevented through use of vaccine. Mortality risk greatest in elderly and persons with underlying medical conditions.

Source: Parents' Guide to Childhood Immunizations, available at www.cdc.gov/vaccines/pubs/parents-guide/default.htm, http://www.cdc.gov/flu/news/flu-vaccine-saved-lives.htm, http://www.cdc.gov/mmwr/Preview/mmwrhtml/00047135.htm

As a result

- *Evidence-based practice advises that vaccine-related risk is less than disease-related risk. Advocating that patients of all ages be protected against vaccine-preventable disease (VPD) is one of the most important primary prevention activities.*

Immediate interventions in anaphylaxis in the primary care setting:
- Assess airway, breathing, circulation.
- Place patient in supine position.
- Activate EMS, facilitate transfer to ED.
- Administer IM epinephrine (anterior-lateral thigh).
  - No contraindications to epinephrine use in anaphylaxis regardless of comorbidity or age
- Give H1/H2 blocker PO (H1=Diphenhydramine, H2=Ranitidine).
- IV access, oxygen, monitoring

↓

In the ED, interventions based on initial response:
- Establish airway if compromised.
- Rapid fluid infusion (IV, IO) as needed for compromised circulation.
- Repeat IM epinephrine as needed or consider IV epinephrine infusion
- Bronchodilators based on respiratory compromise
- Systemic corticosteroids
- Glucagon
- Length of observation based on clinical presentation, response to therapy, risk factors for fatal anaphylaxis, access to medical care, reliability.

↓

Determine disposition:
- Based on presentation and response to therapy
  - Home (most common)
    - With patient education on the use of self-injected epinephrine (SIE, EpiPen®), potential biphasic reaction, trigger avoidance. Consider prescriptions for oral antihistamines and systemic corticosteroids
    - Outpatient follow-up referral (allergist or primary care)
  - Admission: General hospital or intensive care unit depending on persistent respiratory and/or circulatory compromise.

Source: Campbell RL, et al. *Ann Allergy Asthma Immunol.* 2014;113:599-608.

Figure 2-10

5. In a community undergoing a disaster, the use of select vaccines will be prioritized. Match the type of disaster with the priority vaccine.

   A. Immunization against tetanus

   B. Immunization against influenza

   C. Immunization against hepatitis A

Type of disaster	Priority vaccine
Uninjured adults and children evacuated to a crowded group setting	B
Adults with multiple deep lacerations from flying debris	A
A community exposed to unsafe water supply after a hurricane	C

6. True or false?

   (T/F) Immune globulin is a concentrated solution of antibodies derived from pooled donated blood.   T

   (T/F) Tdap (tetanus, diphtheria, acellular pertussis [Adacel®, Boostrix®]) vaccine should replace a single dose of Td (tetanus, diphtheria) vaccine for most adults who have not previously received a dose of Tdap in order to provide additional protection against pertussis.   T

   (T/F) Previously unvaccinated adults age 19 through 59 years with diabetes mellitus type 1 or type 2 should be vaccinated against hepatitis B as soon as possible after the diabetes diagnosis is made.   T

7. A 67-year-old man with well-controlled hypertension and dyslipidemia who received one dose of PPSV23 (Pneumovax®) 1 year ago asks about a "new pneumonia shot" he heard about in a TV promotion. You advise that:

   A. He is adequately immunized against pneumococcal disease.

   B. That there is another pneumococcal vaccine available but its use is not advised in older adults due to its adverse effect profile.

   C. He is eligible for a dose of PCV13 (Prevnar®) today to be optimally protected against pneumococcal disease.

   D. In 4 more years, he should receive a second dose of PPSV23.

Table 2-10 (cont.): 2016–2017 Advisory Committee on Immunization Practices (ACIP) Recommendations on Influenza Immunization
The following recommendations apply when considering influenza vaccination of people who have or report a history of egg allergy. 1. People who have experienced only hives following exposure to egg should receive the influenza vaccine. Any licensed and recommended influenza vaccine that is otherwise appropriate for the patient's age and health status may be used. 2. People who report having had reactions to egg involving angioedema, respiratory distress, lightheadedness, or recurrent emesis, or people who required epinephrine or other emergency medical intervention, may similarly receive any licensed and recommended influenza vaccine (e.g., appropriate IIV or RIV3) that is otherwise appropriate for the patient's age and health status. The selected vaccine should be administered in an inpatient or outpatient medical center (including but not necessarily limited to hospitals, clinics, health departments, and physician offices). Vaccine administration should be supervised by a healthcare provider who is able to recognize and manage severe allergic conditions. 3. People who are able to eat lightly-cooked egg (e.g., scrambled egg) without a reaction are unlikely to be allergic. Egg-allergic people might tolerate egg in baked products (e.g., bread or cake). Tolerance to egg-containing foods does not exclude the possibility of egg allergy. Egg allergy can be confirmed by a consistent medical history of adverse reactions to eggs and egg-containing foods, plus skin and/or blood testing for immunoglobulin E directed against egg proteins. 4. Providers should consider observing all patients for 15 minutes after vaccination to decrease the risk of injury should they experience syncope. 5. A previous severe allergic reaction to influenza vaccine, regardless of the component suspected to be responsible, is a contraindication to future receipt of influenza vaccine.

Source: http://www.cdc.gov/mmwr/volumes/65/rr/rr6505a1.htm

Table 2-11: Immunization Reaction:
Discomfort, Erythema at Immunization Injection Site Common, Generally Expected

Immunization	Common reaction (≥25%)	Less common reaction (<25%)	Rare reaction (<10³ to 10⁶)
Anthrax	Soreness, redness, itching at site, myalgia, arthralgia, headache	Fatigue, chills, nausea	Allergic reaction to IZ (rare)
DTaP (diphtheria, tetanus, acellular pertussis)	Soreness, erythema at injection site	Fatigue, poor appetite, GI upset	Seizure, nonstop crying, T≥105°F (41°C), anaphylactic reaction
Haemophilus influenzae type B (Hib)	Erythema at injection site	Fever	
Hepatitis A	Soreness at injection site	Headache, poor appetite	Allergic reaction to IZ (rare)
Hepatitis B	Soreness at injection site	Mild fever	Allergic reaction to IZ (rare)
Inactivated polio virus (IPV)	Soreness at injection site	None reported	None reported
Injectable influenza vaccine (all types)	Soreness, redness at injection site	Aches, mild fever	Allergic reaction to IZ (rare)
Live, attenuated virus influenza vaccine via nasal spray (LAIV, FluMist®)	Transient nasal congestion and discharge, headache; harmless virus shed from nose for 3–10 d post-administration	Fever, vomiting, abdominal pain, myalgias	Allergic reaction to IZ (rare)
Measles, mumps, rubella (MMR)	Fever, arthralgia (1 in 4 adult women who receive vaccine)	Mild rash, lymphadenopathy	Seizure, allergic reaction (rare), potential though not proven teratogen
Meningococcus types A, C, Y, W-135 (Menactra®)	Erythema at injection site	Fever	No serious adverse effects noted
Serogroup B Meningococcal (MenB®)	Soreness, swelling, erythema at injection site, mild generalized malaise	Fainting	Allergic reaction to IZ (rare)
Pneumococcal conjugate vaccine 13 (PCV13, Prevnar®)	Erythema at injection site, T≥100.4°F (38°C), usually in children only	Fussiness, loss of appetite (up to 80%, lasts up to 24–48 h) in children only	None noted to date
Pneumococcal polysaccharide vaccine (Pneumovax®)	Erythema at injection site	Fever, myalgia	Allergic reaction to IZ (rare)
Quadrivalent human papillomavirus, ([Types 6, 11, 16, 18] vaccine [Gardasil®]), bivalent HPV ([Types 16, 18] vaccine [Cervarix®])	Soreness, swelling, erythema at injection site	Generalized body aches, mild fever, headache (1 in 3)	Serious reactions rare (<0.3%) Reports of post-IZ fainting (sitting or supine position for 15 mins post-IZ recommended)
Rotavirus, live, oral, pentavalent vaccine (RotaTeq®) (pediatric only)	Fussiness, fever on day of immunization	Short-term GI upset (diarrhea, less often vomiting)	Serious reactions rare. No observed increase in rate of intussusception
Smallpox (live vaccinia virus vaccine) (special use only)	Vaccine delivery results in weeping lesion that contains live vaccinia virus	Fatigue, headache, myalgia, regional lymphadenopathy, lymphangitis, pruritus, and edema at vaccination site	Viral replication, shedding occurs at vaccination site. Unintended transmission possible immediately after vaccination until scab separates from the skin (~2–3 weeks)
Tdap (tetanus, diphtheria, acellular pertussis for ages 11–64 years) (Adacel®, Boostrix®)	Erythema at injection site	Myalgia, feverish sensation	Allergic reaction to IZ (rare)
Tetanus diphtheria (Td)	Erythema, soreness at injection site	None reported	Allergic reaction to IZ (rare)
Varicella (chickenpox)	Soreness at injection site	Fever, mild rash up to 1 month post-IZ	Seizure, pneumonia
Zoster (shingles, Zostavax®)	Soreness at injection site	Headache (1 in 70)	None reported

Source: www.cdc.gov/vaccines/vac-gen/side-effects.htm

Important additional study resources available through your Fitzgerald Health online learning portal at fhea.com/npexpert

- Resource 2-1: Therapeutic Communication Skills

Bonus questions for this chapter available through your Fitzgerald Health learning portal at fhea.com/npexpert.

Recommended Immunization Schedule for

Children and Adolescents Aged 18 Years or Younger, UNITED STATES, 2017

This schedule includes recommendations in effect as of January 1, 2017. Any dose not administered at the recommended age should be administered at a subsequent visit, when indicated and feasible. The use of a combination vaccine generally is preferred over separate injections of its equivalent component vaccines. Vaccination providers should consult the relevant Advisory Committee on Immunization Practices (ACIP) statement for detailed recommendations, available online at www.cdc.gov/vaccines/hcp/acip-recs/index.html. Clinically significant adverse events that follow vaccination should be reported to the Vaccine Adverse Event Reporting System (VAERS) online (www.vaers.hhs.gov) or by telephone (800-822-7967). Suspected cases of vaccine-preventable diseases should be reported to the state or local health department. Additional information, including precautions and contraindications for vaccination, is available from CDC online (www.cdc.gov/vaccines/hcp/admin/contraindications.html) or by telephone (800-CDC-INFO [800-232-4636]).

The Recommended Immunization Schedule for Children and Adolescents Aged 18 Years or Younger are approved by the

Advisory Committee on Immunization Practices
(www.cdc.gov/vaccines/acip)

American Academy of Pediatrics
(www.aap.org)

American Academy of Family Physicians
(www.aafp.org)

American College of Obstetricians and Gynecologists
(www.acog.org)

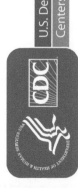

U.S. Department of Health and Human Services
Centers for Disease Control and Prevention

Figure 1. Recommended Immunization Schedule for Children and Adolescents Aged 18 Years or Younger—**United States, 2017.**

(FOR THOSE WHO FALL BEHIND OR START LATE, SEE THE CATCH-UP SCHEDULE [FIGURE 2]).

These recommendations must be read with the footnotes that follow. For those who fall behind or start late, provide catch-up vaccination at the earliest opportunity as indicated by the green bars in Figure 1. To determine minimum intervals between doses, see the catch-up schedule (Figure 2). School entry and adolescent vaccine age groups are shaded in gray.

Vaccine	Birth	1 mo	2 mos	4 mos	6 mos	9 mos	12 mos	15 mos	18 mos	19–23 mos	2–3 yrs	4–6 yrs	7–10 yrs	11–12 yrs	13–15 yrs	16 yrs	17–18 yrs
Hepatitis B[1] (HepB)	1st dose	←— 2nd dose —→			←————————— 3rd dose —————————→												
Rotavirus[2] (RV) RV1 (2-dose series); RV5 (3-dose series)			1st dose	2nd dose	See footnote 2												
Diphtheria, tetanus, & acellular pertussis[3] (DTaP: <7 yrs)			1st dose	2nd dose	3rd dose			←— 4th dose —→				5th dose					
Haemophilus influenzae type b[4] (Hib)			1st dose	2nd dose	See footnote 4		3rd or 4th dose, See footnote 4										
Pneumococcal conjugate[5] (PCV13)			1st dose	2nd dose	3rd dose		←— 4th dose —→										
Inactivated poliovirus[6] (IPV: <18 yrs)			1st dose	2nd dose	←————————— 3rd dose —————————→							4th dose					
Influenza[7] (IIV)					Annual vaccination (IIV) 1 or 2 doses								Annual vaccination (IIV) 1 dose only				
Measles, mumps, rubella[8] (MMR)					See footnote 8		←— 1st dose —→					2nd dose					
Varicella[9] (VAR)							←— 1st dose —→					2nd dose					
Hepatitis A[10] (HepA)							←———— 2-dose series, See footnote 10 ————→										
Meningococcal[11] (Hib-MenCY ≥6 weeks; MenACWY-D ≥9 mos; MenACWY-CRM ≥2 mos)							See footnote 11							1st dose		2nd dose	
Tetanus, diphtheria, & acellular pertussis[12] (Tdap: ≥7 yrs)														Tdap			
Human papillomavirus[13] (HPV)														See footnote 13			
Meningococcal B[11]														See footnote 11			
Pneumococcal polysaccharide[5] (PPSV23)												See footnote 5					

Legend:

☐ Range of recommended ages for all children

☐ Range of recommended ages for catch-up immunization

☐ Range of recommended ages for certain high-risk groups

☐ Range of recommended ages for non-high-risk groups that may receive vaccine, subject to individual clinical decision making

☐ No recommendation

NOTE: The above recommendations must be read along with the footnotes of this schedule.

FIGURE 2. Catch-up immunization schedule for persons aged 4 months through 18 years who start late or who are more than 1 month behind—United States, 2017.

The figure below provides catch-up schedules and minimum intervals between doses for children whose vaccinations have been delayed. A vaccine series does not need to be restarted, regardless of the time that has elapsed between doses. Use the section appropriate for the child's age. Always use this table in conjunction with Figure 1 and the footnotes that follow.

Vaccine	Minimum Age for Dose 1	Minimum Interval Between Doses			
		Dose 1 to Dose 2	Dose 2 to Dose 3	Dose 3 to Dose 4	Dose 4 to Dose 5
Children age 4 months through 6 years					
Hepatitis B[1]	Birth	4 weeks	8 weeks *and at least 16 weeks after first dose.* Minimum age for the final dose is 24 weeks.		
Rotavirus[2]	6 weeks	4 weeks	4 weeks[2]		
Diphtheria, tetanus, and acellular pertussis[3]	6 weeks	4 weeks	4 weeks	6 months	6 months[3]
Haemophilus influenzae type b[4]	6 weeks	4 weeks if first dose was administered before the 1st birthday. 8 weeks (as final dose) if first dose was administered at age 12 through 14 months. No further doses needed if first dose was administered at age 15 months or older.	4 weeks[4] if current age is younger than 12 months **and** first dose was administered at younger than age 7 months, **and** at least 1 previous dose was PRP-T (ActHIB, Pentacel, Hiberix) or unknown. OR 8 weeks and age 12 through 59 months (as final dose)[4] · if current age is younger than 12 months **and** first dose was administered at age 7 through 11 months; OR · if current age is 12 through 59 months **and** first dose was administered before the 1st birthday, **and** second dose administered at younger than 15 months; OR if both doses were PRP-OMP (PedvaxHIB; Comvax) **and** were administered before the 1st birthday. No further doses needed if previous dose was administered at age 15 months or older.	8 weeks (as final dose) This dose only necessary for children age 12 through 59 months who received 3 doses before the 1st birthday.	
Pneumococcal[5]	6 weeks	4 weeks if first dose administered before the 1st birthday. 8 weeks (as final dose for healthy children) if first dose was administered at the 1st birthday or after. No further doses needed for healthy children if first dose was administered at age 24 months or older.	4 weeks if current age is younger than 12 months and previous dose given at <7 months old. 8 weeks (as final dose for healthy children) if previous dose given between 7–11 months (wait until at least 12 months old); OR if current age 12 months or older and at least 1 dose was given before age 12 months. No further doses needed for healthy children if previous dose administered at age 24 months or older.	8 weeks (as final dose) This dose only necessary for children aged 12 through 59 months who received 3 doses before age 12 months or for children at high risk who received 3 doses at any age.	
Inactivated poliovirus[6]	6 weeks	4 weeks[6]	4 weeks[6]	6 months[6] (minimum age 4 years for final dose).	
Measles, mumps, rubella[8]	12 months	4 weeks			
Varicella[9]	12 months	3 months			
Hepatitis A[10]	12 months	6 months			
Meningococcal[11] (Hib-MenCY ≥6 weeks; MenACWY-D ≥9 mos; MenACWY-CRM ≥2 mos)	6 weeks	8 weeks[11]	See footnote 11	See footnote 11	
Children and adolescents age 7 through 18 years					
Meningococcal[11] (MenACWY-D ≥9 mos; MenACWY-CRM ≥2 mos)	Not Applicable (N/A)	8 weeks[11]			
Tetanus, diphtheria; tetanus, diphtheria, and acellular pertussis[12]	7 years[12]	4 weeks	4 weeks if first dose of DTaP/DT was administered before the 1st birthday. 6 months (as final dose) if first dose of DTaP/DT or Tdap/Td was administered at or after the 1st birthday.	6 months if first dose of DTaP/DT was administered before the 1st birthday.	
Human papillomavirus[13]	9 years	Routine dosing intervals are recommended.[13]			
Hepatitis A[10]	N/A	6 months			
Hepatitis B[1]	N/A	4 weeks	8 weeks **and at least 16 weeks after first dose.**		
Inactivated poliovirus[6]	N/A	4 weeks	4 weeks[6]	6 months[6]	
Measles, mumps, rubella[8]	N/A	4 weeks			
Varicella[9]	N/A	3 months if younger than age 13 years. 4 weeks if age 13 years or older.			

NOTE: The above recommendations must be read along with the footnotes of this schedule.

Figure 3. Vaccines that might be indicated for children and adolescents aged 18 years or younger based on medical indications

VACCINE ▼ INDICATION ▶	Pregnancy	Immunocompromised status (excluding HIV infection)	HIV infection CD4+ count (cells/μL): <15% of total CD4 cell count	HIV infection CD4+ count (cells/μL): ≥15% of total CD4 cell count	Kidney failure, end-stage renal disease, on hemodialysis	Heart disease, chronic lung disease	CSF leaks/ cochlear implants	Asplenia and persistent complement component deficiencies	Chronic liver disease	Diabetes
Hepatitis B[1]	Routine schedule	Routine schedule	Routine schedule	Routine schedule	Routine schedule	Routine schedule	Routine schedule	Routine schedule	Routine schedule	Routine schedule
Rotavirus[2]	No recommendation	Precaution; SCID*: Contraindicated	Precaution	Precaution	Routine schedule	Routine schedule	Routine schedule	Routine schedule	Routine schedule	Routine schedule
Diphtheria, tetanus, & acellular pertussis[3] (DTaP)	No recommendation	Routine schedule	Routine schedule	Routine schedule	Routine schedule	Routine schedule	Routine schedule	Routine schedule	Routine schedule	Routine schedule
Haemophilus influenzae type b[4]	No recommendation	Additional doses may be necessary	Additional doses may be necessary	Additional doses may be necessary	Routine schedule	Routine schedule	Routine schedule	Additional doses may be necessary	Routine schedule	Routine schedule
Pneumococcal conjugate[5]	No recommendation	Additional doses may be necessary	Additional doses may be necessary	Additional doses may be necessary	Additional doses may be necessary	Routine schedule	Additional doses may be necessary	Additional doses may be necessary	Routine schedule	Routine schedule
Inactivated poliovirus[6]	Additional risk factor	Routine schedule	Routine schedule	Routine schedule	Routine schedule	Routine schedule	Routine schedule	Routine schedule	Routine schedule	Routine schedule
Influenza[7]	Routine schedule	Routine schedule	Routine schedule	Routine schedule	Routine schedule	Routine schedule	Routine schedule	Routine schedule	Routine schedule	Routine schedule
Measles, mumps, rubella[8]	Contraindicated	Contraindicated	Contraindicated	Routine schedule	Routine schedule	Routine schedule	Routine schedule	Routine schedule	Routine schedule	Routine schedule
Varicella[9]	Contraindicated	Contraindicated	Contraindicated	Routine schedule	Routine schedule	Routine schedule	Routine schedule	Routine schedule	Routine schedule	Routine schedule
Hepatitis A[10]	Additional risk factor	Routine schedule	Routine schedule	Routine schedule	Routine schedule	Routine schedule	Routine schedule	Routine schedule	Additional doses may be necessary	Routine schedule
Meningococcal ACWY[11]	Additional risk factor	Routine schedule	Additional doses may be necessary	Additional doses may be necessary	Routine schedule	Routine schedule	Routine schedule	Additional doses may be necessary	Routine schedule	Routine schedule
Tetanus, diphtheria, & acellular pertussis[12] (Tdap)	Additional doses may be necessary	Routine schedule	Routine schedule	Routine schedule	Routine schedule	Routine schedule	Routine schedule	Routine schedule	Routine schedule	Routine schedule
Human papillomavirus[13]	No recommendation	Additional doses may be necessary	Additional doses may be necessary	Additional doses may be necessary	Routine schedule	Routine schedule	Routine schedule	Routine schedule	Routine schedule	Routine schedule
Meningococcal B[11]	No recommendation	Additional risk factor	Additional risk factor	Additional risk factor	Additional risk factor	Additional risk factor	Additional risk factor	Additional doses may be necessary	Additional risk factor	Additional risk factor
Pneumococcal polysaccharide[5]	Additional risk factor	Additional doses may be necessary	Additional doses may be necessary	Additional doses may be necessary	Additional doses may be necessary	Additional doses may be necessary	Additional doses may be necessary	Additional doses may be necessary	Additional doses may be necessary	Additional doses may be necessary

- Vaccination according to the routine schedule recommended
- Recommended for persons with an additional risk factor for which the vaccine would be indicated
- Vaccination is recommended, and additional doses may be necessary based on medical condition. See footnotes.
- No recommendation
- Contraindicated
- Precaution for vaccination

*Severe Combined Immunodeficiency

NOTE: The above recommendations must be read along with the footnotes of this schedule.

Footnotes — Recommended Immunization Schedule for Children and Adolescents Aged 18 Years or Younger, UNITED STATES, 2017

For further guidance on the use of the vaccines mentioned below, see: www.cdc.gov/vaccines/hcp/acip-recs/index.html.

For vaccine recommendations for persons 19 years of age and older, see the Adult Immunization Schedule.

Additional information

- For information on contraindications and precautions for the use of a vaccine and for additional information regarding that vaccine, vaccination providers should consult the ACIP General Recommendations on Immunization and the relevant ACIP statement, available online at www.cdc.gov/vaccines/hcp/acip-recs/index.html.
- For purposes of calculating intervals between doses, 4 weeks = 28 days. Intervals of 4 months or greater are determined by calendar months.
- Vaccine doses administered ≤4 days before the minimum interval or minimum age should not be counted as valid doses and should be repeated as age-appropriate. The repeat dose should be spaced after the invalid dose by the recommended minimum interval. For further details, see Table 1, *Recommended and minimum ages and intervals between vaccine doses*, in MMWR, *General Recommendations on Immunization and Reports / Vol. 60 / No. 2*, available online at www.cdc.gov/mmwr/pdf/rr/rr6002.pdf.
- Information on travel vaccine requirements and recommendations is available at wwwnc.cdc.gov/travel/.
- For vaccination of persons with primary and secondary immunodeficiencies, see Table 13, *Vaccination of persons with primary and secondary immunodeficiencies*, in *General Recommendations on Immunization* (ACIP), available at www.cdc.gov/mmwr/pdf/rr/rr6002.pdf; and Immunization in Special Clinical Circumstances, (American Academy of Pediatrics). In: Kimberlin DW, Brady MT, Jackson MA, Long SS, eds. *Red Book: 2015 report of the Committee on Infectious Diseases. 30th ed.* Elk Grove Village, IL: American Academy of Pediatrics, 2015:68-107.
- The National Vaccine Injury Compensation Program (VICP) is a no-fault alternative to the traditional legal system for resolving vaccine injury petitions. Created by the National Childhood Vaccine Injury Act of 1986, it provides compensation to people found to be injured by certain vaccines. All vaccines within the recommended childhood immunization schedule are covered by VICP except for pneumococcal polysaccharide vaccine (PPSV23). For more information; see www.hrsa.gov/vaccinecompensation/index.html.

1. Hepatitis B (HepB) vaccine. (Minimum age: birth)

Routine vaccination:

At birth:
- Administer monovalent HepB vaccine to all newborns within 24 hours of birth.
- For infants born to hepatitis B surface antigen (HBsAg)-positive mothers, administer HepB vaccine and 0.5 mL of hepatitis B immune globulin (HBIG) within 12 hours of birth. These infants should be tested for HBsAg and antibody to HBsAg (anti-HBs) at age 9 through 12 months (preferably at the next well-child visit) or 1 to 2 months after completion of the HepB series if the series was delayed.
- If mother's HBsAg status is unknown, within 12 hours of birth, administer HepB vaccine regardless of birth weight. For infants weighing less than 2,000 grams, administer HBIG in addition to HepB vaccine within 12 hours of birth. Determine mother's HBsAg status as soon as possible and, if mother is HBsAg-positive, also administer HBIG to infants weighing 2,000 grams or more as soon as possible, but no later than age 7 days.

Doses following the birth dose:
- The second dose should be administered at age 1 or 2 months. Monovalent HepB vaccine should be used for doses administered before age 6 weeks.
- Infants who did not receive a birth dose should receive 3 doses of a HepB-containing vaccine on a schedule of 0, 1 to 2 months, and 6 months, starting as soon as feasible (see figure 2).
- Administer the second dose 1 to 2 months after the first dose (minimum interval of 4 weeks); administer the third dose at least 8 weeks after the second dose AND at least 16 weeks after the **first** dose. The final (third or fourth) dose in the HepB vaccine series should be administered **no earlier than age 24 weeks.**
- Administration of a total of 4 doses of HepB vaccine is permitted when a combination vaccine containing HepB is administered after the birth dose.

Catch-up vaccination:
- Unvaccinated persons should complete a 3-dose series.
- A 2-dose series (doses separated by at least 4 months) of adult formulation Recombivax HB is licensed for use in children aged 11 through 15 years.
- For other catch-up guidance, see Figure 2.

2. Rotavirus (RV) vaccines. (Minimum age: 6 weeks for both RV1 [Rotarix] and RV5 [RotaTeq])

Routine vaccination:

Administer a series of RV vaccine to all infants as follows:
1. If Rotarix is used, administer a 2-dose series at ages 2 and 4 months.
2. If RotaTeq is used, administer a 3-dose series at ages 2, 4, and 6 months.
3. If any dose in the series was RotaTeq or vaccine product is unknown for any dose in the series, a total of 3 doses of RV vaccine should be administered.

Catch-up vaccination:
- The maximum age for the first dose in the series is 14 weeks, 6 days; vaccination should not be initiated for infants aged 15 weeks, 0 days, or older.
- The maximum age for the final dose in the series is 8 months, 0 days.
- For other catch-up guidance, see Figure 2.

3. Diphtheria and tetanus toxoids and acellular pertussis (DTaP) vaccine. (Minimum age: 6 weeks. Exception: DTaP-IPV [Kinrix, Quadracel]: 4 years)

Routine vaccination:
- Administer a 5-dose series of DTaP vaccine at ages 2, 4, 6, 15 through 18 months, and 4 through 6 years. The fourth dose may be administered as early as age 12 months, provided at least 6 months have elapsed since the third dose.
- Inadvertent administration of fourth DTaP dose early: If the fourth dose of DTaP was administered at least 4 months after the third dose of DTaP and the child was 12 months of age or older, it does not need to be repeated.

Catch-up vaccination:
- The fifth dose of DTaP vaccine is not necessary if the fourth dose was administered at age 4 years or older.
- For other catch-up guidance, see Figure 2.

4. Haemophilus influenzae type b (Hib) conjugate vaccine. (Minimum age: 6 weeks for PRP-T [ActHIB, DTaP-IPV/Hib [Pentacel], Hiberix, and Hib-MenCY (MenHibrix)], PRP-OMP [PedvaxHIB])

Routine vaccination:
- Administer a 2- or 3-dose Hib vaccine primary series and a booster dose (dose 3 or 4, depending on vaccine used in primary series) at age 12 through 15 months to complete a full Hib vaccine series.
- The primary series with ActHIB, MenHibrix, Hiberix, or Pentacel consists of 3 doses and should be administered at ages 2, 4, and 6 months. The primary series with PedvaxHIB consists of 2 doses and should be administered at ages 2 and 4 months; a dose at age 6 months is not indicated.
- One booster dose (dose 3 or 4, depending on vaccine used in primary series) of any Hib vaccine should be administered at age 12 through 15 months.
- For recommendations on the use of MenHibrix in patients at increased risk for meningococcal disease, refer to the meningococcal vaccine footnotes and also to *MMWR* February 28, 2014 / 63(RR01):1-13, available at www.cdc.gov/mmwr/PDF/rr/rr6301.pdf.

For further guidance on the use of the vaccines mentioned below, see: www.cdc.gov/vaccines/hcp/acip-recs/index.html.

Catch-up vaccination:
- If dose 1 was administered at ages 12 through 14 months, administer a second (final) dose at least 8 weeks after dose 1, regardless of Hib vaccine used in the primary series.
- If both doses were PRP-OMP (PedvaxHIB or COMVAX) and were administered before the first birthday, the third (and final) dose should be administered at age 12 through 59 months and at least 8 weeks after the second dose.
- If the first dose was administered at age 7 through 11 months, administer the second dose at least 4 weeks later and a third (and final) dose at age 12 through 15 months or 8 weeks after second dose, whichever is later.
- If first dose is administered before the first birthday and second dose administered at younger than 15 months, a third (and final) dose should be administered 8 weeks later.
- For unvaccinated children aged 15–59 months, administer only 1 dose.
- For other catch-up guidance, see Figure 2. For catch-up guidance related to MenHibrix, see the meningococcal vaccine footnotes and also *MMWR* February 28, 2014 / 63(RR01):1–13, available at www.cdc.gov/mmwr/PDF/rr/rr6301.pdf.

Vaccination of persons with high-risk conditions:
Children aged 12 through 59 months who are at increased risk for Hib disease, including chemotherapy recipients and those with anatomic or functional asplenia (including sickle cell disease), human immunodeficiency virus (HIV) infection, immunoglobulin deficiency, or early component complement deficiency, who have received either no doses or only 1 dose of Hib vaccine before age 12 months, should receive 2 additional doses of Hib vaccine, 8 weeks apart; children who received 2 or more doses of Hib vaccine before age 12 months should receive 1 additional dose.
- For patients younger than age 5 years undergoing chemotherapy or radiation treatment who received a Hib vaccine dose(s) within 14 days of starting therapy or during therapy, repeat the dose(s) at least 3 months following therapy completion.
- Recipients of hematopoietic stem cell transplant (HSCT) should be revaccinated with a 3-dose regimen of Hib vaccine starting 6 to 12 months after successful transplant, regardless of vaccination history; doses should be administered at least 4 weeks apart.
- A single dose of any Hib-containing vaccine should be administered to unimmunized* children and adolescents 15 months of age and older undergoing an elective splenectomy; if possible, vaccine should be administered at least 14 days before procedure.
- Hib vaccine is not routinely recommended for patients 5 years or older. However, 1 dose of Hib vaccine should be administered to unimmunized* persons aged 5 years or older who have anatomic or functional asplenia (including sickle cell disease) and unimmunized* persons 5 through 18 years of age with HIV infection.
  Patients who have not received a primary series and booster dose or at least 1 dose of Hib vaccine after 14 months of age are considered unimmunized.

5. **Pneumococcal vaccines. (Minimum age: 6 weeks for PCV13, 2 years for PPSV23)**
Routine vaccination with PCV13:
- Administer a 4-dose series of PCV13 at ages 2, 4, and 6 months and at age 12 through 15 months.
Catch-up vaccination with PCV13:
- Administer 1 dose of PCV13 to all healthy children aged 24 through 59 months who are not completely vaccinated for their age.
- For other catch-up guidance, see Figure 2.
Vaccination of persons with high-risk conditions with PCV13 and PPSV23:
- All recommended PCV13 doses should be administered prior to PPSV23 vaccination if possible.
- For children aged 2 through 5 years with any of the following conditions: chronic heart disease (particularly cyanotic congenital heart disease and cardiac failure); chronic lung disease (including asthma if treated with high-dose oral corticosteroid therapy); diabetes mellitus; cerebrospinal fluid leak; cochlear implant; sickle cell disease and other hemoglobinopathies; anatomic or functional asplenia; HIV infection; chronic renal failure; nephrotic syndrome; diseases associated with treatment with immunosuppressive drugs or radiation therapy, including malignant neoplasms, leukemias, lymphomas, and Hodgkin disease; solid organ transplantation; or congenital immunodeficiency:
  1. Administer 1 dose of PCV13 if any incomplete schedule of 3 doses of PCV13 was received previously.
  2. Administer 2 doses of PCV13 at least 8 weeks apart if unvaccinated or any incomplete schedule of fewer than 3 doses of PCV13 was received previously.
  3. The minimum interval between doses of PCV13 is 8 weeks.
  4. For children with no history of PPSV23 vaccination, administer PPSV23 at least 8 weeks after the most recent dose of PCV13.
- For children aged 6 through 18 years who have cerebrospinal fluid leak; cochlear implant; sickle cell disease and other hemoglobinopathies; anatomic or functional asplenia; congenital or acquired immunodeficiencies; HIV infection; chronic renal failure; nephrotic syndrome; diseases associated with treatment with immunosuppressive drugs or radiation therapy, including malignant neoplasms, leukemias, lymphomas, and Hodgkin disease; generalized malignancy; solid organ transplantation; or multiple myeloma:
  1. If neither PCV13 nor PPSV23 has been received previously, administer 1 dose of PCV13 now and 1 dose of PPSV23 at least 8 weeks later.
  2. If PCV13 has been received previously but PPSV23 has not, administer 1 dose of PPSV23 at least 8 weeks after the most recent dose of PCV13.
  3. If PPSV23 has been received but PCV13 has not, administer 1 dose of PCV13 at least 8 weeks after the most recent dose of PPSV23.
- For children aged 6 through 18 years with chronic heart disease (particularly cyanotic congenital heart disease and cardiac failure), chronic lung disease (including asthma if treated with high-dose oral corticosteroid therapy), diabetes mellitus, alcoholism, or chronic liver disease, who have not received PPSV23, administer 1 dose of PPSV23. If PCV13 has been received previously, then PPSV23 should be administered at least 8 weeks after any prior PCV13 dose.
- A single revaccination with PPSV23 should be administered 5 years after the first dose to children with sickle cell disease or other hemoglobinopathies; anatomic or functional asplenia; congenital or acquired immunodeficiencies; HIV infection; chronic renal failure; nephrotic syndrome; diseases associated with treatment with immunosuppressive drugs or radiation therapy, including malignant neoplasms, leukemias, lymphomas, and Hodgkin disease; generalized malignancy; solid organ transplantation; or multiple myeloma.

6. **Inactivated poliovirus vaccine (IPV). (Minimum age: 6 weeks)**
Routine vaccination:
- Administer a 4-dose series of IPV at ages 2, 4, 6 through 18 months, and 4 through 6 years. The final dose in the series should be administered on or after the fourth birthday and at least 6 months after the previous dose.
Catch-up vaccination:
- In the first 6 months of life, minimum age and minimum intervals are only recommended if the person is at risk of imminent exposure to circulating poliovirus (i.e., travel to a polio-endemic region or during an outbreak).
- If 4 or more doses are administered before age 4 years, an additional dose should be administered at age 4 through 6 years and at least 6 months after the previous dose.
- A fourth dose is not necessary if the third dose was administered at age 4 years or older and at least 6 months after the previous dose.
- If both oral polio vaccine (OPV) and IPV were administered as part of a series, a total of 4 doses should be administered, regardless of the child's current age. If only OPV was administered, and all doses were given prior to age 4 years, 1 dose of IPV should be given at 4 years or older, at least 4 weeks after the last OPV dose.
- IPV is not routinely recommended for U.S. residents aged 18 years or older.
- For other catch-up guidance, see Figure 2.

For further guidance on the use of the vaccines mentioned below, see: www.cdc.gov/vaccines/hcp/acip-recs/index.html.

7. **Influenza vaccines. (Minimum age: 6 months for inactivated influenza vaccine [IIV], 18 years for recombinant influenza vaccine [RIV])**

Routine vaccination:

- Administer influenza vaccine annually to all children beginning at age 6 months. For the 2016–17 season, use of live attenuated influenza vaccine (LAIV) is not recommended.

For children aged 6 months through 8 years:

- For the 2016–17 season, administer 2 doses (separated by at least 4 weeks) to children who are receiving influenza vaccine for the first time or who have not previously received ≥2 doses of trivalent or quadrivalent influenza vaccine before July 1, 2016. For additional guidance, follow dosing guidelines in the 2016–17 ACIP influenza vaccine recommendations (see *MMWR* August 26, 2016;65(5):1–54, available at www.cdc.gov/mmwr/volumes/65/rr/pdfs/rr6505.pdf).
- For the 2017–18 season, follow dosing guidelines in the 2017–18 ACIP influenza vaccine recommendations.

For persons aged 9 years and older:

- Administer 1 dose.

8. **Measles, mumps, and rubella (MMR) vaccine. (Minimum age: 12 months for routine vaccination)**

Routine vaccination:

- Administer a 2-dose series of MMR vaccine at ages 12 through 15 months and 4 through 6 years, provided at least 4 weeks have elapsed since the first dose. Administer 1 dose of MMR vaccine to infants aged 6 through 11 months before departure from the United States for international travel. These children should be revaccinated with 2 doses of MMR vaccine, the first at age 12 through 15 months (12 months if the child remains in an area where disease risk is high), and the second dose at least 4 weeks later.
- Administer 2 doses of MMR vaccine to children aged 12 months and older before departure from the United States for international travel. The first dose should be administered on or after age 12 months and the second dose at least 4 weeks later.

Catch-up vaccination:

- Ensure that all school-aged children and adolescents have had 2 doses of MMR vaccine; the minimum interval between the 2 doses is 4 weeks.

9. **Varicella (VAR) vaccine. (Minimum age: 12 months)**

Routine vaccination:

- Administer a 2-dose series of VAR vaccine at ages 12 through 15 months and 4 through 6 years. The second dose may be administered before age 4 years, provided at least 3 months have elapsed since the first dose. If the second dose was administered at least 4 weeks after the first dose, it can be accepted as valid.

Catch-up vaccination:

- Ensure that all persons aged 7 through 18 years without evidence of immunity (see *MMWR* 2007;56[No. RR-4], available at www.cdc.gov/mmwr/pdf/rr/rr5604.pdf) have 2 doses of varicella vaccine. For children aged 7 through 12 years, the recommended minimum interval between doses is 3 months (if the second dose was administered at least 4 weeks after the first dose, it can be accepted as valid); for persons aged 13 years and older, the minimum interval between doses is 4 weeks.

10. **Hepatitis A (HepA) vaccine. (Minimum age: 12 months)**

Routine vaccination:

- Initiate the 2-dose HepA vaccine series at ages 12 through 23 months; separate the 2 doses by 6 to 18 months.
- Children who have received 1 dose of HepA vaccine before age 24 months should receive a second dose 6 to 18 months after the first dose.
- For any person aged 2 years and older who has not already received the HepA vaccine series, 2 doses of HepA vaccine separated by 6 to 18 months may be administered if immunity against hepatitis A virus infection is desired.

Catch-up vaccination:

- The minimum interval between the 2 doses is 6 months.

Special populations:

- Administer 2 doses of HepA vaccine at least 6 months apart to previously unvaccinated persons who live in areas where vaccination programs target older children, or who are at increased risk for infection. This includes persons traveling to or working in countries that have high or intermediate endemicity of infection; men having sex with men; users of injection and non-injection illicit drugs; persons who work with HAV-infected primates or with HAV in a research laboratory; persons with clotting-factor disorders; persons with chronic liver disease; and persons who anticipate close, personal contact (e.g., household or regular babysitting) with an international adoptee during the first 60 days after arrival in the United States from a country with high or intermediate endemicity. The first dose should be administered as soon as the adoption is planned, ideally, 2 or more weeks before the arrival of the adoptee.

11. **Meningococcal vaccines. (Minimum age: 6 weeks for Hib-MenCY [MenHibrix], 2 months for MenACWY-CRM [Menveo], 9 months for MenACWY-D [Menactra], 10 years for serogroup B meningococcal [MenB] vaccines: MenB-4C [Bexsero] and MenB-FHbp [Trumenba])**

Routine vaccination:

- Administer a single dose of Menactra or Menveo vaccine at age 11 through 12 years, with a booster dose at age 16 years.
- For children aged 2 months through 18 years with high-risk conditions, see "Meningococcal conjugate ACWY vaccination of persons with high-risk conditions and other persons at increased risk" and "Meningococcal B

vaccination of persons with high-risk conditions and other persons at increased risk of disease" below.

Catch-up vaccination:

- Administer Menactra or Menveo vaccine at age 13 through 18 years if not previously vaccinated.
- If the first dose is administered at age 13 through 15 years, a booster dose should be administered at age 16 through 18 years, with a minimum interval of at least 8 weeks between doses.
- If the first dose is administered at age 16 years or older, a booster dose is not needed.
- For other catch-up guidance, see Figure 2.

Clinical discretion:

- Young adults aged 16 through 23 years (preferred age range is 16 through 18 years) who are not at increased risk for meningococcal disease may be vaccinated with a 2-dose series of either Bexsero (0, ≥1 month) or Trumenba (0, 6 months) vaccine to provide short-term protection against most strains of serogroup B meningococcal disease. The two MenB vaccines are not interchangeable; the same vaccine product must be used for all doses.
- If the second dose of Trumenba is given at an interval of <6 months, a third dose should be given at least 6 months after the first dose; the minimum interval between the second and third doses is 4 weeks.

Meningococcal conjugate ACWY vaccination of persons with high-risk conditions and other persons at increased risk:

Children with anatomic or functional asplenia (including sickle cell disease), children with HIV infection, or children with persistent complement component deficiency (includes persons with inherited or chronic deficiencies in C3, C5–9, properdin, factor D, factor H, or taking eculizumab [Soliris]):

- **Menveo**
  ○ *Children who initiate vaccination at 8 weeks.* Administer doses at ages 2, 4, 6, and 12 months.
  ○ *Unvaccinated children who initiate vaccination at 7 through 23 months.* Administer 2 primary doses, with the second dose at least 12 weeks after the first dose AND after the first birthday.
  ○ *Children 24 months and older who have not received a complete series.* Administer 2 primary doses at least 8 weeks apart.

- **MenHibrix**
  ○ *Children who initiate vaccination at 6 weeks.* Administer doses at ages 2, 4, 6, and 12 through 15 months.
  ○ If the first dose of MenHibrix is given at or after age 12 months, a total of 2 doses should be given at least 8 weeks apart to ensure protection against serogroups C and Y meningococcal disease.

For further guidance on the use of the vaccines mentioned below, see: www.cdc.gov/vaccines/hcp/acip-recs/index.html.

- **Menactra**
  - o **Children with anatomic or functional asplenia or HIV infection**
    - — *Children 24 months and older who have not received a complete series.* Administer 2 primary doses at least 8 weeks apart. If MenHibrix is administered to a child with asplenia (including sickle cell disease) or HIV infection, do not administer Menactra until age 2 years and at least 4 weeks after the completion of all PCV13 doses.
  - o **Children with persistent complement component deficiency**
    - — *Children 9 through 23 months.* Administer 2 primary doses at least 12 weeks apart.
    - — *Children 24 months and older who have not received a complete series.* Administer 2 primary doses at least 8 weeks apart.
  - o **All high-risk children**
    - — If Menactra is to be administered to a child at high risk for meningococcal disease, it is recommended that Menactra be given either before or at the same time as DTaP.

Meningococcal B vaccination of persons with high-risk conditions and other persons at increased risk of disease:

Children with anatomic or functional asplenia (including sickle cell disease) or children with persistent complement component deficiency (includes persons with inherited or chronic deficiencies in C3, C5-9, properdin, factor D, factor H, or taking eculizumab [Soliris]):

- **Bexsero or Trumenba**
  - o *Persons 10 years or older who have not received a complete series.* Administer a 2-dose series of Bexsero, with doses at least 1 month apart, or a 3-dose series of Trumenba, with the second dose at least 1-2 months after the first and the third dose at least 6 months after the first. The two MenB vaccines are not interchangeable; the same vaccine product must be used for all doses.

For children who travel to or reside in countries in which meningococcal disease is hyperendemic or epidemic, including countries in the African meningitis belt or the Hajj:

- Administer an age-appropriate formulation and series of Menactra or Menveo for protection against serogroups A and W meningococcal disease. Prior receipt of MenHibrix is not sufficient for children traveling to the meningitis belt or the Hajj because it does not contain serogroups A or W.

For children at risk during an outbreak attributable to a vaccine serogroup:

- For serogroup A, C, W, or Y: Administer or complete an age- and formulation-appropriate series of MenHibrix, Menactra, or Menveo.

- For serogroup B: Administer a 2-dose series of Bexsero, with doses at least 1 month apart, or a 3-dose series of Trumenba, with the second dose at least 1-2 months after the first and the third dose at least 6 months after the first. The two MenB vaccines are not interchangeable; the same vaccine product must be used for all doses.

For MenACWY booster doses among persons with high-risk conditions, refer to *MMWR* 2013;62(RR02):1-22, at www.cdc.gov/mmwr/preview/mmwrhtml/rr620a1.htm, *MMWR* June 20, 2014 / 63(24):527-530, at www.cdc.gov/mmwr/pdf/wk/mm6324.pdf, and *MMWR* November 4, 2016 / 65(43):1189-1194, at www.cdc.gov/mmwr/volumes/65/wr/pdfs/mm6543a3.pdf.

For other catch-up recommendations for these persons and complete information on use of meningococcal vaccines, including guidance related to vaccination of persons at increased risk of infection, see meningococcal *MMWR* publications, available at: www.cdc.gov/vaccines/hcp/acip-recs/vacc-specific/mening.html.

12. **Tetanus and diphtheria toxoids and acellular pertussis (Tdap) vaccine. (Minimum age: 10 years for both Boostrix and Adacel)**

Routine vaccination:
- Administer 1 dose of Tdap vaccine to all adolescents aged 11 through 12 years.
- Tdap may be administered regardless of the interval since the last tetanus and diphtheria toxoid-containing vaccine.
- Administer 1 dose of Tdap vaccine to pregnant adolescents during each pregnancy (preferably during the early part of gestational weeks 27 through 36), regardless of time since prior Td or Tdap vaccination.

Catch-up vaccination:
- Persons aged 7 years and older who are not fully immunized with DTaP vaccine should receive Tdap vaccine as 1 dose (preferably the first) in the catch-up series; if additional doses are needed, use Td vaccine. For children 7 through 10 years who receive a dose of Tdap as part of the catch-up series, an adolescent Tdap vaccine dose at age 11 through 12 years may be administered.
- Persons aged 11 through 18 years who have not received Tdap vaccine should receive a dose, followed by tetanus and diphtheria toxoids (Td) booster doses every 10 years thereafter.

- Inadvertent doses of DTaP vaccine:
  - If administered inadvertently to a child aged 7 through 10 years, the dose may count as part of the catch-up series. This dose may count as the adolescent Tdap dose, or the child may receive a Tdap booster dose at age 11 through 12 years.
  - If administered inadvertently to an adolescent aged 11 through 18 years, the dose should be counted as the adolescent Tdap booster.
- For other catch-up guidance, see Figure 2.

13. **Human papillomavirus (HPV) vaccines. (Minimum age: 9 years for 4vHPV [Gardasil] and 9vHPV [Gardasil 9])**

Routine and catch-up vaccination:
- Administer a 2-dose series of HPV vaccine on a schedule of 0, 6-12 months to all adolescents aged 11 or 12 years. The vaccination series can start at age 9 years.
- Administer HPV vaccine to all adolescents through age 18 years who were not previously adequately vaccinated. The number of recommended doses is based on age at administration of the first dose.
- For persons initiating vaccination before age 15, the recommended immunization schedule is 2 doses of HPV vaccine at 0, 6-12 months.
- For persons initiating vaccination at age 15 years or older, the recommended immunization schedule is 3 doses of HPV vaccine at 0, 1-2, 6 months.
- A vaccine dose administered at a shorter interval should be readministered at the recommended interval.
  - In a 2-dose schedule of HPV vaccine, the minimum interval is 5 months between the first and second dose. If the second dose is administered at a shorter interval, a third dose should be administered a minimum of 12 weeks after the second dose and a minimum of 5 months after the first dose.
  - In a 3-dose schedule of HPV vaccine, the minimum intervals are 4 weeks between the first and second dose, 12 weeks between the second and third dose, and 5 months between the first and third dose. If a vaccine dose is administered at a shorter interval, it should be readministered after another minimum interval has been met since the most recent dose.

Special populations:
- For children with history of sexual abuse or assault, administer HPV vaccine beginning at age 9 years.
- Immunocompromised persons*, including those with human immunodeficiency virus (HIV) infection, should receive a 3-dose series at 0, 1-2, and 6 months, regardless of age at vaccine initiation.
- Note: HPV vaccination is not recommended during pregnancy, although there is no evidence that the vaccine poses harm. If a woman is found to be pregnant after initiating the vaccination series, no intervention is needed; the remaining vaccine doses should be delayed until after the pregnancy. Pregnancy testing is not needed before HPV vaccination.

*See *MMWR* December 16, 2016;65(49):1405-1408, available at www.cdc.gov/mmwr/volumes/65/wr/pdfs/mm6549a5.pdf.

CS270457-C

Recommended Immunization Schedule for Adults Aged 19 Years or Older, United States, 2017

In February 2017, the *Recommended Immunization Schedule for Adults Aged 19 Years or Older, United States, 2017* became effective, as recommended by the Advisory Committee on Immunization Practices (ACIP) and approved by the Centers for Disease Control and Prevention (CDC). The 2017 adult immunization schedule was also reviewed and approved by the following professional medical organizations:

- American College of Physicians (www.acponline.org)
- American Academy of Family Physicians (www.aafp.org)
- American College of Obstetricians and Gynecologists (www.acog.org)
- American College of Nurse-Midwives (www.midwife.org)

CDC announced the availability of the 2017 adult immunization schedule at www.cdc.gov/vaccines/schedules/hcp/index.html in the *Morbidity and Mortality Weekly Report (MMWR)*.[1] The schedule is published in its entirety in the *Annals of Internal Medicine*.[2]

The adult immunization schedule describes the age groups and medical conditions and other indications for which licensed vaccines are recommended. The 2017 adult immunization schedule consists of:

- Figure 1. Recommended immunization schedule for adults by age group
- Figure 2. Recommended immunization schedule for adults by medical condition and other indications
- Footnotes that accompany each vaccine containing important general information and considerations for special populations
- Table. Contraindications and precautions for vaccines routinely recommended for adults

Consider the following information when reviewing the adult immunization schedule:

- The figures in the adult immunization schedule should be read with the footnotes that contain important general information and information about vaccination of special populations.
- When indicated, administer recommended vaccines to adults whose vaccination history is incomplete or unknown.
- Increased interval between doses of a multi-dose vaccine does not diminish vaccine effectiveness; therefore, it is not necessary to restart the vaccine series or add doses to the series because of an extended interval between doses.
- Adults with immunocompromising conditions should generally avoid live vaccines, e.g., measles, mumps, and rubella vaccine. Inactivated vaccines, e.g., pneumococcal or inactivated influenza vaccines, are generally acceptable.
- Combination vaccines may be used when any component of the combination is indicated and when the other components of the combination vaccine are not contraindicated.
- The use of trade names in the adult immunization schedule is for identification purposes only and does not imply endorsement by the ACIP or CDC.

Details on vaccines recommended for adults and complete ACIP statements are available at www.cdc.gov/vaccines/hcp/acip-recs/index.html. Additional CDC resources include:

- A summary of information on vaccination recommendations, vaccination of persons with immunodeficiencies, preventing and managing adverse reactions, vaccination contraindications and precautions, and other information can be found in *General Recommendations on Immunization* at www.cdc.gov/mmwr/preview/mmwrhtml/rr6002a1.htm.

- Vaccine Information Statements that explain benefits and risks of vaccines are available at www.cdc.gov/vaccines/hcp/vis/index.html.
- Information and resources regarding vaccination of pregnant women are available at www.cdc.gov/vaccines/adults/rec-vac/pregnant.html.
- Information on travel vaccine requirements and recommendations is available at wwwnc.cdc.gov/travel/destinations/list.
- *CDC Vaccine Schedules App* for clinicians and other immunization service providers to download is available at www.cdc.gov/vaccines/schedules/hcp/schedule-app.html.
- *Recommended Immunization Schedule for Children and Adolescents Aged 18 Years or Younger* is available at www.cdc.gov/vaccines/schedules/hcp/index.html.

Report suspected cases of reportable vaccine-preventable diseases to the local or state health department.

Report all clinically significant post-vaccination reactions to the Vaccine Adverse Event Reporting System at www.vaers.hhs.gov or by telephone, 800-822-7967. All vaccines included in the 2017 adult immunization schedule except herpes zoster and 23-valent pneumococcal polysaccharide vaccines are covered by the Vaccine Injury Compensation Program. Information on how to file a vaccine injury claim is available at www.hrsa.gov/vaccinecompensation or by telephone, 800-338-2382.

Submit questions and comments regarding the 2017 adult immunization schedule to CDC through www.cdc.gov/cdc-info or by telephone, 800-CDC-INFO (800-232-4636), in English and Spanish, 8:00am–8:00pm ET, Monday–Friday, excluding holidays.

The following acronyms are used for vaccines recommended for adults:

HepA	hepatitis A vaccine
HepA-HepB	hepatitis A and hepatitis B vaccines
HepB	hepatitis B vaccine
Hib	*Haemophilus influenzae* type b conjugate vaccine
HPV vaccine	human papillomavirus vaccine
HZV	herpes zoster vaccine
IIV	inactivated influenza vaccine
LAIV	live attenuated influenza vaccine
MenACWY	serogroups A, C, W, and Y meningococcal conjugate vaccine
MenB	serogroup B meningococcal vaccine
MMR	measles, mumps, and rubella vaccine
MPSV4	serogroups A, C, W, and Y meningococcal polysaccharide vaccine
PCV13	13-valent pneumococcal conjugate vaccine
PPSV23	23-valent pneumococcal polysaccharide vaccine
RIV	recombinant influenza vaccine
Td	tetanus and diphtheria toxoids
Tdap	tetanus toxoid, reduced diphtheria toxoid, and acellular pertussis vaccine
VAR	varicella vaccine

[1] *MMWR Morb Mortal Wkly Rep.* 2017;66(5). Available at www.cdc.gov/mmwr/volumes/66/wr/mm6605e2.htm?s_cid=mm6605e2_w.

[2] *Ann Intern Med.* 2017;166:209-218. Available at annals.org/aim/article/doi/10.7326/M16-2936.

U.S. Department of Health and Human Services
Centers for Disease Control and Prevention

Figures 1 and 2 should be read with the footnotes that contain important general information and considerations for special populations.

Figure 1. Recommended immunization schedule for adults aged 19 years or older by age group, United States, 2017

Vaccine	19–21 years	22–26 years	27–59 years	60–64 years	≥ 65 years
Influenza[1]	1 dose annually				
Td/Tdap[2]	Substitute Tdap for Td once, then Td booster every 10 yrs				
MMR[3]	1 or 2 doses depending on indication				
VAR[4]	2 doses				
HZV[5]				1 dose	
HPV–Female[6]	3 doses	3 doses			
HPV–Male[6]	3 doses	3 doses			
PCV13[7]				1 dose	
PPSV23[7]	1 or 2 doses depending on indication				1 dose
HepA[8]	2 or 3 doses depending on vaccine				
HepB[9]	3 doses				
MenACWY or MPSV4[10]	1 or more doses depending on indication				
MenB[10]	2 or 3 doses depending on vaccine				
Hib[11]	1 or 3 doses depending on indication				

Recommended for adults who meet the age requirement, lack documentation of vaccination, or lack evidence of past infection

Recommended for adults with additional medical conditions or other indications

No recommendation

Figure 2. Recommended immunization schedule for adults aged 19 years or older by medical condition and other indications, United States, 2017

Vaccine	Pregnancy[1-6,9]	Immunocompromised (excluding HIV infection)[3-7,11]	HIV infection CD4+ count (cells/µL)[3-7,9-11] <200	HIV infection CD4+ count (cells/µL)[3-7,9-11] ≥200	Asplenia, persistent complement deficiencies[7,10,11]	Kidney failure, end-stage renal disease, on hemodialysis[7,9]	Heart or lung disease, chronic alcoholism[7]	Chronic liver disease[7-9]	Diabetes[7,9]	Healthcare personnel[3,4,9]	Men who have sex with men[6,8,9]
Influenza[1]	1 dose annually										
Td/Tdap[2]	1 dose Tdap each pregnancy	Substitute Tdap for Td once, then Td booster every 10 yrs									
MMR[3]	contraindicated	contraindicated	contraindicated		1 or 2 doses depending on indication						
VAR[4]	contraindicated	contraindicated	contraindicated		2 doses						
HZV[5]	contraindicated	contraindicated	contraindicated		1 dose						
HPV–Female[6]		3 doses through age 26 yrs			3 doses through age 26 yrs						
HPV–Male[6]		3 doses through age 26 yrs			3 doses through age 21 yrs						3 doses through age 26 yrs
PCV13[7]					1 dose						
PPSV23[7]					1, 2, or 3 doses depending on indication						
HepA[8]					2 or 3 doses depending on vaccine						
HepB[9]					3 doses						
MenACWY or MPSV4[10]					1 or more doses depending on indication						
MenB[10]					2 or 3 doses depending on vaccine						
Hib[11]		3 doses post-HSCT recipients only			1 dose						

Legend:
- Recommended for adults who meet the age requirement, lack documentation of vaccination, or lack evidence of past infection
- Recommended for adults with additional medical conditions or other indications
- Contraindicated
- No recommendation

Footnotes. Recommended immunization schedule for adults aged 19 years or older, United States, 2017

1. Influenza vaccination

General information

- All persons aged 6 months or older who do not have a contraindication should receive annual influenza vaccination with an age-appropriate formulation of inactivated influenza vaccine (IIV) or recombinant influenza vaccine (RIV).
- In addition to standard-dose IIV, available options for adults in specific age groups include: high-dose or adjuvanted IIV for adults aged 65 years or older, intradermal IIV for adults aged 18 through 64 years, and RIV for adults aged 18 years or older.
- Notes: Live attenuated influenza vaccine (LAIV) should not be used during the 2016–2017 influenza season. A list of currently available influenza vaccines is available at www.cdc.gov/flu/protect/vaccine/vaccines.htm.

Special populations

- Adults with a history of egg allergy who have only hives after exposure to egg should receive age-appropriate IIV or RIV.
- Adults with a history of egg allergy other than hives, e.g., angioedema, respiratory distress, lightheadedness, or recurrent emesis, or who required epinephrine or another emergency medical intervention, may receive age-appropriate IIV or RIV. The selected vaccine should be administered in an inpatient or outpatient medical setting and under the supervision of a healthcare provider who is able to recognize and manage severe allergic conditions.
- Pregnant women and women who might become pregnant in the upcoming influenza season should receive IIV.

2. Tetanus, diphtheria, and acellular pertussis vaccination

General information

- Adults who have not received tetanus and diphtheria toxoids and acellular pertussis vaccine (Tdap) or for whom pertussis vaccination status is unknown should receive 1 dose of Tdap followed by a tetanus and diphtheria toxoids (Td) booster every 10 years. Tdap should be administered regardless of when a tetanus or diphtheria toxoid-containing vaccine was last received.
- Adults with an unknown or incomplete history of a 3-dose primary series with tetanus and diphtheria toxoid-containing vaccines should complete the primary series that includes 1 dose of Tdap. Unvaccinated adults should receive the first 2 doses at least 4 weeks apart and the third dose 6–12 months after the second dose.
- Notes: Information on the use of Td or Tdap as tetanus prophylaxis in wound management is available at www.cdc.gov/mmwr/preview/mmwrhtml/rr5517a1.htm.

Special populations

- Pregnant women should receive 1 dose of Tdap during each pregnancy, preferably during the early part of gestational weeks 27–36, regardless of prior history of receiving Tdap.

3. Measles, mumps, and rubella vaccination

General information

- Adults born in 1957 or later without acceptable evidence of immunity to measles, mumps, or rubella (defined below) should receive 1 dose of measles, mumps, and rubella vaccine (MMR) unless they have a medical contraindication to the vaccine, e.g., pregnancy or severe immunodeficiency.
- Notes: Acceptable evidence of immunity to measles, mumps, or rubella in adults is: born before 1957, documentation of receipt of MMR, or laboratory evidence of immunity or disease. Documentation of healthcare provider-diagnosed disease without laboratory confirmation is not acceptable evidence of immunity.

Special populations

- Pregnant women who do not have evidence of immunity to rubella should receive 1 dose of MMR upon completion or termination of pregnancy and before discharge from the healthcare facility; non-pregnant women of childbearing age without evidence of rubella immunity should receive 1 dose of MMR.
- Adults with primary or acquired immunodeficiency including malignant conditions affecting the bone marrow or lymphatic system, systemic immunosuppressive therapy, or cellular immunodeficiency should not receive MMR.
- Adults with human immunodeficiency virus (HIV) infection and CD4+ T-lymphocyte count ≥200 cells/μl for at least 6 months who do not have evidence of measles, mumps, or rubella immunity should receive 2 doses of MMR at least 28 days apart. Adults with HIV infection and CD4+ T-lymphocyte count <200 cells/μl should not receive MMR.
- Adults who work in healthcare facilities should receive 2 doses of MMR at least 28 days apart; healthcare personnel born before 1957 who are unvaccinated or lack laboratory evidence of measles, mumps, or rubella immunity, or laboratory confirmation of disease should be considered for vaccination with 2 doses of MMR at least 28 days apart for measles or mumps, or 1 dose of MMR for rubella.
- Adults who are students in postsecondary educational institutions or plan to travel internationally should receive 2 doses of MMR at least 28 days apart.
- Adults who received inactivated (killed) measles vaccine or measles vaccine of unknown type during years 1963–1967 should be revaccinated with 1 or 2 doses of MMR.
- Adults who were vaccinated before 1979 with either inactivated mumps vaccine or mumps vaccine of unknown type who are at high risk for mumps infection, e.g., work in a healthcare facility, should be considered for revaccination with 2 doses of MMR at least 28 days apart.

4. Varicella vaccination

General information

- Adults without evidence of immunity to varicella (defined below) should receive 2 doses of single-antigen varicella vaccine (VAR) 4–8 weeks apart, or a second dose if they have received only 1 dose.
- Persons without evidence of immunity for whom VAR should be emphasized are: adults who have close contact with persons at high risk for serious complications, e.g., healthcare personnel and household contacts of immunocompromised persons; adults who live or work in an environment in which transmission of varicella zoster virus is likely, e.g., teachers, childcare workers, and residents and staff in institutional settings; adults who live or work in environments in which varicella transmission can occur, e.g., college students, residents and staff members of correctional institutions, and military personnel; non-pregnant women of childbearing age; adolescents and adults living in households with children; and international travelers.
- Notes: Evidence of immunity to varicella in adults is: U.S.-born before 1980 (for pregnant women and healthcare personnel, U.S.-born before 1980 is not considered evidence of immunity); documentation of 2 doses of VAR at least 4 weeks apart; history of varicella or herpes zoster diagnosis or verification of varicella or herpes zoster disease by a healthcare provider; or laboratory evidence of immunity or disease.

Special populations

- Pregnant women should be assessed for evidence of varicella immunity. Pregnant women who do not have evidence of immunity should receive the first dose of VAR upon completion or termination of pregnancy and before discharge from the healthcare facility, and the second dose 4–8 weeks after the first dose.
- Healthcare institutions should assess and ensure that all healthcare personnel have evidence of immunity to varicella.
- Adults with malignant conditions, including those that affect the bone marrow or lymphatic system or who receive systemic immunosuppressive therapy, should not receive VAR.

5. Herpes zoster vaccination

General information

- Adults aged 60 years or older should receive 1 dose of herpes zoster vaccine (HZV), regardless of whether they had a prior episode of herpes zoster.

Special populations

- Adults aged 60 years or older with chronic medical conditions may receive HZV unless they have a medical contraindication, e.g., pregnancy or severe immunodeficiency.
- Adults with malignant conditions, including those that affect the bone marrow or lymphatic system or who receive systemic immunosuppressive therapy, should not receive HZV.
- Adults with human immunodeficiency virus (HIV) infection and CD4+ T-lymphocyte count <200 cells/μl should not receive HZV.

6. Human papillomavirus vaccination

General information

- Adult females through age 26 years and adult males through age 21 years who have not received any human papillomavirus (HPV) vaccine should receive a 3-dose series of HPV vaccine at 0, 1–2, and 6 months. Males aged 22 through 26 years may be vaccinated with a 3-dose series of HPV vaccine at 0, 1–2, and 6 months.
- Adult females through age 26 years and adult males through age 21 years (and males aged 22 through 26 years who may receive HPV vaccination) who initiated the HPV vaccination series before age 15 years and received 2 doses at least 5 months apart are considered adequately vaccinated and do not need an additional dose of HPV vaccine.
- Adult females through age 26 years and adult males through age 21 years (and males aged 22 through 26 years who may receive HPV vaccination) who initiated the HPV vaccination series before age 15 years and received only 1 dose, or 2 doses less than 5 months apart, are not considered adequately vaccinated and should receive 1 additional dose of HPV vaccine.
- Notes: HPV vaccination is routinely recommended for children at age 11 or 12 years. For adults who had initiated but did not complete the HPV vaccination series, consider their age at first HPV vaccination (described above) and other factors (described below) to determine if they have been adequately vaccinated.

Special populations

- Men who have sex with men through age 26 years who have not received any HPV vaccine should receive a 3-dose series of HPV vaccine at 0, 1–2, and 6 months.
- Adult females and males through age 26 years with immunocompromising conditions (described below), including those with human immunodeficiency virus (HIV) infection, should receive a 3-dose series of HPV vaccine at 0, 1–2, and 6 months.
- Pregnant women are not recommended to receive HPV vaccine, although there is no evidence that the vaccine poses harm. If a woman is found to be pregnant after initiating the HPV vaccination series, delay the remaining doses until after the pregnancy. No other intervention is needed. Pregnancy testing is not needed before administering HPV vaccine.
- Notes: Immunocompromising conditions for which a 3-dose series of HPV vaccine is indicated are primary or secondary immunocompromising conditions that might reduce cell-mediated or humoral immunity, e.g., B-lymphocyte antibody deficiencies, complete or partial T-lymphocyte defects, HIV infection, malignant neoplasm, transplantation, autoimmune disease, and immunosuppressive therapy.

- Adults with human immunodeficiency virus (HIV) infection and CD4+ T-lymphocyte count ≥200 cells/μl may receive 2 doses of VAR 3 months apart. Adults with HIV infection and CD4+ T-lymphocyte count <200 cells/μl should not receive VAR.

7. Pneumococcal vaccination

General information

- Adults who are immunocompetent and aged 65 years or older should receive 13-valent pneumococcal conjugate vaccine (PCV13) followed by 23-valent pneumococcal polysaccharide vaccine (PPSV23) at least 1 year after PCV13.
- Notes: Adults are recommended to receive 1 dose of PCV13 and 1, 2, or 3 doses of PPSV23 depending on indication. When both PCV13 and PPSV23 are indicated, PCV13 should be administered first; PCV13 and PPSV23 should not be administered during the same visit. If PPSV23 has previously been administered, PCV13 should be administered at least 1 year after PPSV23. When two or more doses of PPSV23 are indicated, the interval between PPSV23 doses should be at least 5 years. Supplemental information on pneumococcal vaccine timing for adults aged 65 years or older and adults aged 19 years or older at high risk for pneumococcal disease (described below) is available at www.cdc.gov/vaccines/vpd-vac/pneumo/downloads/adult-vax-clinician-aid.pdf. No additional doses of PPSV23 are indicated for adults who received PPSV23 at age 65 years or older. When indicated, PCV13 and PPSV23 should be administered to adults whose pneumococcal vaccination history is incomplete or unknown.

Special populations

- Adults aged 19 through 64 years with chronic heart disease including congestive heart failure and cardiomyopathies (excluding hypertension); chronic lung disease including chronic obstructive lung disease, emphysema, and asthma; chronic liver disease including cirrhosis; alcoholism; or diabetes mellitus; or who smoke cigarettes should receive PPSV23. At age 65 years or older, they should receive PCV13 and another dose of PPSV23 at least 1 year after PCV13 and at least 5 years after the most recent dose of PPSV23.
- Adults aged 19 years or older with immunocompromising conditions or anatomical or functional asplenia (described below) should receive PCV13 and a dose of PPSV23 at least 8 weeks after PCV13, followed by a second dose of PPSV23 at least 5 years after the first dose of PPSV23. If the most recent dose of PPSV23 was administered before age 65 years, at age 65 years or older, administer another dose of PPSV23 at least 8 weeks after PCV13 and at least 5 years after the most recent dose of PPSV23.
- Adults aged 19 years or older with cerebrospinal fluid leak or cochlear implant should receive PCV13 followed by PPSV23 at least 8 weeks after PCV13. If the most recent dose of PPSV23 was administered before age 65 years, at age 65 years or older, administer another dose of PPSV23 at least 8 weeks after PCV13 and at least 5 years after the most recent dose of PPSV23.
- Notes: Immunocompromising conditions that are indications for pneumococcal vaccination are congenital or acquired immunodeficiency including B- or T-lymphocyte deficiency, complement deficiencies, and phagocytic disorders excluding chronic granulomatous disease; human immunodeficiency virus (HIV) infection; chronic renal failure and nephrotic syndrome; leukemia, lymphoma, Hodgkin disease, generalized malignancy, and multiple myeloma; solid organ transplant; and iatrogenic immunosuppression including long-term systemic corticosteroid and radiation therapy. Anatomical or functional asplenia that are indications for pneumococcal vaccination are sickle cell disease and other hemoglobinopathies, congenital or acquired asplenia, splenic dysfunction, and splenectomy. Pneumococcal vaccines should be given at least 2 weeks before immunosuppressive therapy or an elective splenectomy, and as soon as possible to adults who are diagnosed with HIV infection.

8. Hepatitis A vaccination

General information

- Adults who seek protection from hepatitis A virus infection may receive a 2-dose series of single antigen hepatitis A vaccine (HepA) at either 0 and 6–12 months (Havrix) or 0 and 6–18 months (Vaqta). Adults may also receive a combined hepatitis A and hepatitis B vaccine (HepA-HepB) (Twinrix) as a 3-dose series at 0, 1, and 6 months. Acknowledgment of a specific risk factor by those who seek protection is not needed.

Special populations

- Adults with any of the following indications should receive a HepA series: have chronic liver disease, receive clotting factor concentrates, men who have sex with men, use injection or non-injection drugs, or work with hepatitis A virus-infected primates or in a hepatitis A research laboratory setting.
- Adults who travel in countries with high or intermediate levels of endemic hepatitis A infection or anticipate close personal contact with an international adoptee, e.g., reside in the same household or regularly babysit, from a country with high or intermediate level of endemic hepatitis A infection within the first 60 days of arrival in the United States should receive a HepA series.

9. Hepatitis B vaccination

General information

- Adults who seek protection from hepatitis B virus infection may receive a 3-dose series of single-antigen hepatitis B vaccine (HepB) (Engerix-B, Recombivax HB) at 0, 1, and 6 months. Adults may also receive a combined hepatitis A and hepatitis B vaccine (HepA-HepB) (Twinrix) at 0, 1, and 6 months. Acknowledgment of a specific risk factor by those who seek protection is not needed.

Special populations

- Adults at risk for hepatitis B virus infection by sexual exposure should receive a HepB series, including sex partners of hepatitis B surface antigen (HBsAg)-positive persons, sexually active persons who are not in a mutually monogamous relationship, persons seeking evaluation or treatment for a sexually transmitted infection, and men who have sex with men (MSM).
- Adults at risk for hepatitis B virus infection by percutaneous or mucosal exposure to blood should receive a HepB series, including adults who are recent or current users of injection drugs, household contacts of HBsAg-positive persons, residents and staff of facilities for developmentally disabled persons, incarcerated, healthcare and public safety workers at risk for exposure to blood or blood-contaminated body fluids, younger than age 60 years with diabetes mellitus, and age 60 years or older with diabetes mellitus at the discretion of the treating clinician.
- Adults with chronic liver disease including, but not limited to, hepatitis C virus infection, cirrhosis, fatty liver disease, alcoholic liver disease, autoimmune hepatitis, and an alanine aminotransferase (ALT) or aspartate aminotransferase (AST) level greater than twice the upper limit of normal should receive a HepB series.
- Adults with end-stage renal disease including those on pre-dialysis care, hemodialysis, peritoneal dialysis, and home dialysis should receive a HepB series. Adults on hemodialysis should receive a 3-dose series of 40 µg Recombivax HB at 0, 1, and 6 months or a 4-dose series of 40 µg Engerix-B at 0, 1, 2, and 6 months.
- Adults with human immunodeficiency virus (HIV) infection should receive a HepB series.
- Pregnant women who are at risk for hepatitis B virus infection during pregnancy, e.g., having more than one sex partner during the previous six months, been evaluated or treated for a sexually transmitted infection, recent or current injection drug use, or had an HBsAg-positive sex partner, should receive a HepB series.
- International travelers to regions with high or intermediate levels of endemic hepatitis B virus infection should receive a HepB series.
- Adults in the following settings are assumed to be at risk for hepatitis B virus infection and should receive a HepB series: sexually transmitted disease treatment facilities, HIV testing and treatment facilities, facilities providing drug-abuse treatment and prevention services, healthcare settings targeting services to persons who inject drugs, correctional facilities, healthcare settings targeting services to MSM, hemodialysis facilities and end-stage renal disease programs, and institutions and nonresidential day care facilities for developmentally disabled persons.

10. Meningococcal vaccination

Special populations

- Adults with anatomical or functional asplenia or persistent complement component deficiencies should receive a 2-dose primary series of serogroups A, C, W, and Y meningococcal conjugate vaccine (MenACWY) at least 2 months apart and revaccinate every 5 years. They should also receive a series of serogroup B meningococcal vaccine (MenB) with either a 2-dose series of MenB-4C (Bexsero) at least 1 month apart or a 3-dose series of MenB-FHbp (Trumenba) at 0, 1–2, and 6 months.
- Adults with human immunodeficiency virus (HIV) infection who have not been previously vaccinated should receive a 2-dose primary series of MenACWY at least 2 months apart and revaccinate every 5 years. Those who previously received 1 dose of MenACWY should receive a second dose at least 2 months after the first dose. Adults with HIV infection are not routinely recommended to receive MenB because meningococcal disease in this population is caused primarily by serogroups C, W, and Y.
- Microbiologists who are routinely exposed to isolates of *Neisseria meningitidis* should receive 1 dose of MenACWY and revaccinate every 5 years if the risk for infection remains, and either a 2-dose series of MenB-4C at least 1 month apart or a 3-dose series of MenB-FHbp at 0, 1–2, and 6 months.
- Adults at risk because of a meningococcal disease outbreak should receive 1 dose of MenACWY if the outbreak is attributable to serogroup A, C, W, or Y, or either a 2-dose series of MenB-4C at least 1 month apart or a 3-dose series of MenB-FHbp at 0, 1–2, and 6 months if the outbreak is attributable to serogroup B.
- Adults who travel to or live in countries with hyperendemic or epidemic meningococcal disease should receive 1 dose of MenACWY and revaccinate every 5 years if the risk for infection remains. MenB is not routinely indicated because meningococcal disease in these countries is generally not caused by serogroup B.
- Military recruits should receive 1 dose of MenACWY and revaccinate every 5 years if the increased risk for infection remains.
- First-year college students aged 21 years or younger who live in residence halls should receive 1 dose of MenACWY if they have not received MenACWY at age 16 years or older.
- Young adults aged 16 through 23 years (preferred age range is 16 through 18 years) who are healthy and not at increased risk for serogroup B meningococcal disease (described above) may receive either a 2-dose series of MenB-4C at least 1 month apart or a 2-dose series of MenB-FHbp at 0 and 6 months for short-term protection against most strains of serogroup B meningococcal disease.
- For adults aged 56 years or older who have not previously received serogroups A, C, W, and Y meningococcal vaccine and need only 1 dose, meningococcal polysaccharide serogroups A, C, W, and Y vaccine (MPSV4) is preferred. For adults who previously received MenACWY or anticipate receiving multiple doses of serogroups A, C, W, and Y meningococcal vaccine, MenACWY is preferred.
- Notes: MenB-4C and MenB-FHbp are not interchangeable, i.e., the same vaccine should be used for all doses to complete the series. There is no recommendation for MenB revaccination at this time. MenB may be administered at the same time as MenACWY but at a different anatomic site, if feasible.

11. *Haemophilus influenzae* type b vaccination

Special populations

- Adults who have anatomical or functional asplenia or sickle cell disease, or are undergoing elective splenectomy should receive 1 dose of *Haemophilus influenzae* type b conjugate vaccine (Hib) if they have not previously received Hib. Hib should be administered at least 14 days before splenectomy.
- Adults with a hematopoietic stem cell transplant (HSCT) should receive 3 doses of Hib in at least 4 week intervals 6–12 months after transplant regardless of their Hib history.
- Notes: Hib is not routinely recommended for adults with human immunodeficiency virus infection because their risk for *Haemophilus influenzae* type b infection is low.

Table. Contraindications and precautions for vaccines recommended for adults aged 19 years or older*

The Advisory Committee on Immunization Practices (ACIP) recommendations and package inserts for vaccines provide information on contraindications and precautions related to vaccines. Contraindications are conditions that increase chances of a serious adverse reaction in vaccine recipients and the vaccine should not be administered when a contraindication is present. Precautions should be reviewed for potential risks and benefits for vaccine recipient. For a person with a severe allergy to latex, e.g., anaphylaxis, vaccines supplied in vials or syringes that contain natural rubber latex should not be administered unless the benefit of vaccination clearly outweighs the risk for a potential allergic reaction. For latex allergies other than anaphylaxis, vaccines supplied in vials or syringes that contain dry, natural rubber or natural rubber latex may be administered.

Contraindications and precautions for vaccines routinely recommended for adults

Vaccine	Contraindications	Precautions
All vaccines routinely recommended for adults	• Severe reaction, e.g., anaphylaxis, after a previous dose or to a vaccine component	• Moderate or severe acute illness with or without fever

Additional contraindications and precautions for vaccines routinely recommended for adults

Vaccine	Additional Contraindications	Additional Precautions
IIV[1]		• History of Guillain-Barré Syndrome within 6 weeks after previous influenza vaccination • Egg allergy other than hives, e.g., angioedema, respiratory distress, lightheadedness, or recurrent emesis; or required epinephrine or another emergency medical intervention (IIV may be administered in an inpatient or outpatient medical setting and under the supervision of a healthcare provider who is able to recognize and manage severe allergic conditions)
RIV[1]		• History of Guillain-Barré Syndrome within 6 weeks after previous influenza vaccination
LAIV[1]	• LAIV should not be used during 2016–2017 influenza season	• LAIV should not be used during 2016–2017 influenza season
Tdap/Td	• For pertussis-containing vaccines: encephalopathy, e.g., coma, decreased level of consciousness, or prolonged seizures, not attributable to another identifiable cause within 7 days of administration of a previous dose of a vaccine containing tetanus or diphtheria toxoid or acellular pertussis	• Guillain-Barré Syndrome within 6 weeks after a previous dose of tetanus toxoid-containing vaccine • History of Arthus-type hypersensitivity reactions after a previous dose of tetanus or diphtheria toxoid-containing vaccine. Defer vaccination until at least 10 years have elapsed since the last tetanus toxoid-containing vaccine • For pertussis-containing vaccine, progressive or unstable neurologic disorder, uncontrolled seizures, or progressive encephalopathy (until a treatment regimen has been established and the condition has stabilized)
MMR[2]	• Severe immunodeficiency, e.g., hematologic and solid tumors, chemotherapy, congenital immunodeficiency or long-term immunosuppressive therapy[3], human immunodeficiency virus (HIV) infection with severe immunocompromise • Pregnancy	• Recent (within 11 months) receipt of antibody-containing blood product (specific interval depends on product)[4] • History of thrombocytopenia or thrombocytopenic purpura • Need for tuberculin skin testing[5]
VAR[2]	• Severe immunodeficiency, e.g., hematologic and solid tumors, chemotherapy, congenital immunodeficiency or long-term immunosuppressive therapy[3]; HIV infection with severe immunocompromise • Pregnancy	• Recent (within 11 months) receipt of antibody-containing blood product (specific interval depends on product)[4] • Receipt of specific antiviral drugs (acyclovir, famciclovir, or valacyclovir) 24 hours before vaccination (avoid use of these antiviral drugs for 14 days after vaccination)
HZV[2]	• Severe immunodeficiency, e.g., hematologic and solid tumors, chemotherapy, congenital immunodeficiency or long-term immunosuppressive therapy[3]; HIV infection with severe immunocompromise • Pregnancy	• Receipt of specific antiviral drugs (acyclovir, famciclovir, or valacyclovir) 24 hours before vaccination (avoid use of these antiviral drugs for 14 days after vaccination)
HPV vaccine		• Pregnancy
PCV13	• Severe allergic reaction to any vaccine containing diphtheria toxoid	

1. For additional information on use of influenza vaccines among persons with egg allergy, see: CDC. Prevention and control of seasonal influenza with vaccines: recommendations of the Advisory Committee on Immunization Practices—United States, 2016–17 influenza season. MMWR 2016;65(RR-5):1–54. Available at www.cdc.gov/mmwr/volumes/65/rr/rr650a1.htm.
2. MMR may be administered together with VAR or HZV on the same day. If not administered on the same day, separate live vaccines by at least 28 days.
3. Immunosuppressive steroid dose is considered to be daily receipt of 20 mg or more prednisone or equivalent for two or more weeks. Vaccination should be deferred for at least 1 month after discontinuation of immunosuppressive steroid therapy. Providers should consult ACIP recommendations for complete information on the use of specific live vaccines among persons on immune-suppressing medications or with immune suppression because of other reasons.
4. Vaccine should be deferred for the appropriate interval if replacement immune globulin products are being administered. See: CDC. General recommendations on immunization: recommendations of the Advisory Committee on Immunization Practices (ACIP). MMWR 2011;60(No. RR-2). Available at www.cdc.gov/mmwr/preview/mmwrhtml/rr6002a1.htm.
5. Measles vaccination may temporarily suppress tuberculin skin reactivity. Measles-containing vaccine may be administered on the same day as tuberculin skin testing, or should be postponed for at least 4 weeks after vaccination.

* Adapted from: CDC. Table 6. Contraindications and precautions to commonly used vaccines. General recommendations on immunization: recommendations of the Advisory Committee on Immunization Practices (ACIP). MMWR 2011;60(No. RR-2):40–41 and from: Hamborsky J, Kroger A, Wolfe S, eds. Epidemiology and prevention of vaccine preventable diseases. 13th ed. Washington, DC: Public Health Foundation, 2015. Available at www.cdc.gov/vaccines/pubs/pinkbook/index.html.

Acronyms of vaccines recommended for adults

HepA	hepatitis A vaccine	LAIV	live attenuated influenza vaccine
HepA-HepB	hepatitis A and hepatitis B vaccines	MenACWY	serogroups A, C, W, and Y meningococcal conjugate vaccine
HepB	hepatitis B vaccine		
Hib	Haemophilus influenzae type b conjugate vaccine	MenB	serogroup B meningococcal vaccine
HPV vaccine	human papillomavirus vaccine	MMR	measles, mumps, and rubella vaccine
HZV	herpes zoster vaccine	MPSV4	serogroups A, C, W, and Y meningococcal polysaccharide vaccine
IIV	inactivated influenza vaccine		
PCV13	13-valent pneumococcal conjugate vaccine		
PPSV23	23-valent pneumococcal polysaccharide vaccine		
RIV	recombinant influenza vaccine		
Td	tetanus and diphtheria toxoids		
Tdap	tetanus toxoid, reduced diphtheria toxoid, and acellular pertussis vaccine		
VAR	varicella vaccine		

Resources for Additional Study

Books:

Fitzgerald, M. A. (2017) Health Promotion and Disease Prevention, <u>Nurse Practitioner Certification Examination and Practice Preparation</u>, 5th Edition, Philadelphia, PA: F. A. Davis.

Internet:

The Centers for Disease Control and Prevention website, www.cdc.gov (immunizations, infectious disease, including hepatitis; travel medicine, disease updates)

http://www.cdc.gov/vaccines/hcp/acip-recs/index.html

Chapter 3: Secondary Prevention: Detecting Preclinical Disease

Table 3-1: Key Concepts in Secondary Prevention	
What it is	**What it is not**
Early case finding of *asymptomatic disease* via the use of a screening test • Abnormal screening test typically requires additional diagnostics to rule in or rule out disease.	Differential diagnosis Follow-up in established disease

Table 3-2: Secondary Prevention Principles	
Principle	**Comment**
Prevalence of the disease sufficient to justify screening.	Routine mammography in women but not men
The health problem has significant effect on quality and/or quantity of life.	Target diseases for secondary prevention include hypertension, type 2 diabetes mellitus, dyslipidemia, and certain cancers.
The target disease has a long asymptomatic period. The natural history of the disease, or how the disease unfolds without intervention, is known.	Treatment is available for the target disease. Providing treatment alters the disease's natural history.
A population-acceptable screening test is available.	The test should be safe, available at moderate cost, and have reasonable sensitivity and specificity.

Source: www.clevelandclinicmeded.com/medicalpubs/diseasemanagement/preventive-medicine/principles-of-screening

1. A 51-year-old woman of European ancestry who has had no primary care for more than 10 years presents to your practice. She has a 40 pack-year cigarette smoking history, currently smoking 1 PPD and reports drinking about 3–4, 12 oz (0.35 L) beers per month. Her history is otherwise unremarkable as is her physical examination. You order the following screening test:

    A. Hemoglobin electrophoresis.

    B. Mammography.

    C. Chest x-ray.

    D. Fasting serum triglycerides.

Table 3-3: Calculating Pack-year History to Quantify Tobacco Use	
Calculation formula	**Examples**
Number of packs-per-day (PPD) × the number of years smoked	2 PPD × 30 years=60 pk-y hx 0.5 PPD × 10 years=5 pk-y hx

2. A 65-year-old Native American man presents for a "physical." He feels well, denies tobacco or alcohol use, and has not seen a healthcare provider in more than 10 years. The patient states, "I am a really healthy person. I would not come in except my wife and daughter told me I should have a checkup." As part of today's visit, he should be screened for:

   A. Pancreatic cancer.

   B. Hemolytic anemia.

   C. Hepatic sclerosis.

   D. Visual defect.

3. A 30-year-old woman of Asian ancestry presents for a routine health visit. She is in good health and reports she is concerned about her personal breast and ovarian cancer risk and asks about *BRCA* gene mutation testing. You advise the following:

   A. *BRCA* gene mutation testing should be offered to all women who request this evaluation.

   B. A standardized screening questionnaire for *BRCA* gene mutation such as FHS-7 should be administered today to determine if *BRCA* gene mutation testing is warranted.

   C. She is not a candidate for this test due to her ethnicity.

   D. A referral to genetic counseling for guidance on *BRCA* gene mutation testing should be ordered.

See Table 3-10: U.S. Preventive Services Task Force: Genetic Risk Assessment and *BRCA* Mutation Testing for Breast and Ovarian Cancer Susceptibility for additional guidance

4. Suicide: True or false?

   (T/F) Males represent nearly 80% of all completed suicides. T

   (T/F) When compared with male suicide attempts, female attempts at suicide are approximately 2–3 times more common. T

   (T/F) The highest rate of completed suicide is found in teenage males. F

   (T/F) Inquiring about suicidal ideation could precipitate the act. F

Table 3-4: U.S. Suicide Statistics, Breakdown by Gender/Ethnicity/Age Group						
All ages combined			**Elderly (75+ y)**		**Youth (15–24 y)**	
Group	Number of suicides	Rate of suicide per 100,000	Elderly suicides	Elderly suicide rate per 100,000	Youth suicides	Youth suicide rate per 100,000
Nation	42,773	13.3	3,583	21.4	5,079	11.4
Men	33,113	*20.7*	3,106	*38.8*	4,089	*18.2*
Women	9,660	*5.8*	477	*4.0*	990	*4.6*
Whites	35,398	16.7	3,286	24.3	3,495	13.9
Hispanic	3,244	6.4	131	-	719	7.5
Blacks	2,326	5.9	73	-	517	7.5
White Men	27,368	25.8	2,865	*44.0*	2,842	22.4
White Women	8,030	7.5	421	4.5	653	5.4
Hispanic Men	2,582	10.3	117	20.6	562	11.5
Hispanic Women	662	2.5	14	-	157	3.4
Black Men	1,871	9.7	63	11.0	426	12.3
Black Women	455	2.1	10	-	91	2.7

Source: www.cdc.gov/violenceprevention/pdf/Suicide-DataSheet-a.pdf and
http://www.cdc.gov/nchs/data/hestat/suicide/rates_1999_2014.pdf

5. Ms. Kane is a 25-year-old woman who presents with finger-shaped ecchymotic areas on her right shoulder that are an incidental finding during a physical examination. She denies abuse or assault. The NP's most appropriate response is:

   A. "Your bruises look as if they were caused by someone grabbing you."

   B. "Was this an accident?"

   C. "I notice the bruises are in the shape of a hand."

   D. "How did you fall?"

For information on reporting elder abuse, please see http://www.ncea.aoa.gov
For information on reporting child abuse, please see
https://www.childwelfare.gov/responding/reporting.cfm

6. Mr. Jacobs is a 65-year-old man with COPD and a 60 pack-year history who is currently smoking 1.5 packs of cigarettes per day. He is reading a pamphlet in your office about smoking cessation. You ask him if he has any questions and he states, "I don't plan to quit smoking. My health is pretty good." According to the Transtheoretical Model of Change, he is most likely in which of the following stages?

A. Precontemplation

B. Contemplation

C. Preparation

D. Minimization

Table 3-5: Prochaska and DiClemente: Stages of Change		
The NP must maintain the attitude that the patient is capable of changing and achieving a given health goal. Change occurs dynamically and often unpredictably. A commonly used change framework is based on the work of Prochaska and DiClemente, who note five stages of preparation and maintenance for change. This is an example of a transtheoretical model that assesses an individual's readiness to act on a new healthier behavior, and provides strategies, or processes of change, to guide the individual through the stages of change to action and maintenance.		
Stage	**Comment**	**Healthcare provider action**
Precontemplation	The patient is not interested in change and might not be aware that the problem exists, or minimizes the problem's impact.	Help patient to move toward thinking about changing the unhealthy behavior.
Contemplation	The patient is considering change and looking at its positive and negative aspects. At the same time, the person often reports feeling "stuck" with the problem.	Help the patient to examine benefits and barriers to change.
Preparation	The patient exhibits some change behaviors or thoughts and often reports feeling that he or she does not have the tools to proceed.	Assist patient in finding and using tools to help with change, continuing to work to lower barriers to change.
Action	The patient is ready to go forth with change, often takes concrete steps to change but is inconsistent with carrying through.	Work with the patient on use of tools, encouraging the healthy behavior change, praising the positive, acknowledging reverting back to former behavior as a common but not insurmountable problem.
Maintenance/relapse	The patient learns to continue the change and has adopted and embraced the healthy habit. At the same time, relapse can occur and the person learns to deal with backsliding.	Continued positive reinforcement for the behavior change, put backsliding into perspective of a common but not insurmountable problem.

Source: Prochaska, J.O., Redding, C.A., and Evers, K.E. The Transtheoretical Model and Stages of Change. In: Health Behavior and Health Education: Theory, Research, and Practice, 2nd ed. Glanz, K., Lewis, F.M., and Rimer, B.K. (editors). San Francisco, CA: Jossey-Bass. 1997.

7. Mr. Jacobs further states, "I am too old to quit now. Why bother?" The NP's most appropriate response is:

    A. Since you have COPD, you really should quit smoking.

    B. You know your lungs will get more damaged if you continue to smoke.

    C. Tell me what you mean by, "I am too old to quit."

    D. I can provide medication that will help you to quit smoking.

Table 3-6: "The 5 As:" Ask, Advise, Assess, Assist, and Arrange: Successful intervention begins with identifying tobacco users and appropriate interventions based upon the patient's willingness to quit	
Ask	Identify and document tobacco use status for every patient at every visit.
Advise	In a clear, strong, and personalized manner, urge every tobacco user to quit.
Assess	Is the tobacco user willing to make a quit attempt at this time?
Assist	For the patient willing to make a quit attempt, use counseling and pharmacotherapy to help him or her quit.
Arrange	Schedule follow-up contact, in person or by telephone, preferably within the first week after the quit date.

Source: http://www.ahrq.gov/professionals/clinicians-providers/guidelines-recommendations/tobacco/5steps.html

Table 3-7 Leading Causes of Death by Age Group		
Age group (years)	**Rank**	**Cause of death**
15–34	First	Unintentional injury
	Second	Suicide
	Third	Homicide
35–44	First	Unintentional injury
	Second	Malignant neoplasms
	Third	Heart disease
45–64	First	Malignant neoplasms
	Second	Heart disease
	Third	Unintentional injury
65+	First	Heart disease
	Second	Malignant neoplasms
	Third	Chronic, lower respiratory disease*
Overall leading causes of death by total deaths reported		
First	Heart disease (611,105)	
Second	Malignant neoplasms (584,881)	
Third	Chronic, lower respiratory disease (149,205)	

*Chronic, lower respiratory disease refers to COPD, pneumonia, and flu
Source: http://www.cdc.gov/injury/wisqars/leadingcauses.html

Table 3-8: Leading Sites of New Cancer Cases and Deaths 2016 Estimates			
Estimated New Cases		Estimated Deaths	
Male	Female	Male	Female
Lung & bronchus 117,920	Lung & bronchus 106,470	Lung & bronchus 85,920	Lung & bronchus 72,160
Prostate 180,890	Breast 246,660	Prostate 26,120	Breast 40,450
Colon & rectum 70,820	Colon & rectum 63,670	Colon & rectum 26,020	Colon & rectum 23,170
All sites 841,390	All sites 843,820	All sites 314,290	All sites 281,400

Source:
http://www.cancer.org/acs/groups/content/@research/documents/document/acspc-047068.pdf,
http://www.cancer.org/acs/groups/content/@research/documents/document/acspc-047066.pdf

Test-taking tip:
When guidelines have conflicting information, focus on the commonalities, not the differences.

8. According to current nationally-recognized recommendations, are the following cancer screenings indicated?

(Y/N) Annual digital rectal exam as colorectal cancer screening in a 63-year-old man ~NO~

(Y/N) An initial liquid-based Pap test with HPV cotesting in a 19-year-old woman who is one year post-coitarche ~NO~

(Y/N) Endometrial biopsy in a 52-year-old woman who is two years post-LMP and who denies vaginal bleeding ~No~

(Y/N) Annual prostate specific antigen testing in an 81-year-old man who has hypertension and benign prostatic hypertrophy ~No~

(Y/N) Lung cancer screening with low-dose CT (LDCT) for a 60-year-old who is generally in good health who has a 35 pack-year cigarette smoking history who quit smoking 5 years ago ~Yes~

Table 3-9: The US Preventive Services Task Force (USPSTF) Recommendations on Using Prostate-specific Antigen (PSA)–Based Screening for Prostate Cancer

The US Preventive Services Task Force (USPSTF) recommends against prostate-specific antigen (PSA)–based screening for prostate cancer. This is a grade D recommendation, suggesting that there is moderate or high certainty that the service has no net benefit or that the harms outweigh the benefits. This recommendation applies to men in the US population who do not have symptoms that are highly suspicious for prostate cancer, regardless of age, race, or family history.

The USPSTF did not evaluate the use of the PSA test as part of a diagnostic strategy in men with symptoms that are highly suspicious for prostate cancer. This recommendation also does not consider the use of the PSA test for surveillance after diagnosis and/or treatment of prostate cancer.

Source: www.uspreventiveservicestaskforce.org/prostatecancerscreening/prostatefinalrs.htm

---

Table 3-10: U.S. Preventive Services Task Force: Genetic Risk Assessment and *BRCA* Mutation Testing for Breast and Ovarian Cancer Susceptibility
Summary of Recommendations / Supporting Documents

Summary of Recommendations

The U.S. Preventive Services Task Force (USPSTF) recommends against routine genetic counseling or breast cancer susceptibility gene (*BRCA*) testing for women whose family history is not associated with an increased risk for potentially harmful mutations in breast cancer susceptibility gene 1 (*BRCA1*) or breast cancer susceptibility gene 2 (*BRCA2*).

Rating: D Recommendation.

Rationale: The USPSTF found fair evidence that women without certain specific family history patterns, termed here "increased risk family history" (i.e., those having a relative with a *known* deleterious mutation in *BRCA1* or *BRCA2* genes); have a low risk for developing breast or ovarian cancer associated with *BRCA1* or *BRCA2* mutations. Thus, the benefit to routine testing of these women for *BRCA1* or *BRCA2* mutations, or routine referral for genetic counseling, would be few to none.

The USPSTF recommends that primary care providers screen women who have first- or second-degree family members with breast, ovarian, tubal, or peritoneal cancer with 1 of several screening tools designed to identify a family history that may be associated with an increased risk for potentially harmful mutations in *BRCA1* or *BRCA2* genes. Women with positive screening results via the use of an appropriate screening tool such as Ontario Family History Assessment Tool, Manchester Scoring System, Referral Screening Tool, Pedigree Assessment Tool, and FHS-7 should receive genetic counseling done by a suitably-trained healthcare provider and, if indicated after counseling, *BRCA* testing. **Rating: B Recommendation.**

Rationale: The USPSTF found fair evidence that women with certain specific family history patterns (increased risk family history) have an increased risk for developing breast or ovarian cancer associated with *BRCA1* or *BRCA2* mutations. The USPSTF determined that these women would benefit from genetic counseling that allows informed decision-making about testing and further prophylactic treatment. This counseling should be done by suitably-trained healthcare providers. There is insufficient evidence to determine the benefits of chemoprevention or intensive screening in improving health outcomes in these women if they test positive for deleterious *BRCA1* or *BRCA2* mutations. However, there is fair evidence that prophylactic surgery for these women significantly decreases breast and ovarian cancer incidence. Thus, the potential benefits of referral and discussion of testing and prophylactic treatment for these women may be substantial.

The USPSTF recognizes that each risk assessment tool has limitations and found insufficient comparative evidence to recommend one tool over another. The USPSTF also found insufficient evidence to support a specific risk threshold for referral of testing.

Source: BRCA-related Cancer: Risk Assessment, Genetic Counseling, and Genetic Testing (2013).
http://www.uspreventiveservicestaskforce.org/Page/Document/RecommendationStatementFinal/brca-related-cancer-risk-assessment-genetic-counseling-and-genetic-testing

Table 3-11: American Cancer Society Cancer Detection Guidelines

Cancer site	Population	Test or procedure	Comment
Breast	Women, age ≥20 years	Breast cancer screening (general)	All women should become familiar with the potential benefits, limitations, and harms associated with breast cancer screening.
		Clinical breast examination (CBE)	Does not recommend CBE for breast cancer screening among average-risk women at any age.
		Mammography	Begin annual mammography at age 45 years. Perform annually to age 54 years, then biennially for as long as a woman is in good health and has a life expectancy of at least 10 years.
		MRI	Women at high risk (greater than 20% lifetime risk*, with *BRCA* mutation, or has first-degree relative of *BRCA* carrier) should get an MRI and a mammogram every year. Women at moderately increased risk (15–20% lifetime risk) should talk with their healthcare providers about the benefits and limitations of adding MRI screening to their yearly mammogram. An estimated 2% of all women in the USA will fall into a category in which MRI breast screening is recommended. Yearly MRI screening is not recommended for women whose lifetime risk of breast cancer is less than 15%. *Lifetime risk can be determined by BRCAPRO or other models that are largely dependent on family history.
Colorectal	Men and women, age ≥50 years	Guaiac-based fecal occult blood test (gFOBT) or fecal immunochemical test (FIT) *or*	Annually, starting at age 50 years FOBT as it is sometimes done in healthcare providers' offices, with the single stool sample collected on a fingertip during a digital rectal examination, is not an adequate substitute for the recommended at-home procedure of collecting two samples from 2–3 consecutive specimens (depending on manufacturer's instructions). Toilet-bowl FOBT tests also are not recommended. In comparison with guaiac-based tests for the detection of occult blood, immunochemical tests are more patient-friendly, and are likely to be equal or better in sensitivity and specificity. There is no justification for repeating FOBT in response to an initial positive finding. Colonoscopy should be done if any test results are positive.
		Flexible sigmoidoscopy, *or*	Every 5 years, starting at age 50 years Colonoscopy should be done if results are positive.
		Double-contrast barium enema (DCBE), *or*	DCBE every 5 years, starting at age 50 years Colonoscopy should be done if results are positive.
		Colonoscopy, *or*	Colonoscopy every 10 years, starting at age 50
		CT colonography	CT colonography (virtual colonoscopy) every 5 years Colonoscopy should be done if results are positive.
		Additional recommendations	Patients should talk to their healthcare provider about earlier or more frequent screening if they have the following colorectal risk factors: A personal history of colorectal cancer or adenomatous polyps, inflammatory bowel disease, Crohn's disease or ulcerative colitis, a strong family history (first-degree relative [parent, sibling, or child] age <60 years or in 2 or more first-degree relatives of any age) of colorectal cancer or polyps, a family history of colon cancer or adenomatous polyps in a first-degree relative age ≥60 years, or a known family history of hereditary colorectal cancer syndromes, such as familial adenomatous polyposis (FAP) or hereditary non-polyposis colon cancer (HNPCC).

Continued…

Table 3-11 (cont.): American Cancer Society Cancer Detection Guidelines

Cancer site	Population	Test or procedure	Comment
Endometrial	Women, at menopause	Endometrial biopsy in select situations	At the time of menopause, all women should be informed about risks and symptoms of endometrial cancer and strongly encouraged to report any unexpected vaginal bleeding, discharge, or spotting to their healthcare provider. Abnormal vaginal bleeding is a presenting sign in >90% of women with endometrial carcinoma. For women who have hereditary non-polyposis colon cancer (HNPCC), annual screening should be offered for endometrial cancer with endometrial biopsy beginning at age 35 years.
Lung	Persons at high risk for lung cancer based on age, smoking history	Low-dose computed tomography (LDCT)	For individuals ages 55 to 74 years in fairly good health with a ≥30 pack-year smoking history and who currently smoke or it has been ≤15 years since quitting, annual screening for lung cancer with LDCT until the age of 74 years as long as patient is in good health. At least 80% of all lung cancer cases (majority, non-small cell lung cancer [NSCLC]) in USA associated with tobacco use. Strongly suggest that all adults who receive screening enter an organized screening program that has experience in LDCT.
Cancer-related checkup	Men and women, age ≥20 years	Periodic health examination	On the occasion of a periodic health examination, the cancer-related checkup should include health counseling, and depending on a person's age and gender, might include exams for cancers of the thyroid, oral cavity, skin, lymph nodes, testes, and ovaries, as well as for some non-malignant (non-cancerous) diseases.

Source: American Cancer Society Cancer Screening Guidelines, available at
www.cancer.org/Healthy/FindCancerEarly/CancerScreeningGuidelines/index

Table 3-12: Additional Breast Cancer Screening Guidelines

Association/society	Guidelines
The US Preventive Services Task Force (USPSTF)	The USPSTF recommends biennial screening for women age 50–74 years. The USPSTF concludes that the current evidence is insufficient to assess the additional benefits and harms of screening mammography in women 75 years and older. The USPSTF recommends against teaching breast self-examination (BSE) and concludes that the current evidence is insufficient to assess the additional benefits and harms of CBE beyond screening mammography in women 40 years or older.
American College of Obstetricians and Gynecologists	Women 40 years and older should have annual screening mammography. All women ages 40 years and older should have CBEs annually as part of the physical examination, while women ages 29–39 years should have CBE every 1–3 years. Despite a lack of definitive data for or against BSE, it has the potential to detect palpable breast cancer and can be recommended, particularly for high-risk patients. Breast self-awareness should be encouraged (defined as a woman's awareness of the normal appearance and feel of her breasts).
American Geriatrics Society	For women in average-better health, with an estimated life expectancy of 5 or more years, it is appropriate to offer screening mammography every 1–2 years up to age 85 years. The recommendation should include an individualized review of the potential benefits and harms of screening and patients' personal preferences. Mammography screening beyond the age of 85 years should be reserved for those women most likely to benefit by virtue of excellent health and functional status, and for those who feel strongly that they will benefit from such screening, either in peace of mind or improved quality of life. CBE should be performed periodically. BSE is neither endorsed nor discouraged.

Sources: http://www.uspreventiveservicestaskforce.org/uspstf/uspsbrca.htm,
ACOG. Practice bulletin No. 122: Breast Cancer Screening. *Obstet Gynecol.* 2011;118(2 Pt
1):372-382, http://www.consultantlive.com/geriatrics/content/article/10162/1563530

Table 3-13: Guideline Recommendations for Cervical Cancer Screening

Screening before age 21 years should be avoided because women younger than 21 years are at very low risk of cancer. Screening these women may lead to unnecessary and harmful evaluation and treatment. Although the rate of HPV infection is high among sexually active adolescents, invasive cervical cancer is very rare in women younger than 21 years. *The immune system clears the HPV infection within one to two years among most adolescent women. Because the adolescent cervix is immature, there is a higher incidence of HPV-related precancerous lesions (called dysplasia). However, the large majority of cervical dysplasias in adolescents resolve on their own without treatment. A significant increase in premature births has recently been documented among women who have been treated with excisional procedures for dysplasia.*

Recommendation	ACOG	ACS	USPSTF
Cervical cancer screening should begin at age 21 years. Recommends against screening for cervical cancer in women younger than 21 years.	X	X	X
In women ages 21 to 29 years, a Pap test should be done every 3 years.	X[a]	X[b]	X[c]
Women between the ages of 30 and 65 years should have both a Pap test and HPV test every 5 years, or a Pap test alone every 3 years.	X[d]	X[e]	X
Women with certain risk factors may need more frequent screening, including those who have HIV, are immunosuppressed, or were exposed to diethylstilbestrol (DES) *in utero*.	X[f]	X	NR
Recommends against screening women age 65 years and older who have had adequate negative cytology results and are not otherwise at high risk for cervical cancer.	X	X[g]	X
Women with a history of CIN 2 or CIN 3 should continue to have testing for at least 20 years after the abnormality was found.	X	X	NR
Women who have had a total hysterectomy (including removal of the cervix) should stop cervical cancer screening unless the surgery was done as a treatment for cervical cancer or pre-cancer (i.e., CIN 2 or CIN 3).	X	X	X
Women who have had a hysterectomy without the removal of the cervix should continue to follow the standard guidelines.	NR	X	NR
Women who have been vaccinated against HPV should follow the same screening guidelines.	X	X	NR

ACOG, American Congress of Obstetricians and Gynecologists; ACS, American Cancer Society; USPSTF, US Preventive Services Task Force; NR, no recommendation
a. Either standard PAP or liquid-based cytology.
b. HPV should not be carried out in this age group unless there has been an abnormal Pap test result.
c. Recommends against screening with HPV testing, alone or in combination with cytology, in women younger than 30 years
d. For women 30 years and older who have had 3 consecutive negative cervical cytology test results.
e. Pap test and HPV test every 5 years is preferred.
f. Including those who have been treated for cervical intraepithelial neoplasia (CIN) 2, CIN 3, or cervical cancer.
g. Screening can be stopped in those 65 years and older who have had regular screening in the previous 10 years and not had any serious pre-cancers (like CIN 2 or CIN 3) found in the past 20 years.

Sources: ACOG. Available at: http://www.acog.org/Patients/FAQs/Cervical-Cancer-Screening.
American Cancer Society Cervical Cancer Detection Guidelines, available at www.cancer.org/healthy/findcancerearly/cancerscreeningguidelines/american-cancer-society-guidelines-for-the-early-detection-of-cancer.
USPTF, http://www.uspreventiveservicestaskforce.org/uspstf/uspscerv.htm

Important additional study resources available through your Fitzgerald Health online learning portal at fhea.com/npexpert

- Resource 3-1: Updated Guidelines for Detection and Treatment of Latent and Active Tuberculosis
- Resource 3-2: Epidemiologic Terms

Table 3-14: Behavior Change: An Overview
Assumptions:
• Change is not linear.
• Relapse is expected and anticipated.
• Ambivalence is expected.
• The patient is involved in the problem.
• The patient is willing to take action.
NP responsibility:
• Assess stage of change.
• Intervene when the patient is at an appropriate stage of change.
Questions to assess readiness
• "Have you or are you thinking about…_____?" (insert behavior change, e.g., quitting smoking)
• "What thoughts have you had about…_____?" (insert behavior change, e.g., quitting smoking)

Bonus questions for this chapter available through your Fitzgerald Health learning portal at fhea.com/npexpert.

Resources for Additional Study

Books:

Desai, S. (2009) <u>Clinician's Guide to Laboratory Medicine: Pocket</u>, Houston, TX: MD2B.

Fitzgerald, M. A. (2017) Health Promotion and Disease Prevention, <u>Nurse Practitioner Certification Examination and Practice Preparation</u>, 5th Edition, Philadelphia, PA: F. A. Davis.

Ferri, F. (2014) <u>Ferri's Best Test: A Practical Guide to Clinical Laboratory Medicine and Diagnostic Imaging</u>, 3rd Edition, St. Louis, MO: Elsevier Health Sciences.

Internet:

The Centers for Disease Control and Prevention, www.cdc.gov

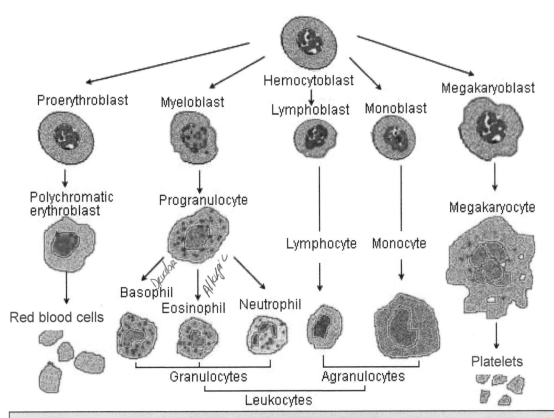

Table 4-1: Anemia Defined

A complex of signs and symptoms characterized by decreases in numbers of red blood cells (RBCs) or hemoglobin (Hb) content caused by blood loss, deficient erythropoiesis, excessive hemolysis, or a combination of these changes. *Anemia occurs when the insult is severe enough to disturb normal homeostatic mechanisms and exceed reserves.*

Cause	Mechanism	Comment
Acute blood loss	In adult ≥1 L blood loss before clinically significant drop in hemoglobin. Uncommon in primary care	Hemorrhage most likely cause of sudden, dangerous drop in Hct and Hb. Can usually be ruled in/out by health history and/or physical examination.
Chronic blood loss	Chronic from erosive gastritis, menorrhagia, GI malignancy, others	Iron from RBC wasted via blood loss cannot be recycled. Clinically significant blood loss can be as little as a few mL/d.
Reduced RBC production	Nutritional deficit (vitamin B_{12}, folic acid, iron deficiency), anemia of chronic disease (ACD), bone marrow suppression, reduced erythropoietin production (chronic renal failure)	Also associated with the use of select medications that prevent micronutrient absorption including chronic PPI use (vitamin B_{12} and iron malabsorption), metformin (vitamin B_{12} malabsorption)
Premature destruction	Hemolysis, shortened RBC lifespan (normal RBC lifespan= 90–120 d)	Hemolysis is a relatively uncommon reason for anemia. Shortened RBC lifespan is part of mechanism in anemia of chronic disease.

Table 4-2: Hemogram Evaluation in Anemia

Lab test	Comment

What are hematocrit, hemoglobin, and RBC values?	Values should be proportionately decreased.
	Normally, hemoglobin to hematocrit (H & H) ratio=1:3
	  - 10 g/dL (100 g/L)=30%
	  - 12 g/dL (120 g/L)=36%
	  - 15 g/dL (150 g/L)=45%

What is the red blood cell size? (RBC size remains unchanged during RBC's 90–120-day lifespan.)	Wintrobe's classification of anemia by evaluation of mean corpuscle volume (MCV).
	  - Microcytic: Small cell with MCV<80 fL
	  - Normocytic: Normal size cell with MCV=80–96 fL
	  - Macrocytic: Abnormally large cell with MCV>96 fL

What is the red blood cells' hemoglobin content? (RBC color remains unchanged during RBC's 90–120-day lifespan.)	Reflected by mean cell hemoglobin (MCH), mean cell hemoglobin concentration (MCHC)
	  - Hemoglobin: Source of the cell's color (-chromic)
	    Hemoglobin comprises about 90% of the RBC volume.
	Normochromic=Normal color=MCHC=31–37 g/dL (310–370 g/L)
	Hypochromic=Pale=MCHC<31 g/dL (310 g/L)

What is the RDW (RBC distribution width)?	An index of variation in RBC size (NL=11.5–15%) (0.115–0.15 proportion) Abnormal value=Greater than 15% (>0.15 proportion), indicating that new cells differ in size (larger or smaller) when compared with older cells - This is one of the earliest laboratory indicators of an evolving microcytic or macrocytic anemia.

What is the reticulocyte percentage?	The body's normal response to anemia is to attempt correction via increasing the number of young RBCs (reticulocytes).
	  - In healthy person, reticulocyte percentage=1–2%
	  - NL response to anemia is reticulocytosis (>2%) _2%_
	  - Since the reticulocyte MCV>96 fL, marked reticulocytosis can cause RDW to increase transiently.

In an evolving microcytic anemia, as MCV decreases	In an evolving macrocytic anemia, as MCV increases
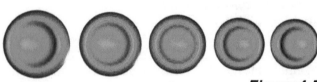 RDW increases _Figure 4-5_	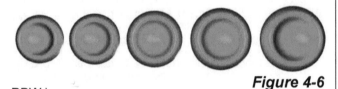 RDW increases _Figure 4-6_

Sources: Cash, J. (2014) <u>Family Practice Guidelines</u>, 3rd Edition, New York, NY: Springer Publishing.
Desai, S. (2009) <u>Clinician's Guide to Laboratory Medicine: Pocket</u>, Houston, TX: MD2B.
Ferri, F. (2014) <u>Ferri's Best Test: A Practical Guide to Clinical Laboratory Medicine and Diagnostic Imaging</u>, 3rd Edition, St. Louis, MO: Elsevier Health Sciences.
Fitzgerald, M. A. (2017) Hematologic and Immunologic Disorders, <u>Nurse Practitioner Certification Examination and Practice Preparation</u>, 5th Edition, Philadelphia, PA: F. A. Davis.
All available at fhea.com

metformin – B12

Table 4-3: Identifying Anemia		
Anemia type	**Description**	**Example**
Normocytic (MCV=80–96 fL) normochromic anemia with NL RDW **Most common etiology: Acute blood loss or anemia of chronic disease (ACD) (select chronic inflammatory diseases, particularly with poor control)**	Hb=↓ Hct=↓ RBC=↓ MCV=NL MCHC=NL RDW=NL Cells made under ordinary conditions with sufficient hemoglobin. This yields cells that are normal size (normocytic), normal color (normochromic), and about the same size (NL RDW).	*72-year-old man with an acute GI bleed (acute blood loss)* *32-year-old woman with newly-diagnosed systemic lupus erythematosus (ACD)* Hb=10.1 g/dL (12–14 g) ↓ (101 g/L [120–140 g/L]) Hct=32% (36–43%) ↓ (0.32 proportion [0.36–0.43 proportion]) RBC=3.2 million/mm^3 (4.2–5.4 mil) ↓ MCV=82 fL (81–96 fL) NL MCHC=34.8 g/dL (31–37 g/dL) NL (348 g/L [310–370 g/L]) RDW=12.1% (11.5–15%) NL (0.121 proportion [0.115–0.15 proportion])
Microcytic (MCV<80 fL) hypochromic anemia with elevated RDW **Most common etiology: Iron deficiency anemia (IDA, chronic low volume blood loss as most common IDA etiology in adults. 85% of iron in body recycled from old RBCs.)**	Hb=↓ Hct=↓ RBC=↓ MCV=↓ MCHC=↓ RDW=↑ Small cell (microcytic) due to insufficient hemoglobin (hypochromic), with new cells smaller than old cells (elevated RDW) Next step test= Ferritin for estimate of iron stores	*68-year-old man with erosive gastritis* *48-year-old woman with menorrhagia* Hb=10.1 g/dL (12–14 g/dL) ↓ (101 g/L [120–140 g/L]) Hct=32% (36–43%) ↓ (0.32 proportion [0.36–0.43 proportion]) RBC=3.2 million/mm^3 (4.2–5.4 mil) ↓ MCV=72 fL (81–96 fL) ↓ MCHC=26.8 g/dL (31–37 g/dL) ↓ (268 g/L [310–370 g/L]) RDW=18.1% (11.5–15%) ↑ (0.181 proportion [0.115–0.15 proportion])
Microcytic (MCV<80 fL) hypochromic anemia with NL RDW **Most common etiology: Alpha or beta thalassemia minor (also known as thalassemia trait)** At-risk ethnic groups for alpha thalassemia minor: Asian, African ancestry (A, A, A) At-risk ethnic groups for beta thalassemia minor: African, Mediterranean, Middle Eastern ancestry (B, A, M, M E)	Hb=↓ Hct=↓ RBC=↑ MCV=↓ MCHC=↓ RDW=NL Through inherited genetic variation (not considered a disease state), small (microcytic), pale (hypochromic) cells that are all around the same size (NL RDW) Next step test= Hemoglobin electrophoresis for evaluation of hemoglobin variants	*27-year-old man of African ancestry with beta thalassemia minor* Hb=11.6 g (14–16 g) ↓ (116 g/L [140–160 g/L]) Hct=36.7% (42–48%) ↓ (0.367 proportion [0.42–0.48 proportion]) RBC=6.38 million/mm^3 (4.7–6.10 mil) ↑ MCV=69.5 fL (81–99 fL) ↓ MCH=22 pg (27–33 pg) ↓ RDW=13.8% (11.5–15%) NL (0.138 proportion [0.115–0.15 proportion]) *CBC results reflect younger adult male norms.*

Continued...

Notes:

Table 4-3 (cont.): Identifying Anemia		
Anemia type	**Description**	**Example**

Macrocytic, (MCV>96 fL) normochromic anemia with elevated RDW
Most common etiology: Pernicious anemia, dietary-induced vitamin B$_{12}$ deficiency (uncommon), folate deficiency anemia (uncommon) -
	Hb=↓
	Hct=↓
	RBC=↓
	MCV=↑
	MCHC=NL
	RDW=↑
	
	Abnormally large (macrocytic) cells due to altered RNA:DNA ratio, hemoglobin content WNL (normochromic), new cells larger than old cells (elevated RDW)
	Next step test= Vitamin B$_{12}$ and folate
		72-year-old woman with untreated pernicious anemia
		Hb=8.2 g/dL (12–14 g/dL) ↓
		  (82 g/L [120–140 g/L])
		Hct=25% (36–43%) ↓
		  (0.25 proportion [0.36–0.43 proportion])
		RBC=2.7 million/mm^3 (4.2–5.4 mil) ↓
		MCV=125.5 fL (81–99 fL) ↑
		MCH=31 pg (27–33 pg) NL
		RDW=18.8% (11.5–15%) ↑
		  (0.188 proportion [0.115–0.15 proportion])

Drug-induced macrocytosis usually without anemia
Most common etiology: Excessive alcohol ≥5 drinks per day in male, ≥3 drinks per day in female), use of select medications, such as carbamazepine (Tegretol®), valproic acid (Depakote®), phenytoin (Dilantin®), zidovudine (AZT®), others
1 drink=12 oz (0.35 L) of beer, 5 oz (0.15 L) of wine, 1.5 oz (0.04 L) of 80-proof liquor
	Hb=WNL
	Hct=WNL
	RBC=WNL
	MCV=↑
	MCHC=NL
	RDW=NL
	
	Abnormally large (macrocytic) cells due to altered RNA:DNA ratio, hemoglobin content WNL (normochromic), new cells usually same size as old cells (NL RDW)
	Reversible when use of offending medication is discontinued but usually not a reason to curtail the drug's use, except for excessive alcohol intake
		32-year-old woman who is taking phenytoin
		38-year-old woman who drinks 5 glasses of wine a day
		Hb=12 g/dL (12–14 g/dL) NL
		  (120 g/L [120–140 g/L])
		Hct=37% (36–43%) NL
		  (0.37 proportion [0.36–0.43 proportion])
		RBC=4.2 million/mm^3 (4.2–5.4 mil) NL
		MCV=105.5 fL (81–99 fL) ↑
		MCH=31 pg (27–33 pg) NL
		RDW=12.8% (11.5–15%) NL
		  (0.128 proportion [0.115–0.15 proportion])

Table 4-4: Intervention in Anemia	
Intervention	**Comment**
Treat the underlying cause.	For this to be effective, etiology of anemia must be accurately determined. In severe and/or chronic anemia, consider multiple causes.
Replace needed micronutrients, such as iron and select vitamins.	Micronutrient requirements increase in reticulocytosis.
Epoetin alfa (EPO®, Procrit®) as indicated. Biologically identical to endogenous erythropoietin, induces erythropoiesis	Helpful in severe anemia, particularly presence of advancing renal failure. Erythropoietin supply is diminished in advancing renal failure, usually beginning when glomerular filtration rate (GFR)<49 mL/min (normal GFR=90–120 mL/min).

Source: Fitzgerald, M. A. (2017) Hematologic and immunologic disorders, <u>Nurse Practitioner Certification Examination and Practice Preparation</u>, 5th Edition, Philadelphia, PA: F. A. Davis.

What is the most common type of anemia?	
In childhood?	*iron deficiency*
During pregnancy?	*Iron deficiency*
In women during reproductive years?	*Iron deficiency*
In the elderly?	*Anemia chronic*

1. You advise a person who follows a vegan diet to supplement with:

    A. Vitamin A.

    B. Iron.

    C. Vitamin B_{12}.

    D. Folic acid.

2. A 78-year-old woman presents with fatigue, spoon-shaped nails and the following laboratory results.

    Hb=9 g/dL (11.8–14 g/dL) (90 g/L [118–140 g/L])

    Hct=28.1% (35.4–42%) (0.281 proportion [0.354–0.42 proportion])

    RBC=2.4 million/mm^3 (3.2–4.3 million/mm^3)

    MCV=70 fL (80–96 fL)

    MCHC=24.2 g/dL (31–37 g/dL) (242 g/L [310–370 g/L])

    RDW=19% (11–15%) (0.19 proportion [0.11–0.15 proportion])

    Iron deficiency

A critical causative diagnosis to consider as origin of her anemia is:

    A. Gastrointestinal blood loss.

    B. Micronutrient malabsorption.

    C. Chronic ileitis.

    D. Folic acid deficiency.

3. Which of the following represents the optimal advice to a patient who is taking oral iron therapy to maximize the medication's effectiveness?

    A. Take your medication with an antacid.

    B. Take your medication on an empty stomach.

    C. Take your medication after the largest meal of the day.

    D. Take your medication with a large glass of milk.

4. A 68-year-old woman presents with a 6-month history of increasingly severe peripheral numbness and oral irritation. Hemogram results are as follows. *B~12*

   Hb=6.2 g/dL (12–14 g/dL) (62 g/L [120–140 g/L])

   Hct=20% (36–42%) (0.2 proportion [0.36–0.42 proportion]) ↓

   RBC=2.1 million/mm³ (4.2–5.4 million/mm³) ↓

   MCV=132 fL (80–96 fL) ↑

   MCHC=32.4 g/dL (31–37 g/dL) (324 g/L [310–370 g/L])

   RDW=19% (11–15%) (0.19 proportion [0.11–0.15 ↑ proportion])

Physical exam reveals pale conjunctiva, a grade 2/6 systolic ejection murmur over the precordium without radiation, and a smooth, red tongue. The most likely cause of this anemia is:

   A. Vitamin B₁₂ deficiency. *—big beefy tongue*

   B. Iron deficiency.

   C. Hemolysis.

   D. Chronic disease.

5. The heart murmur noted in the above-mentioned patient has not been present on previous examination. As a result, you consider that this is likely a _____ murmur and will resolve with anemia treatment.

   A. Pathologic

   B. Hemic *— innocent —*

   C. Venous hum

   D. Congenital

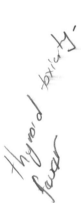
thyroid toxicity fever

6. A 65-year-old woman with rheumatoid arthritis who is on optimized therapy and continues to have significant symptoms presents with the following hemogram.

    Hb=10.1 g/dL (12–14 g/dL) (101 g/L [120–140 g/L]) ↓

    Hct=32% (36–42%) (0.32 proportion [0.36–0.42 proportion]) ↓

    RBC=3.2 million/mm^3 (4.2–5.4 million/mm^3) ↓

    MCV=82 fL (80–96 fL) WNL

    RDW=12.8% (11–15%) (0.128 proportion [0.11–0.15 WNL proportion])

    Reticulocytes=0.7% (1–2%) (0.007 proportion [0.01–0.02 ↓ proportion])

These findings are most consistent with:

    A. Iron deficiency anemia.

    B. Folate deficiency anemia.

    C. Anemia of chronic disease.

    D. Alpha thalassemia minor.

[handwritten: RA chronic inflammatory disease]

7. You see Maria, a 32-year-old well woman of Mediterranean ancestry. Hemogram results are as follows:

    Hb=10.6 g/dL (12–14 g/dL) (106 g/L [120–140 g/L]) ↓

    Hct=32% (36–42%) (0.32 proportion [0.36–0.42 proportion]) ↓

    RBC=5.2 million/mm^3 (3.2–4.3 million/mm^3) ↑

    MCV=71 fL (80–96 fL) ↓

    MCHC=25.2 g/dL (31–37 g/dL) (252 g/L [310–370 g/L]) ↓

    RDW=12% (<15%) (0.12 proportion [<0.15 proportion]) WNL

These findings are most consistent with:

    A. Iron deficiency anemia.

    B. Cooley's anemia.

    C. Beta thalassemia minor.

    D. Acute blood loss.

[handwritten: small pale cells a lots of them N]

8. Match the best next test to order in an adult with anemia based on hemogram results.

    A. MCV ↓, MCHC ↓, RDW ↑ *[handwritten: iron defi — feritin — iron store]*

    B. MCV ↓, MCHC ↓, RDW NL *[handwritten: thalasimia - B.]*

    C. MCV ↑, MCHC NL, RDW ↑ *[handwritten: B12 and folate]*

Ferritin *[iron deficiency]*	A
Vitamin B$_{12}$ and folate *[B]*	C
Hemoglobin electrophoresis	B

9. The use of all of the following nutritional supplements is potentially associated with increased bleeding risk except:

A. Ginseng. ✓

B. Gingko. ✓

C. Fish oil ✓

D. Coenzyme Q10.

10. Primary care of Sarah, a 27-year-old woman with beta thalassemia minor, should include:

A. Prescribing a low-dose iron supplement to counteract microcytosis.

B. An evaluation of hemoglobin electrophoresis every 5 years.

C. Advising taking a multivitamin with high-dose folate supplementation daily.

D. Offering genetic counseling prior to pregnancy.

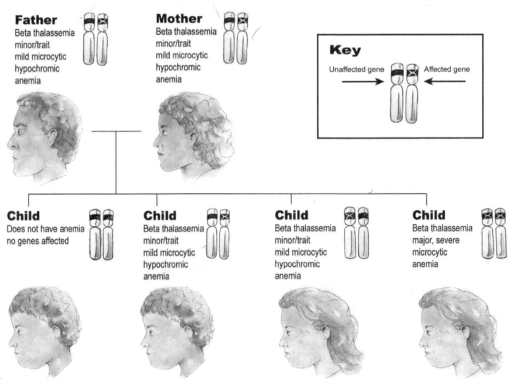

1 in 4 Risk with Each Pregnancy
Beta Thalassemia - Reflects risk with each pregnancy

Father
Beta thalassemia minor/trait mild microcytic hypochromic anemia

Mother
Beta thalassemia minor/trait mild microcytic hypochromic anemia

Key
Unaffected gene → ← Affected gene

Child
Does not have anemia no genes affected

Child
Beta thalassemia minor/trait mild microcytic hypochromic anemia

Child
Beta thalassemia minor/trait mild microcytic hypochromic anemia

Child
Beta thalassemia major, severe microcytic anemia

Figure 4-26

1 in 4 Risk with Each Pregnancy

Sickle Cell - Reflects risk with each pregnancy

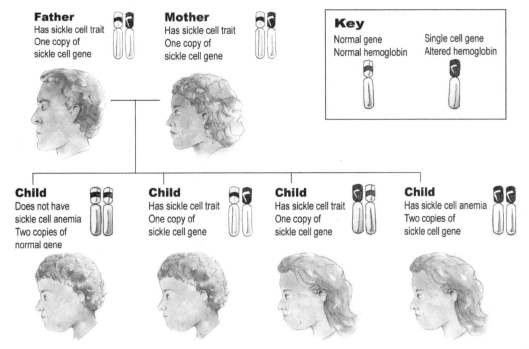

Father
Has sickle cell trait
One copy of
sickle cell gene

Mother
Has sickle cell trait
One copy of
sickle cell gene

Key

Normal gene
Normal hemoglobin

Single cell gene
Altered hemoglobin

Child
Does not have
sickle cell anemia
Two copies of
normal gene

Child
Has sickle cell trait
One copy of
sickle cell gene

Child
Has sickle cell trait
One copy of
sickle cell gene

Child
Has sickle cell anemia
Two copies of
sickle cell gene

Figure 4-27

Bonus questions for this chapter available through your Fitzgerald Health learning portal at fhea.com/npexpert.

Resources for Additional Study

Books:

Cash, J. (2014) <u>Family Practice Guidelines</u>, 3rd Edition, New York, NY: Springer Publishing.

Desai, S. (2009) <u>Clinician's Guide to Laboratory Medicine: Pocket</u>, Houston, TX: MD2B.

Ferri, F. (2014) <u>Ferri's Best Test: A Practical Guide to Clinical Laboratory Medicine and Diagnostic Imaging</u>, 3rd Edition, St. Louis, MO: Elsevier Health Sciences.

Fitzgerald, M. A. (2017) Hematologic and Immunologic Disorders, <u>Nurse Practitioner Certification Examination and Practice Preparation</u>, 5th Edition, Philadelphia, PA: F. A. Davis.

Audio programs:

Fitzgerald, M. A. <u>Analysis of the WBC Count and Differential</u>, North Andover, MA: Fitzgerald Health Education Associates.

Fitzgerald, M. A. <u>Assessment of Hepatic Function</u>, North Andover, MA: Fitzgerald Health Education Associates.

Fitzgerald, M. A. <u>Assessment and Intervention in Common Anemias</u>, North Andover, MA: Fitzgerald Health Education Associates.

Fitzgerald, M. A. <u>Challenging Case Studies in Laboratory Diagnosis</u>, North Andover, MA: Fitzgerald Health Education Associates.

Fitzgerald, M. A. <u>Drug-drug and Drug-nutrient Interactions: A Focus on Common Problems</u>, North Andover, MA: Fitzgerald Health Education Associates.

Fitzgerald, M. A. <u>Evaluation in Immunologic and Autoimmune Disorders</u>, North Andover, MA: Fitzgerald Health Education Associates.

Fitzgerald, M. A. <u>Evaluation and Intervention in Thyroid Disorders</u>, North Andover, MA: Fitzgerald Health Education Associates.

Fitzgerald, M. A. <u>Evaluation of Renal Function</u>, North Andover, MA: Fitzgerald Health Education Associates.

Fitzgerald, M. A. <u>Laboratory Monitoring During Drug Therapy</u>, North Andover, MA: Fitzgerald Health Education Associates.

Chapter 5: Eye, Ear, Nose, and Throat Disorders

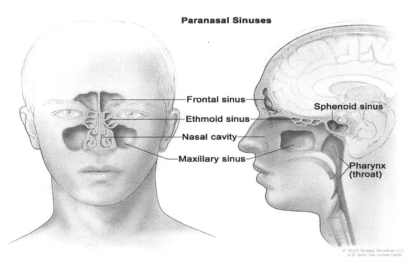

Paranasal Sinuses

Frontal sinus
Ethmoid sinus
Nasal cavity
Maxillary sinus
Sphenoid sinus
Pharynx (throat)

Figure 5-1

Table 5-1: Acute Rhinosinusitis (ARS): Defining the Terms	
Acute rhinosinusitis (ARS)	Inflammation of the mucosal lining of nasal passages and paranasal sinuses lasting up to 4 weeks, caused by allergens, environmental irritants, and/or infection (viruses [majority], bacteria, and fungi).
Acute bacterial rhinosinusitis (ABRS or ABS)	Secondary bacterial infection of paranasal sinuses, usually following viral URI; relatively uncommon in adults and children. ***Less than 2% of viral URIs are complicated by ABRS. In the majority, ABRS will resolve without antimicrobial therapy.***

Source: Clinical Infectious Diseases Advance Access, available at
http://cid.oxfordjournals.org

Table 5-2: Principles of Empiric Antimicrobial Therapy: Applicable to choice of intervention in all infectious disease to help optimize treatment success and minimize development of resistant pathogens	
Empiric antimicrobial therapy	**Questions to ask prior to choosing an antimicrobial**
The decision-making process in which the clinician chooses the agent based on patient characteristics and site of infection	What is/are the most likely pathogen(s) causing this infection? What is the spectrum of a given antimicrobial's activity? What is the likelihood of a resistant pathogen? What is the danger if there is treatment failure? What is the optimal safe antimicrobial dose? What is the duration of the shortest but effective course of therapy?

Table 5-3: Causative Pathogens in ABRS (ABS)

Organism	Description	Resistance
S. pneumoniae Most common bacterial pathogen in ABRS, acute otitis media (AOM), community-acquired pneumonia (CAP)	Gram-positive diplococci, ABRS causative organism in adults=38%, children=21–33%	≥25% drug-resistant (DRSP) via altered protein-binding sites that limit certain antibiotic's ability to bind to the pathogen
H. influenzae Common pathogen in ABRS, AOM, CAP, particularly with recurrent infection, tobacco use	Gram-negative bacillus, ABRS causative organism in adults=36%, children=31–32%	≥30% penicillin-resistant via production of beta-lactamase that cleaves beta-lactam ring in most penicillins including amoxicillin, ampicillin. Most cephalosporins are stable in the presence of beta-lactamase.
M. catarrhalis Less common pathogen in ABRS, AOM, uncommon cause of CAP	Gram-negative coccus, ABRS causative organism in adults=16%, children=8–11%	≥90% penicillin-resistant via beta-lactamase production

In treating ABRS, an antimicrobial with activity against Gram-positive pathogens (*S. pneumoniae,* consider DRSP risk) and Gram-negative pathogens (*H. influenzae, M. catarrhalis,* consider beta-lactamase production rates) should be chosen.

Algorithm for the Management of Acute Bacterial Rhinosinusitis

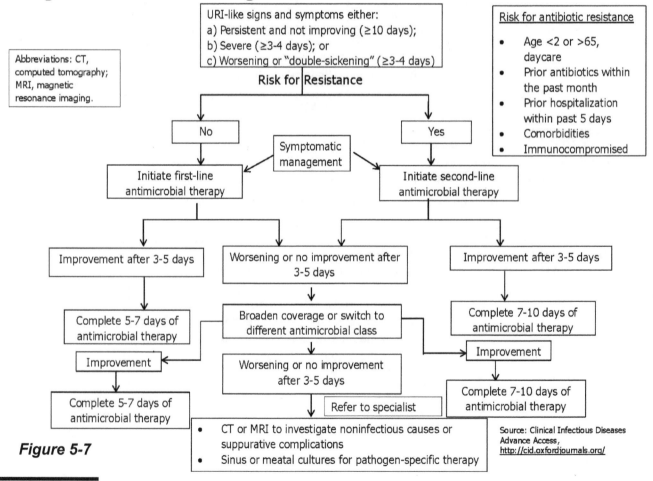

Figure 5-7

Table 5-4: Symptomatic Treatment in ABRS
Saline nasal irrigations
Intranasal corticosteroids when ABRS is accompanied by allergic rhinitis

Source: Chow, A. et al., IDSA Clinical Practice Guideline for Acute Bacterial Rhinosinusitis in Children and Adults, available at https://www.idsociety.org/uploadedFiles/IDSA/Guidelines-Patient_Care/PDF_Library/IDSA%20Clinical%20Practice%20Guideline%20for%20Acute%20Bacterial%20Rhinosinusitis%20in%20Children%20and%20Adults.pdf

Table 5-5: Antimicrobial Regimens for Acute Bacterial Rhinosinusitis in Adults

Indication	Daily dose	Comments
Initial empiric therapy	First-line • Amoxicillin-clavulanate 500 mg/125 mg PO TID, or 875 mg/125 mg PO BID Second-line • Amoxicillin-clavulanate 2000 mg/125 mg PO BID • or • Doxycycline 100 mg PO BID or 200 mg PO daily	High-dose (HD, 3–4 g/d) amoxicillin needed against drug-resistant *Streptococcus pneumoniae* (DRSP) Clavulanate as a beta-lactamase inhibitor, allows amoxicillin to have activity against beta-lactamase–producing organisms, such as *H. influenzae, M. catarrhalis* Doxycycline: DRSP treatment failure risk, activity against Gram-negative organisms, stable in presence of beta-lactamase. Doxycycline=Pregnancy risk category D
In beta-lactam allergy (Allergy to antimicrobials with beta-lactam ring, such as penicillins, cephalosporins)	Doxycycline 100 mg PO BID or 200 mg PO daily • or Levofloxacin 500 mg PO daily* • or Moxifloxacin 400 mg PO daily*	Respiratory fluoroquinolones (FQ): Activity against DRSP, Gram-negative organisms, stable in presence of beta-lactamase Major rationale for the use of respiratory FQ is the presence of DRSP risk. See FDA advisory on limiting FQ use.
Risk for antibiotic resistance or failed initial therapy	Amoxicillin-clavulanate 2000 mg/125 mg PO BID • or Levofloxacin 500 mg PO daily* • or Moxifloxacin 400 mg PO daily*	All options with activity against DRSP, Gram-negative organisms, stable in presence of and/or active against beta-lactamase

Source: Chow, A. et al., IDSA Clinical Practice Guideline for Acute Bacterial Rhinosinusitis in Children and Adults, available at https://www.idsociety.org/uploadedFiles/IDSA/Guidelines-Patient_Care/PDF_Library/IDSA%20Clinical%20Practice%20Guideline%20for%20Acute%20Bacterial%20Rhinosinusitis%20in%20Children%20and%20Adults.pdf

*The U.S. FDA is advising that the serious side effects associated with fluoroquinolone antibacterial drugs generally outweigh the benefits for patients with acute sinusitis, acute bronchitis, and uncomplicated urinary tract infections who have other treatment options. For patients with these conditions, fluoroquinolones should be reserved for those who do not have alternative treatment options. See *http://www.fda.gov/Drugs/DrugSafety/ucm500143.htm for additional information.

Table 5-6: CYP450 Drug-metabolizing Isoenzymes: A potential source of drug-drug interactions

Definition	Clinical example
Subtrate Utilizes a specific enzymatic pathway EXIT *Figure 5-10* A medication or substance that is metabolized by the isoenzyme, utilizing this enzyme in order to be modified so it can reach drug site of action and/or be eliminated	CYP450 3A4 substrates: Sildenafil (Viagra®), atorvastatin, simvastatin, venlafaxine (Effexor®), alprazolam (Xanax®), many others ***About 50% of all prescription medications are CYP450 3A4 substrates.***
Inhibitor Blocks a specific enzymatic pathway, keeps substrate from exiting. EXIT STOP *Figure 5-11* Blocks the activity of the isoenzyme, limiting substrate excretion, allowing increase in substrate levels, and possible risk of substrate-induced toxicity	Erythro-, clarithromycin=CYP450 3A4 inhibitors Concomitant use of one of these antibiotics with any of the aforementioned CYP450 3A4 substrates (sildenafil, atorvastatin, simvastatin, venlafaxine, alprazolam, many others) results in an increase in substrate levels, potentially leading to substrate-induced toxicity.

Continued...

Table 5-6 (cont.): CYP450 Drug-metabolizing Isoenzymes: A potential source of drug-drug interactions	
	Clinical example
Inducer Pushes the substrate out the exit pathway. *Figure 5-12* Accelerates the activity of the isoenzyme so that substrate is pushed out the exit pathway, leading to a reduction in substrate level	St. John's wort=CYP450 3A4 inducer Concomitant use of St. John's wort and 3A4 substrate can lead to reduced target drug levels and diminished therapeutic effect, possible treatment failure Medications of particular concern include select antiretrovirals, combined oral contraceptives, and cyclosporine

Source: P450 Drug Interaction Table: Abbreviated "Clinically Relevant" Table, available at
medicine.iupui.edu/clinpharm/DDIs/ClinicalTable.aspx

1. You see a 47-year-old man in urgent care who has hypertension, dyslipidemia, and depression. He states, "I am on a big list of medications but I am not sure of all the names." He also has a history of penicillin allergy with a hive-form reaction. He has not taken a systemic antimicrobial in more than a year and denies recent hospitalization. When developing a treatment plan for acute bacterial rhinosinusitis, you consider prescribing the following course of an oral antimicrobial.

   A. A 5-day course of clarithromycin. —

   B. A 7-day course of doxycycline.

   C. A 10-day course of amoxicillin-clavulanate.

   D. A 7-day course of moxifloxacin.

2. Sandra is a 45-year-old well woman diagnosed with a left-sided unilateral acute otitis media 10 days ago and treated with an antimicrobial. She is seen today with a report of resolution of ear pain, but with persistent sensation of ear fullness and diminished ability to discriminate speech in the affected ear. Anticipated findings on today's physical examination include:

   A. Erythema of the ear canal.

   B. Weber test lateralizing to the affected ear.

   C. Discomfort on tragus pull.

   D. Anterior cervical lymphadenopathy on the affected side.

3. For Sandra, which of the following represents the best advice for this point in her AOM therapy?

   A. She should have a second course of antimicrobial therapy.

   B. A short course of an oral corticosteroid should be prescribed.

   C. The sensation of ear fullness is an anticipated finding.

   D. She should be seen by an otolaryngology specialist.

Conductive vs. Sensorineural Hearing Loss

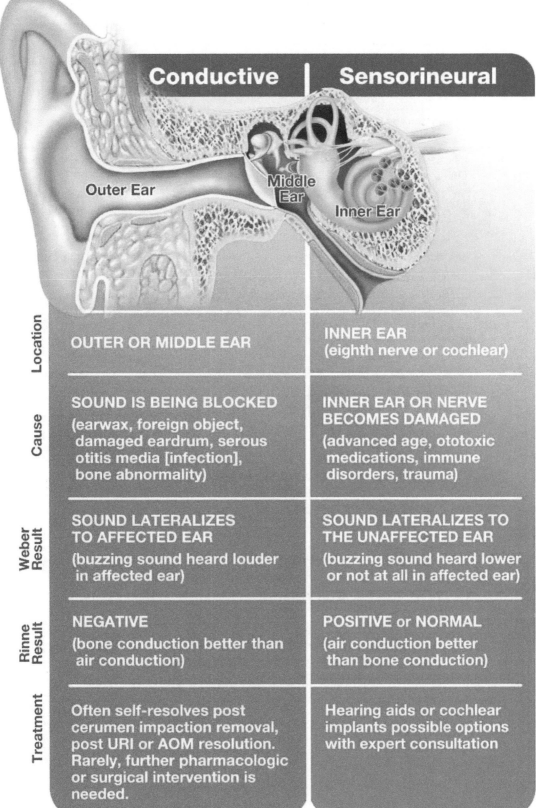

	Conductive	Sensorineural
Location	OUTER OR MIDDLE EAR	INNER EAR (eighth nerve or cochlear)
Cause	SOUND IS BEING BLOCKED (earwax, foreign object, damaged eardrum, serous otitis media [infection], bone abnormality)	INNER EAR OR NERVE BECOMES DAMAGED (advanced age, ototoxic medications, immune disorders, trauma)
Weber Result	SOUND LATERALIZES TO AFFECTED EAR (buzzing sound heard louder in affected ear)	SOUND LATERALIZES TO THE UNAFFECTED EAR (buzzing sound heard lower or not at all in affected ear)
Rinne Result	NEGATIVE (bone conduction better than air conduction)	POSITIVE or NORMAL (air conduction better than bone conduction)
Treatment	Often self-resolves post cerumen impaction removal, post URI or AOM resolution. Rarely, further pharmacologic or surgical intervention is needed.	Hearing aids or cochlear implants possible options with expert consultation

Figure 5-14

Table 5-7: Allergic Rhinitis (AR) Treatment:
A Combination Approach

Allergic rhinitis (AR) is an inflammatory, IgE-mediated disease due to genetic and environmental interactions and characterized by nasal congestion, rhinorrhea (nasal drainage), sneezing, intraocular and/or nasal itching

Risk factors for allergic disorders, pattern of symptoms, allergic comorbidities, and physical exam help differentiate between AR, common cold, and ABRS.

AR issue	Intervention	Comment
Allergen avoidance/ environmental control	1st-line therapy in any allergic disorder	Patient education to avoid the allergen whenever possible
Controller therapy to prevent symptoms	Intranasal corticosteroids as 1st-line controller therapy. • Examples- Fluticasone propionate (Flonase®), triamcinolone (Nasacort AQ®) Leukotriene modifiers (LTM) should not be offered as 1st-line controller therapy. • Example- Montelukast (Singulair®)	Mechanism of action- Prevention of inflammatory mediators Intranasal corticosteroids significantly more effective when compared to LTM due to suppression of more inflammatory mediators, onset of action within 2–7 days of use. LTM- Best as add-on therapy if symptoms not adequately controlled with intranasal corticosteroids
Reliever therapy to relieve acute symptoms	2nd-generation oral antihistamines preferred over 1st-generation antihistamines due to more favorable adverse effect profile. • Examples- Loratadine (Claritin®), Cetirizine (Zyrtec®) Intranasal antihistamine- An option for nasal symptom relief • Intranasal antihistamine example- Azelastine (Astelin®, Astepro®) Ocular antihistamine- Helpful in managing allergic conjunctivitis signs and symptoms • Examples- Olopatadine (Patanol®, Pataday®), azelastine (Optivar®), bepotastine (Bepreve®)	Mechanism of action- Block histamine-1 receptor sites. Limited benefit with nasal congestion. Oral 1st-generation antihistamines (diphenhydramine [Benadryl®], chlorpheniramine [Chlor-Trimeton®], others) clinically effective but not favored over 2nd-generation oral antihistamines. Significant potential to cause sedation, impair performance, and exert anticholinergic effects. Due to adverse effects, not 1st-line therapy. Adverse effects particularly problematic in the older adult. Found in OTC URI and AR medications labeled to "dry runny nose" and in most OTC sleep aids.
Immunotherapy	Immunotherapy (sublingual or subcutaneous) for patients with allergic rhinitis who have inadequate response to symptoms with pharmacologic therapy with or without environmental controls. Usually requires specialty referral.	Mechanism of action- Restore tolerance to allergen by reducing its tendency to induce IgE production
Acupuncture	Provide or refer to a clinician who can offer acupuncture, for patients with allergic rhinitis who are interested in nonpharmacologic therapy	No current evidence to support herbal therapy.

Source: American Academy of Otolaryngology Clinical Practice Guideline: Allergic Rhinitis Executive Summary, available at http://oto.sagepub.com/content/152/2/197.full

4. Hank is a 58-year-old man who presents with a chief complaint of bilateral itchy eyes occurring intermittently throughout the year. Exam reveals 20/30 vision OD (right eye), OS (left eye), OU (both eyes) with corrective lenses, bilateral hyperemic bulbar and palpebral conjunctiva, and a small amount of rope-like pale yellow discharge. These findings are most consistent with:

    A. Bacterial conjunctivitis.

    B. Blepharoconjunctivitis.

    C. Allergic conjunctivitis.

    D. Dry-eye syndrome.

5. The most appropriate treatment option for Hank is the use of:

    A. Ocular antimicrobial.

    B. Lubricating eye solution.

    C. Ocular antihistamine.

    D. Systemic decongestant.

6. Appropriate pharmacologic management options for allergic rhinitis in a 29-year-old woman who is a home daycare provider includes all of the following except:

    A. Short-term use of a decongestant nasal spray.

    B. Oral chlorpheniramine.

    C. Flunisolide nasal spray.

    D. Oral loratadine.

7. Edgar is a 75-year-old man with a 60 pack-year history of cigarette smoking and COPD who presents with a chief complaint of a "sore" on the base of his tongue. This lesion has been present for a number of months, remaining relatively stable in size and is not painful. Physical examination reveals a painless ulcerated lesion with indurated margin and is accompanied by a firm, nontender submandibular node. His current medications include inhaled corticosteroids with a long-acting beta$_2$-agonist. This clinical scenario is most consistent with:

    A. Syphilitic chancre.

    B. Aphthous stomatitis.

    C. Squamous cell carcinoma.

    D. Oral candidiasis.

Table 5-8: Cranial Nerves

I	II	III	IV	V	VI	VII	VIII	IX	X	XI	XII
Olfactory	Optic	Oculomotor	Trochlear	Trigeminal	Abducens	Facial	Acoustic	Glossopharyngeal	Vagus	Spinal accessory	Hypoglossal
Smell	Vision	Eyelid and eyeball movement	Innervates superior oblique, turns eye downward and laterally	Chewing, face and mouth, touch and pain	Turns eye laterally	Controls most facial expressions, secretion of tears and saliva, taste	Hearing, equilibrium, sensation	Taste, senses carotid blood pressure	Senses aortic blood pressure, slows heart rate, stimulates digestive organs, taste	Controls trapezius and sternocleido mastoid, controls swallowing movements	Controls tongue movements
Oh	Oh	Oh	To	Touch	And	Feel	A	Great	Vein	Ah	Heaven!
On	Old	Olympus	Towering	Tops	A	Finn	And	German	Viewed	Some	Hops!
Oh	Oh	Oh	Tiny	Tim	And	Fat	Albert	Give	Vincent	A (Some)	Hand (Help)

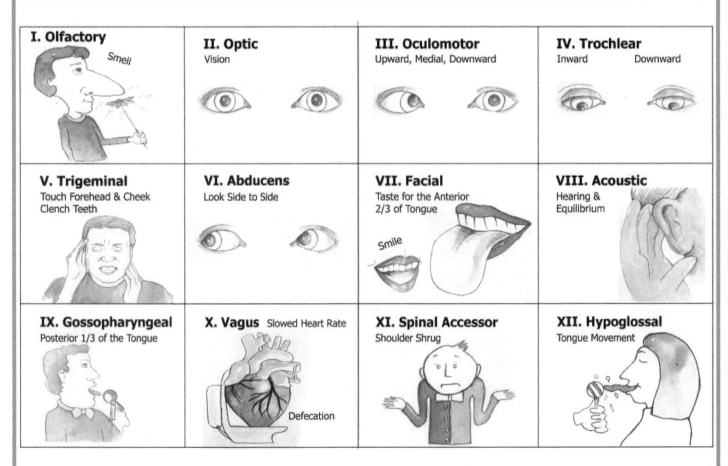

I. Olfactory — Smell

II. Optic — Vision

III. Oculomotor — Upward, Medial, Downward

IV. Trochlear — Inward, Downward

V. Trigeminal — Touch Forehead & Cheek Clench Teeth

VI. Abducens — Look Side to Side

VII. Facial — Taste for the Anterior 2/3 of Tongue — Smile

VIII. Acoustic — Hearing & Equilibrium

IX. Gossopharyngeal — Posterior 1/3 of the Tongue

X. Vagus — Slowed Heart Rate — Defecation

XI. Spinal Accessor — Shoulder Shrug

XII. Hypoglossal — Tongue Movement

Figure 5-20

8. The function of which of the following cranial nerves is being tested with the following patient requests?
   A. CN I
   B. CN XI
   C. CN III
   D. CN VII
   E. CN XII

Puff out your cheeks.	√II
Do you recognize this scent?	I
Without moving your head, follow my finger with your eyes.	·III
Shrug your shoulders.	✗ I
Stick out your tongue.	✗II

9. Matthew is a 29-year-old man who presents with a 6-hour history of sudden onset of inability to raise his eyebrow or smile on the right side. He also reports decreased lacrimation in the right eye and difficulty closing the right eyelid. The rest of his health history and physical examination is otherwise unremarkable. This likely represents paralysis of cranial nerve (CN):
   A. III.
   B. VIII.
   C. IV.
   D. VII.

10. Which of the following is the most appropriate next step in Matthew's care?
   A. Emergent referral for neuroimaging
   B. Initiating a course of oral corticosteroids
   C. Prescribing a short course of high-dose antiviral therapy
   D. Referral to a neurology specialist within the next 24–48 hours

Table 5-9: When to Measure Visual Acuity "The vital signs of the eye"	
Clinical situation	**Comment**
With comprehensive physical examination in adult or child	Typically done in office with Snellen chart. Refer to eye care specialist for additional evaluation if patient fails test. Have patient use appropriate vision aid (contact lens, eye glasses) if normally used.
With any eye complaint	If significant change from baseline, refer to eye care specialist for additional evaluation, particularly if findings are of new onset. A patient presenting with the triad of red eye, painful eye, and new-onset vision change should be promptly referred to ophthalmology.

Source: Goolsby, M.J. & Grubbs, L. (2014) The eye. <u>Advanced Assessment: Interpreting Findings and Formulating Differential Diagnoses</u>, 3rd Edition. Philadelphia, PA: F. A. Davis.

11. You see a 55-year-old woman who presents for a health maintenance visit. She has longstanding myopia and newer-onset presbyopia, both corrected with eyeglasses. She is normotensive and without ocular complaint. You anticipate the following on today's eye exam:

    A. Retinal arteries wider than veins.

    B. Equal, sluggish pupillary response.

    C. Sharp disc margins.

    D. Lid ectropion.

12. Which of the following is most likely to be found on the funduscopic exam in the person with angle-closure glaucoma?

    A. A deeply-cupped optic disc

    B. Arteriovenous nicking

    C. Papilledema

    D. Hemorrhagic lesions

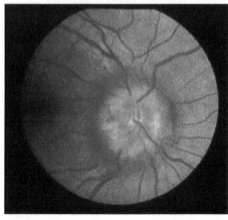

Figure 5-29

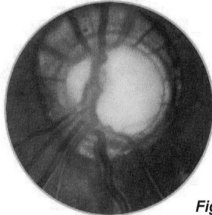

Figure 5-30

13. Match each vision alteration with the most likely etiology.

    A. Macular degeneration

    B. Untreated open-angle glaucoma

    C. Proliferative diabetic retinopathy

Peripheral vision loss 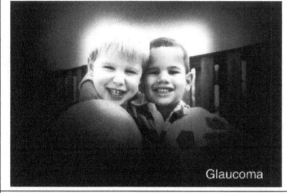 *Figure 5-31*	B Untreated open-angle
Floating spots in visual field 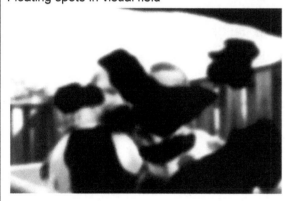 *Figure 5-32*	Proliferative diabetic retinopath
Central vision loss 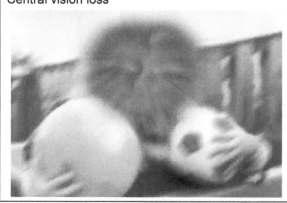 *Figure 5-33*	A Macular

14. Match the following select ophthalmologic tests with the appropriate indication.

  A. Amsler grid test

  B. Snellen chart

  C. Slit-lamp examination

  D. Tonometry

Indication	
Evaluation of anterior eye structures, including cornea, conjunctiva, sclera, and iris	C
General visual acuity screen	B
Early detection of macular degeneration	A
Measurement of intraocular pressure, glaucoma screening test	D

15. During a clinical encounter with a 78-year-old man who has presbycusis, the NP considers that communication will be enhanced by all of the following except:

  A. Maintaining eye contact with the patient.

  B. Ensuring the patient can see the NP's face clearly.

  C. Playing soft music in the background.

  D. Providing adequate illumination in the exam room.

Table 5-10: Age-related Changes and Conditions that Result in Changes of the Senses			
Condition	Etiology	Result	Comment
Presbyopia	Hardening of lens	Close vision problems	Nearly all ≥45-yo need reading glasses or other similar correction.
Senile cataracts	Lens clouding	Progressive vision dimming, distance vision problems, close vision usually retained and often initially improves	Risk factors: Tobacco use, poor nutrition, sun exposure, systemic corticosteroid therapy Potentially correctable with surgery, lens implant
Open-angle glaucoma	Painless, gradual onset of increased intraocular pressure leading to optic atrophy	Loss of peripheral vision if untreated, avoidable with appropriate and ongoing intervention	≥80% of all glaucoma Periodic screening with tonometry, assessment of visual fields Treatment with topical miotics, beta-blockers, others, or surgery effective in vision preservation
Angle-closure glaucoma	Sudden increase in intraocular pressure	Usually unilateral, acutely red, painful eye with vision change including halos around lights; eyeball firm when compared to other	Immediate referral to ophthalmology care for rapid pressure reduction via medication, possible surgery
Age-related maculopathy (macular degeneration)	Thickening, sclerotic changes in retinal basement membrane complex	Painless vision changes including distortion of central vision. On funduscopic examination, drusen (soft yellow deposits in the macular region) often visible	Aside from aging, risk factors include tobacco use, sun exposure, and fm hx. Dry form: Given few treatment options, prevention should be the goal. Develops over decades. No treatment available Wet form: Laser treatment for photocoagulation to obliterate neovascular membrane; intravitreal injection of anti-vascular growth factor. Develops relatively quickly, usually over months.
Anosmia, hyposmia	Neural degeneration	Diminished sense of smell, with resulting decline in fine taste discrimination	Accelerated by tobacco use
Presbycusis	Loss of 8th cranial nerve sensitivity	Difficulty with conversation in noisy environment Person can hear but cannot understand what is said.	Accelerated by excessive noise exposure Hearing aids helpful
Cerumen impaction	Conductive hearing loss	General diminution of hearing	Cerumen removal helpful in improving hearing

Sources:
www.merckmanuals.com/professional/geriatrics/approach_to_the_geriatric_patient/physic
al_changes_with_aging.html
www.merckmanuals.com/professional/ear_nose_and_throat_disorders.html

Table 5-11: Treatment of Common Bacterial EENT Infections

Site of infection	Common pathogens	Recommended antimicrobial	Comment
Suppurative conjunctivitis (non-gonococcal, non-chlamydial)	S. aureus, S. pneumoniae, H. influenzae Outbreaks due to S. pneumoniae	Primary: Ophthalmic treatment with FQ ocular solution (cipro-, levo-, moxifloxacin) Alternative: Ophthalmic treatment with polymyxin B with trimethoprim solution	Most S. pneumoniae are resistant to tobramycin, gentamicin Viral conjunctivitis ("pinkeye," usually caused by adenovirus), often self-limiting Relieve irritative symptoms with use of cold artificial tear solution.
Otitis externa (swimmer's ear)	Pseudomonas spp., anaerobes, S. epidermidis Acute infection often S. aureus Fungi rare etiology	For milder disease: Acetic acid with propylene glycol and hydrocortisone (VoSoL) drops For moderate to severe disease: Otic drops with ciprofloxacin with hydrocortisone	Systemic (oral or injectable) antimicrobial seldom needed. Ear canal cleansing important. Decrease risk of reinfection by use of eardrops of 1:2 mixture of white vinegar and rubbing alcohol after swimming. Do not use neomycin-containing product if punctured TM is suspected.
Malignant otitis externa in person w/DM, HIV/AIDS, on chemo-therapy	Pseudomonas spp. in >95%	Oral ciprofloxacin for early disease suitable for outpatient therapy Other options are available if inpatient therapy warranted in severe disease	Risk for osteomyelitis of the skull or TMJ. MRI or CT imaging to rule out osteomyelitis often indicated. ENT consult with surgical débridement should be considered. Obtain cultures of ear drainage or results of surgical debridement. Parenteral antimicrobial therapy often warranted for severe disease.
Exudative pharyngitis	Group A, C, G Streptococcus, viral, HHV-6, N. gonorrhoeae, F. necrophorum	1st-line: Penicillin V PO × 10 d or benzathine penicillin IM × 1 dose if adherence an issue Alternative: Second-generation cephalosporin × 4–6 d, azithromycin × 5 d, clarithromycin × 10 d (all PO) Up to 35% of S. pyogenes isolates resistant to macrolides	Vesicular, ulcerative pharyngitis usually viral Only 10% of adult pharyngitis due to group A Streptococcus (GAS). More common in children, teens, younger adults. Major rationale to treat GAS is prevention of rheumatic fever and eradication of organism to reduce transmission. No treatment recommended for asymptomatic group A Streptococcus carrier. For recurrent culture-proven S. pyogenes infection, consider coinfection w/beta-lactamase–producing organism; treat w/amoxicillin-clavulanate or clindamycin.

Source: Gilbert, D.N., Chambers, H.F., Eliopoulos, G.M., Saag, M.S., Pavia, A.T. (2016) The Sanford Guide to Antimicrobial Therapy (46th ed.). Sperryville, VA: Antimicrobial Therapy, Inc.

Important additional study resources available through your Fitzgerald Health online learning portal at fhea.com/npexpert

- Resource 5-1: Treatment Options in Glaucoma

- Resource 5-2: Middle Ear Conditions: History, findings, treatment, and images of normal findings, otitis media with effusion, acute otitis media

- Resource 5-3: Clinical Presentation Ophthalmologic Emergency: Trauma, anterior uveitis, acute angle-closure glaucoma

Bonus questions for this chapter available through your Fitzgerald Health learning portal at fhea.com/npexpert.

Resources for Additional Study

Books:

Fitzgerald, M. A. (2017) Eye, Ear, Nose, and Throat Disorders, <u>Nurse Practitioner Certification Examination and Practice Preparation</u>, 5th Edition, Philadelphia, PA: F. A. Davis.

Audio programs:

Fitzgerald, M. A. <u>Bacterial Pharyngitis, Conjunctivitis, Acute Otitis Media: A Focus on the Latest Treatment Recommendations</u>, North Andover, MA: Fitzgerald Health Education Associates.

Fitzgerald, M. A. <u>Prescribing for the Elder</u>, North Andover, MA: Fitzgerald Health Education Associates.

Yates, C. M. <u>Allergic Rhinitis: A Focus on Assessment and Intervention</u>, North Andover, MA: Fitzgerald Health Education Associates.

Video programs:

McDevitt, L., Tombasco, M. <u>Expert Exam: ENT Skills for Primary and Acute Care Practitioners</u>, North Andover, MA: Fitzgerald Health Education Associates.

Wright, W. L. <u>Expert Exam: The Primary Care Neurologic Exam</u>, North Andover, MA: Fitzgerald Health Education Associates.

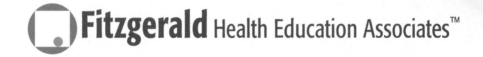

Chapter 6: Commonly Encountered Dermatologic Disorders

Figures from this chapter are available through your
Fitzgerald Health online learning portal at
www.fhea.com/npexpert.

Assessment and intervention for acne vulgaris is found in the adolescent portion of the program.

Table 6-1: Dermatology Assessment Tips Assess the entire patient, not simply the skin problem. Consider whether there is transmission/contagion risk.	
Is the patient otherwise well without systemic symptoms and other signs?	When otherwise well, likely condition limited to the skin with few to minor symptoms, such as rosacea, keratosis pilaris, seborrheic dermatitis.
Is the patient miserable (highly symptomatic) but not systemically ill (without additional signs and symptoms)?	When miserable but not systemically ill, often uncomfortable with itch, burning, pain, or the like Examples include scabies, herpes zoster (shingles), others
Is the patient systemically ill with constitutional signs and symptoms (fever, fatigue, loss of appetite, unintended weight loss, malaise, and/or others)?	When systemically ill, especially with constitutional signs and symptoms, often has the dermatologic manifestation of a systemic disease, such as varicella, transepidermal necrosis, Lyme disease, systemic lupus erythematosus, others
Are there primary lesions only? Primary and secondary lesions?	Where is the oldest lesion, and when did it occur? Where is the newest lesion, and when did it occur? This allows the examiner to assess the evolution of the skin lesions.

Table 6-2: Primary vs. Secondary Skin Lesions		
Type	**Defined**	**Example**
Primary	Result from a disease process Has not been altered by outside manipulation, treatment, natural course of disease	Vesicle: Fluid-filled lesion, diameter <1 cm, noted in varicella (chickenpox), herpes zoster (shingles), herpes simplex type 1 and type 2
Secondary	Lesions altered by outside manipulation, treatment, natural course of disease	Crust: Raised lesion caused by dried serum and blood remnants, develops when vesicle ruptures

Table 6-3: Description of Primary Skin Lesions
Learn the language of dermatology.

Lesion size	Description	Example
<1 cm	Flat, nonpalpable discoloration (macule)	Freckle
	Solid elevation (papule)	Raised nevus
	Papule with indented center (umbilicated)	Molluscum contagiosum
	Vesicle-like lesion with purulent content (pustule)	Impetigo
>1 cm	Flat, nonpalpable area of skin discoloration, larger than macule (patch)	Vitiligo
	Raised lesion, same or different color from surrounding skin, can result from a coalescence of papules (plaque)	Psoriasis vulgaris
	Fluid-filled >1 cm (bulla)	2nd degree burn
Any size	Raised, encapsulated, fluid-filled lesion (cyst)	Intradermal cyst
	Circumscribed area of skin edema (wheal)	Hive (urticaria)
	Flat red-purple discoloration that does not blanch with pressure (purpura, petechiae when <1 cm)	Purpura, petechiae

Sources: Habif, T. (2011) Skin Disease, 3rd Edition, St. Louis, MO: Elsevier Health Sciences.

Barankin, B. (2006) Derm Notes: Clinical Dermatology Pocket Guide, Philadelphia, PA: F. A. Davis.

Habif, T. (2012) Dermatology DDxDeck, 2nd Edition, St. Louis, MO: Elsevier Health Sciences.

Table 6-4: Description of Secondary Skin Lesions

Lesion size	Description	Dermatologic term	Example
Any size	Usually linear, raised, often covered with crust	Excoriation	Scratch marks over a pruritic primary lesion
	Skin thickening usually found over pruritic or friction areas	Lichenification	Callus
	Raised superficial lesions that flake with ease	Scales	Dandruff
>1 cm	Loss of epidermis	Erosion	Area beneath an opened bulla or vesicle
	Loss of epidermis and dermis	Ulcer	Arterial ulcer, syphilitic chancre
	Narrow linear crack into epidermis, exposing dermis	Fissure	Athlete's foot

Table 6-5: Pulling Together the Concepts: Varicella (Chickenpox) vs. Zoster (Shingles)		
	Varicella (chickenpox)	**Zoster (shingles)**
At-risk population	Usually in nonimmune or unimmunized older child or young adult. Infants vulnerable since vaccine given at age 1 year	Typically in person age ≥50 years but possible in anyone at any age with history of varicella (chickenpox). Nearly all in USA age ≥40 years with history of varicella (chickenpox)
Transmission/ contagion risk	Transmitted person-to-person by direct contact, inhalation of aerosols from vesicular fluid of skin lesions of acute varicella, or aerosolized respiratory tract secretions	Varicella virus possibly transmitted person-to-person by direct contact, inhalation of aerosols from vesicular fluid of zoster lesions
Systemic presentation	Mildly to moderately systemically ill with myalgia, fever, often quite miserable with itch	Usually not systemically ill but quite miserable with pain, itch
Dermatologic manifestation	2–3 mm vesicles that start on trunk then appear on limbs 2–3 days later. Nonclustered lesions at a variety of stages, including crusts, with reasonably high rate of complication, including bacterial suprainfection of lesions	Vesicles typically in a unilateral dermatomal pattern, slowly resolving with crusting, usually accompanied with pain and/or severe itch. Complications include postherpetic neuralgia, ophthalmologic involvement, and superimposed bacterial infection.
Treatment	Antiviral medication such as acyclovir in early illness (within 24–48 h of eruption), particularly in higher-risk situations such as children with underlying health problems and most adults, helps minimize duration and severity of illness. Avoid aspirin therapy due to Reyes syndrome risk, and NSAIDs due to necrotizing fasciitis risk.	Antiviral medication such as high-dose acyclovir in early illness (within 72 h of eruption) helps minimize duration and severity of illness. Provide appropriate analgesia. Itch often a major issue, treat systemically and locally (ice pack, calamine lotion, avoid clothes rubbing on lesions, others).
Prevention	Providing immunization against varicella (Varivax®) provides approximately 80% lifetime immunity with 1st dose, approximately 99% immunity with 2nd dose.	Providing zoster vaccine (Zostavax®) to eligible patients significantly minimizes the risk of developing shingles.

Sources: http://www.cdc.gov/chickenpox/hcp/index.html,
http://www.cdc.gov/shingles/hcp/index.html

1. Match each dermatologic term with the description.

   A. Annular

   B. Scattered

   C. Confluent or coalescent

   D. Clustered

   E. Linear

Description	Dermatologic term
In streaks such as the typical phytodermatitis caused by exposure to plant oil (urushiol) contained in poison ivy, poison oak, poison sumac	Linear
Occurring in a group without pattern, such as the lesions seen in an outbreak of herpes simplex type 1 (HSV-1, "cold sore")	Clustered
Generalized over body without a specific pattern or distribution, as seen in a viral exanthem such as rubella or roseola	scattered
Multiple lesions blending together, such as the lesions seen in psoriasis vulgaris	Confluent or
In a ring, often seen in the characteristic "Bull's Eye" lesion seen in Lyme disease	Anular

2. A 60-year-old otherwise well man presents with a dermatologic condition. Which of the following conditions requires biopsy to confirm diagnosis?

   A. Scaling flesh-colored lesions in a cluster, ranging in size from 3–10 mm on the dorsal aspect of the hand, present for a number of months, without patient complaint.

   B. Well-demarcated round-to-oval erythematous coin-shaped plaques approximately 10 mm in diameter on the anterior aspects of the lower legs described as being intermittently itchy that has been present for a number of months.

   C. Painless ulcerated lesion approximately 1.5 cm over the sternum that has been present for a number of weeks.

   D. Oval plaque that is approximately 5 cm in diameter with a central wrinkled salmon-colored area and a dark red peripheral zone on the anterior trunk that has been present for 5 days without patient complaint.

Table 6-6: Precancerous Skin Lesions

Condition	Location and description	Comment
Actinic keratoses (AK)	Location: Predominantly on sun-exposed skin. Size ranges from microscopic to several centimeters in diameter. Description: On skin surface, red or brown, scaly, often tender but usually minimally symptomatic. Occasionally flesh-colored, more easily felt by running a finger over the affected area than seen. Clinical diagnosis, biopsy usually not required.	Most common precancerous skin lesion though possibly represents early-stage squamous cell carcinoma. Lesions can remain unchanged, spontaneously resolve, or progress to invasive squamous cell carcinoma. Intervention • Pharmacotherapy options: Topical 5-fluorouracil (5-FU), 5% imiquimod cream, topical diclofenac gel, or photodynamic therapy (PDT) with topical delta-aminolevulinic acid • Tissue destruction options: Cryosurgery (liquid nitrogen), medical-grade laser resurfacing or chemical peel

Sources: Habif, T. (2012) Dermatology DDxDeck, 2nd Edition, St. Louis, MO: Elsevier Health Sciences.

Habif, T. (2011) Skin Disease, 3rd Edition, St. Louis, MO: Elsevier Health Sciences.

Table 6-7: Basal Cell Carcinoma vs. Squamous Cell Carcinoma
Biopsy/excision to confirm diagnosis
Additional assessment, intervention based on results

BCC	SCC
More common	Less common
Sun-exposed areas	Sun-exposed areas
Arises *de novo*	Can arise from actinic keratoses (AK) or *de novo*
Papule, nodule with or without central erosion	Red, conical hard lesions with or without ulceration
Pearly or waxy appearance, usually relatively distinct borders with or without telangiectasia	Less distinct borders
Metastatic risk low, significant tissue destruction risk without treatment	Metastatic risk greater (3–7%), also with significant tissue destruction risk without treatment Greatest metastatic risk=Lesion located on lip, oral cavity, genitalia

Table 6-8: Malignant Melanoma
ABCDE Sensitivity, Specificity with ≥2 features=100% Sensitive, 98% Specific
Biopsy/excision to confirm diagnosis
Additional assessment, intervention based on results

A	Asymmetric
B	Irregular borders
C	Color not uniform (shades of brown, black, red, blue, white)
D	Diameter (usually ≥6 mm)
E	Evolving (new) lesion or change in a longstanding lesion, particularly in a nevus (mole) or other pigmented lesion Elevated (not consistently present)

Source: Whited JD, Grichnick JM. Does the patient have a mole or melanoma? *JAMA.* 1998;279;696-701.

3. Match each treatment option with the relevant condition.

A. Permethrin lotion

B. Medium-potency topical corticosteroid

C. Imiquimod cream

D. Topical ketoconazole

E. Topical metronidazole

Condition	Treatment
Psoriasis vulgaris	B cortico.
Scabies	A Permethrin lotion
Verruca vulgaris	C imiquimod cream
Tinea pedis	D ketoconazole
Rosacea	E topical Metronidazole

4. Identify each condition with the most likely location.

A. Pityriasis rosea

B. Psoriasis vulgaris

C. Actinic keratosis

D. Scabies

E. Eczema

Location	Condition
Antecubital fossa	Eczema
Anterior surface of knees	Psoriasis vulgaris
Sun-exposed areas	Acthic keratosis
Over waistband area	Scabies
Usually preceded by herald patch on the trunk	Pityriasis rosea

5. Ana is a 22-year-old well woman who presents with a four-day history of an intense itch with skin lesions on hands and arms as well as her right cheek. She has used an over-the-counter hydrocortisone cream on the affected area with little effect, and denies any other symptoms or previous history of similar rash. Ana denies recent travel and exposure to new creams, soaps, or medications. She works as a landscaper. When considering a diagnosis of phytodermatitis due to exposure to urushiol (poison ivy, poison oak, poison sumac), you anticipate finding three of the following.

   A. Fever and generalized malaise

   B. Vesicles —

   C. Crusts —

   D. Fissures

   E. Most of the lesions in a linear pattern

6. When evaluating Ana, you note that approximately 20% total body surface area is affected. You consider treatment with:

   A. Topical application of a medium-potency corticosteroid cream.

   B. An oral antihistamine.

   C. A systemic corticosteroid.

   D. A topical antihistamine.

Table 6-9: Treatment of Poison Ivy (Urushiol-induced Contact Dermatitis) Topical vs. Systemic Therapy		
	Topical treatment	**Systemic treatment**
Extent of area affected	Optimal for localized acute contact dermatitis	Preferred when ≥20% of total body surface area is affected, severe rash (i.e., large number of blisters), or if rash impacts face, genitals, hands and/or rash impacts occupational function.
Types of treatment	Mid- or high-potency topical corticosteroids, such as triamcinolone (0.1%, Kenalog®, Aristocort®) or clobestasol (0.05%, Temovate®) For areas of thinner skin (e.g., flexural surfaces, eyelids, face, anogenital region), lower-potency corticosteroids recommended, such as desonide ointment (Desowen®) or consider oral therapy	Prednisone 0.5 to 1 mg/kg/day for 5–7 days (usually provides relief within 12–24 hours); typically significant patient response with this treatment, should be followed by 5–7 additional days with prednisone dose reduced by 50% to minimize risk of recurrence of skin lesion. Total recommended systemic corticosteroid therapy duration=10–14 days.
Considerations	Ointment preferred over cream (allows medication to contact skin longer); skin atrophy risk with higher-potency corticosteroid use	No additional taper needed with short-term (≤14 days) systemic corticosteroid use
Adjunctive therapies	Cool compresses to relieve symptoms; calamine lotion and colloidal oatmeal baths to help dry and soothe oozing lesions OTC analgesics to relieve pain Oral antihistamines typically helpful for management of pruritus	

Source: Usatine RP, Riojas M. Diagnosis and management of contact dermatitis. *Am Fam Physician*. 2010;82:249-55.

Table 6-10: Bacterial Skin Infections		
Condition	**Clinical presentation**	**Likely causative organism(s)**
Impetigo	Nonbullous impetigo- Erythematous macule that rapidly evolves into vesicle or pustule, ruptures, contents dry, leaving a crusted, honey-colored exudate. Bullous impetigo- Bulla contains clear, yellow fluid that turns cloudy, dark yellow. Bulla rupture easily, within 1–3 days, leaving a rim of scale around red, moist base, followed by a brown-lacquered or scalded-skin appearance	*Staphylococcus aureus, Streptococcus pyogenes* Nonbullous impetigo- Often able to be treated with topical antimicrobial such as mupirocin. Requires systemic antimicrobial therapy when extensive or if topical treatment fails. Bullous impetigo- Often requires systemic antimicrobial therapy due to extensive distribution.
Erysipelas	Infection of upper dermis, superficial lymphatics, usually includes heat, redness and discomfort in the region	*Streptococcus pyogenes* Requires systemic antimicrobial therapy.
Cellulitis	Infection of dermis and subcutaneous fat usually includes heat, redness and discomfort in the region.	*Streptococcus pyogenes,* less commonly *Staphylococcus aureus* (MSSA [methicillin-susceptible *S. aureus*], beta-lactamase–producing; MRSA [methicillin-resistant *S. aureus*], resistance via altered protein-binding sites). Requires systemic antimicrobial therapy.
Cutaneous abscess, furuncle, carbuncles	Skin infection involving a hair follicle and surrounding tissue, (usually includes heat, redness and discomfort in the region).	*Staphylococcus aureus* (MRSA, MSSA) Treatment variable according to clinical presentation.

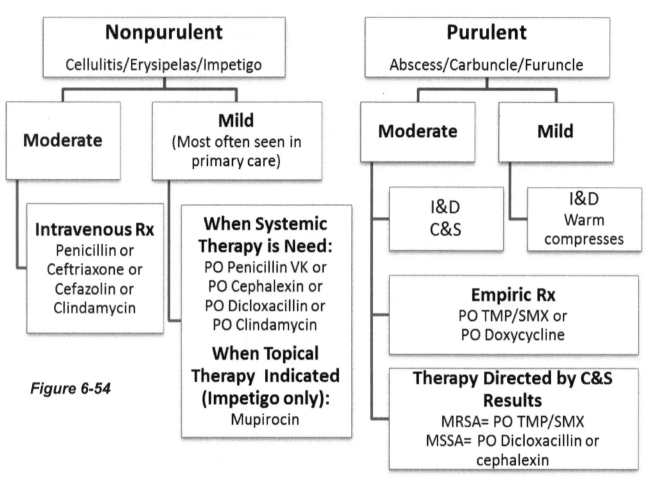

Figure 6-54

Source: Practice Guidelines for the Diagnosis and Management of Skin and Soft Tissue Infections: 2014 Update by the Infectious Diseases Society of America, available at http://cid.oxfordjournals.org/content/early/2014/06/14/cid.ciu296.full.pdf+html

7. True or false?
   (T/F) Across North America, brown recluse spider bites are the most common reason for new-onset ulcerating skin lesions.

Table 6-11: Brown Recluse Spider Bite
"Red, white, and blue" sign- Central blistering with surrounding gray to purple discoloration at bite site surrounded by ring of blanched skin surrounded by large area of redness
Treatment of brown recluse spider bite- Local debridement, elevation, loose immobilization. At time of bite, ice to limit venom spread helpful. Dapsone often prescribed with scant evidence of effectiveness.
Avoidance- Check before putting body part into area where spiders hide (footwear, boxes, other).

Source: http://emedicine.medscape.com/article/772295-overview

8. A 28-year-old woman who works in food service presents with a chief complaint of an on-the-job injury caused when her right forearm was accidently exposed to steam. Approximately 2% body surface area is involved. You assess the injury as a partial thickness (second degree) burn and describe the skin lesion as appearing:

A. Reddened easily blanched with gentle pressure.

B. Red, moist with peeling borders and scattered bulla.

C. Thickened, hypopigmented tissue.

D. Vesicular with hyperpigmentation.

Table 6-12: Types of Burns and Burn Classification	
Burn sources (mechanism of injury)	
Thermal	Caused by a heat source such as a hot item, steam, smoke, etc.
Chemical	Caused by a chemical agent such as an acid or alkali chemical substance.
Electrical	Caused by a form of electrical current such as an AC or DC current
Radiation	Caused by a form of radiation such as sun exposure or cancer treatments
Burn classification	
First degree	• **Superficial burns** (affect only the epidermis) • Appearance: Burn site is red, painful, dry, with no blisters • Causes: Sunburn, scald, flash flame • Treatment: Cold compresses, lotion or ointment, acetaminophen or ibuprofen
Second degree	• **Superficial partial thickness** (upper layers of papillary dermis) or **deep partial thickness** (deeper layers of dermis, including reticular dermis) • Appearance: Red, blistered, may be swollen and painful • Causes: Scalds, flash burns, chemicals • See below for table on management of partial thickness burns
Third degree	• **Full thickness** (epithelium, dermis, underlying fat) • Appearance: Can appear white or charred • Causes: Flame, hot surface, hot liquids, chemical, electric • Referral to burn specialty care advised.

Source: Lloyd ECO, et al. Outpatient burns: prevention and care. *Am Fam Phys.* 2012;85:25-32.

American Burn Association. Guidelines for the operation of burn centers. Available at: http://www.ameriburn.org/Chapter14.pdf

Calculating percentage of total body surface area burned (%TBSA)

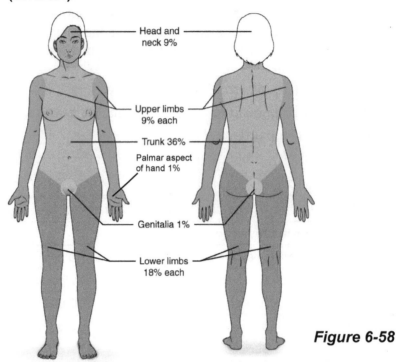

Head and neck 9%

Upper limbs 9% each

Trunk 36%

Palmar aspect of hand 1%

Genitalia 1%

Lower limbs 18% each

Figure 6-58

Source: https://commons.wikimedia.org/wiki/File:513_Degree_of_burns.jpg

Table 6-12 (cont.): Types of Burns	
Management of partial thickness burns **(>95% of burns can be managed in outpatient setting)**	
• Adequate pain control (e.g., acetaminophen or NSAIDs) • Thermal burns: run cool water for 15–20 minutes • Clean wound with sterile water • Leave blisters intact when possible. Debride large blisters with thin walls, that prevent movement of a joint, and/or likely to rupture • Use topical agents and dressing to keep area moist, provide pain control, promote healing, and prevent infection and desiccation	• <u>Topical antimicrobials</u>: Bacitracin, mafenide acetate (Sulfamylon®), mupirocin (Bactroban®), silver sulfadiazine (Silvadene®) • <u>Types of dressings</u>: Wound dressings (Aquacel® Ag, Biobrane®), hydrocolloids (DuoDERM®, Urgotul®), impregnated nonadherent gauze (Xeroform®, Vaseline® gauze), silicone (Mepitel®), and silver-impregnated dressing (Acticoat®) • Pain control 30 min before dressing changes • Ensure adequate hydration • Teach patient/family clean technique for wound care and dressing changes
When to refer to burn center (American Burn Association Criteria)	
• Patients with burns and concomitant trauma in whom burn injury poses greatest risk of morbidity and death • Children at hospitals without qualified personnel or equipment for the care of children • Patients who will require special social, emotional, or rehabilitative intervention • Patients with preexisting medical disorders that could complicate management, prolong recovery, or affect mortality	• Partial and full thickness burns that involve the face, hands, feet, genitalia, perineum, or major joints • Chemical burns • Electrical burns, including lightning injury • Inhalational injury • Partial-thickness burns on more than 10% of total body surface area • Third-degree (full-thickness) burns in any age group

Source: Lloyd ECO, et al. Outpatient burns: prevention and care. *Am Fam Phys.* 2012;85:25-32.

American Burn Association. Guidelines for the operation of burn centers. Available at: http://www.ameriburn.org/Chapter14.pdf

Table 6-13: Sun Safety Information	
Babies <6 months	Avoid sun exposure, dress infants in lightweight long pants, long-sleeved shirts, and brimmed hats that shade the neck to prevent sunburn.
	When adequate clothing and shade are not available, a minimal amount of sunscreen with ≥15 SPF (sun protection factor) can be applied to small areas, such as the infant's face and the back of the hands.
	If an infant gets sunburned, apply cold compresses to affected area.
Children ≥6 months, adults	The first and best line of defense against the sun is covering up. Hat with a three-inch brim or bill facing forward, sunglasses that block 99–100% of ultraviolet rays, cotton clothing with a tight weave
	Stay in shade whenever possible and limit sun exposure during the peak intensity hours (between 10 AM and 4 PM)
	On both sunny and cloudy days, use a sunscreen with an SPF ≥15 that protects against UVB and UVA rays.
	Apply enough sunscreen, about 1 oz (approx. 30 mL) per sitting for the older child and adult.
	Reapply sunscreen every two hours, or after swimming or sweating.
	Use extra caution near water, sand, and snow, as these reflect UV rays and can result in sunburn more quickly.

Source: American Academy of Pediatrics, Summer Safety Tips, available at www.aap.org/en-us/about-the-aap/aap-press-room/news-features-and-safety-tips/Pages/Summer-Safety-Tips.aspx

Bonus questions for this chapter available through your Fitzgerald Health learning portal at fhea.com/npexpert.

Resources for Additional Study

Books:

Barankin, B. (2006) <u>Derm Notes: Clinical Dermatology Pocket Guide</u>, Philadelphia, PA: F. A. Davis.

Fitzgerald, M. A. (2017) Skin Disorders, <u>Nurse Practitioner Certification Examination and Practice Preparation</u>, 5th Edition, Philadelphia, PA: F. A. Davis.

Habif, T. (2012) <u>Dermatology DDxDeck</u>, 2nd Edition, St. Louis, MO: Elsevier Health Sciences.

Habif, T. (2011) <u>Skin Disease</u>, 3rd Edition, St. Louis, MO: Elsevier Health Sciences.

Audio programs:

Czerkasij, V. <u>Atopic Dermatitis: The Latest Research and Treatment Paradigms</u>, North Andover, MA: Fitzgerald Health Education Associates.

Czerkasij, V. <u>Best Practices in Managing Patients with Skin Cancer</u>, North Andover, MA: Fitzgerald Health Education Associates.

Czerkasij, V. <u>The Changing Face of Acne and Rosacea</u>, North Andover, MA: Fitzgerald Health Education Associates.

Czerkasij, V. <u>Essentials of Diagnosis and Intervention in Dermatology</u>, North Andover, MA: Fitzgerald Health Education Associates.

Czerkasij, V. <u>The Golden Years: Understanding and Treating Skin in the Older Adult</u>, North Andover, MA: Fitzgerald Health Education Associates.

Czerkasij, V. <u>Help My Child: Topics, Diagnosis and Treatment of Common Pediatric Dermatologic Conditions</u>, North Andover, MA: Fitzgerald Health Education Associates.

Czerkasij, V. <u>Identifying Cutaneous Manifestations of Internal Disease</u>, North Andover, MA: Fitzgerald Health Education Associates.

Czerkasij, V. <u>Issues of Darkly Pigmented Skin</u>, North Andover, MA: Fitzgerald Health Education Associates.

Czerkasij, V. <u>Latest Advances in Dermatology</u>, North Andover, MA: Fitzgerald Health Education Associates.

Chapter 7: Thyroid Disorders

Key concept in thyroid disease: The thyroid produces two hormones, thyroxine (T_4) and triiodothyronine (T_3). These hormones act as cellular energy release catalysts and influence the function and health of every cell in the body.

Table 7-1: Hypothyroidism Reduced Cellular Energy Release All signs, symptoms reversible with treatment	
Affected area	**Change noted**
Skin	Thick, dry
Reflexes	"Hung up" patellar reflex, slow arc out, slower arc back, overall hyporeflexia
Mentation	"Can't make sense, thoughts too slow"
Weight change	Small gain (5–10 lb [2.25–4.5 kg]), largely fluid
Stool pattern	Constipation
Menstrual issue	Menorrhagia
Heat/cold tolerance	Easily chilled

Table 7-2: Hypothyroidism: Common Etiology	
Condition	**Common etiology**
Hashimoto thyroiditis	Autoimmune in origin
Post-radioactive iodine (RAI) treatment	S/P Graves' disease treatment, thyroid cancer treatment
Select medication use	Lithium, amiodarone, interferon, others

Table 7-3: Hyperthyroidism Excessive Cellular Energy Release All signs, symptoms reversible with treatment.	
Affected area	**Change noted**
Skin	Smooth, silky
Reflexes	Hyperreflexia
Mentation	"Can't make sense, mind racing"
Weight change	Loss (~10 lb [4.5 kg] average)
Stool pattern	Frequent, low volume, loose
Menstrual issue	Oligomenorrhea
Heat/cold tolerance	Heat intolerance

Notes:

Table 7-4: Hyperthyroidism: Common Etiology

Condition	Comment
Graves' disease	Autoimmune in nature. Multisystem presentation including exophthalmus, tachycardia, proximal muscle weakness, goiter
Toxic adenoma	Benign, metabolically active thyroid nodule
Thyroiditis	Viral or autoimmune, postpartum, drug-induced, often transient, usually accompanied by thyroid tenderness
Select medication use	Amiodarone (also hypothyroidism), interferon (also hypothyroidism), others

Table 7-5: Thyroid Test

Test	Evaluates	Comment
Thyroid-stimulating hormone (TSH) NL=0.4–4.0 mIU/L True population distribution=0.5–1.5 mIU/L range with M=1.18 mIU/L	Hypothalamic-pituitary-thyroid axis function, reflects anterior pituitary lobe's ability to detect amount of circulating free thyroxine	*Per American Thyroid Association, single most reliable test to diagnose all common forms of hypo- and hyperthyroidism, particularly in the ambulatory setting. Given TSH's high sensitivity and specificity, when TSH results are WNL, thyroid disease has been ruled out.*
Free T_4 (FT$_4$, free thyroxine) NL=10–27 pmol/L	Unbound, metabolically active portion of thyroxine	Follow-up test to confirm, support the diagnosis of hypo- or hyperthyroidism in the face of an abnormal TSH. About 0.025% of all T_4.
Thyroid peroxidase antibody (TPO Ab) NL<35 IU/mL	A test to help detect autoimmune thyroid disease	Measures an antibody against peroxidase, an enzyme held within the thyroid
Total T_4 (Total thyroxine) NL=4.5–12.0 mcg/dL (57.91–154.44 nmol/L) **Rarely indicated test**	Reflects the total of the protein-bound and free thyroxine	Often altered (increased or decreased) in the absence of thyroid disease but with the use of select medications (exogenous estrogen [HT, COC], methadone) and presence of clinical conditions, such as pregnancy, chronic hepatitis
Free T_3 NL=3.5–7.7 pmol/L (0.2–0.5 ng/dL) **Rarely indicated test**	Unbound, metabolically active portion of triiodothyronine (T_3) When compared to T_4, T_3 is about 4 × more metabolically active.	About 20% of circulating T_3 is from the thyroid, rest as a result of conversion of T_4 to T_3
Total T_3 NL=95–190 ng/dL (1.5–2.9 pmol/L) **Rarely indicated test**	Reflects the total of the protein-bound and free triiodothyronine	See comments on total T_4

Source: Medical Guidelines for Clinical Practice for the Evaluation and Treatment of Hyperthyroidism and Hypothyroidism, available at https://www.aace.com/files/hypo_hyper.pdf

Table 7-6: Thyroid Test Results	
Etiology, test results	**Intervention**

Untreated hypothyroidism
Inadequate thyroxine dose
Low thyroxine (FT_4)=High TSH
Example:
TSH=84 mIU/L ↑
  • NL=0.4–4.0 mIU/L
Free T_4=3 pmol/L ↓
  • NL=10–27 pmol/L
	•Calculating anticipated levothyroxine (Synthroid®, Levoxyl®, generic, a bioidentical hormone) dose, using ideal body weight in obesity, actual body weight in healthy weight, underweight
	  –1.6 mcg/kg/d in adults
	  –1.0 mcg/kg/d in elderly
	  –4.0 mcg/kg/d in children
	  –≥50% increase during pregnancy
	    •Increase levothyroxine dose by ≥33% as soon as pregnancy is confirmed.
	•Check TSH after approximately 8 weeks of therapeutic levothyroxine therapy. Checking sooner leads to errors in clinical decision-making. Most adults will tolerate starting on full dose. Consider titrating up dose over a 1- to 2-month time frame particularly in elder or presence of anxiety, then check TSH after reaching desired dose for time frame listed above.
	•Desiccated thyroid preparations (T_4/T_3 combination, porcine or bovine origin such as Armour® Thyroid, Nature-Throid®, Bio-Throid®, Westhroid®). Not recommended by AACE.
	  –1 grain=60–65 mg thyroid USP=100 mcg levothyroxine. Thyroid USP 60–120 mg/d for typical adult daily dose
	•If TSH too high during hypothyroidism treatment
	  –Dose too low or adherence issues or both
	  –Drug interaction
	    •Levothyroxine should be taken with water on an empty stomach, same time every day.
	    •Should not be taken within 2 hours of cation, such as calcium, iron, aluminum, magnesium, others
	•If TSH too low during hypothyroid treatment
	  –Excessive use or dose is too high or both

Untreated hyperthyroidism
High thyroxine (FT_4)=Low TSH
Example:
TSH<0.15 mIU/L ↓
  • NL=0.4–4.0 mIU/L
Free T_4=79 pmol/L ↑
  • NL=10–27 pmol/L
	At time of diagnosis
	–Beta-adrenergic antagonist with β_1-, β_2-blockade (propranolol, nadolol), if not contraindicated, to counteract tachycardia, tremor Hyperthyroidism treatment (usually in consultation with endocrinology)
	–Antithyroid medication, such as propylthiouracil (PTU), methimazole (Tapazole®). Both drugs carry acute hepatic failure warning.
	–Radioactive iodine (RAI) with end-result of thyroid ablation and hypothyroidism

Subclinical hypothyroidism
Elevated TSH with NL free T_4
Example:
TSH=8.9 mIU/L ↑
  • NL=0.4–4.0 mIU/L
Free T_4=15 pmol/L (NL)
  • NL=10–27 pmol
TPO Ab=76 IU/mL ↑
  • NL<35 IU/mL
	AACE guidelines recommend treatment of patients with TSH>5 mIU/L if:
	-The patient has a goiter or if thyroid antibodies are present.
	-The presence of symptoms compatible with hypothyroidism, infertility, pregnancy, or imminent pregnancy would also favor treatment.

Sources: American Association of Clinical Endocrinologists Subclinical hypothyroidism, available at https://www.aace.com/files/position-statements/subclinical.pdf
Medical Guidelines for Clinical Practice for the Evaluation and Treatment of Hyperthyroidism and Hypothyroidism, available at www.aace.com/files/hypo_hyper.pdf

1. Untreated hyperthyroidism or hypothyroidism or both?

   (Hyper/hypo) Dry skin

   (Hyper/hypo) Fine tremor

   (Hyper/hypo) Hypoactive deep tendon reflexes (DTR)

   (Hyper/hypo) Mental status change

   (Hyper/hypo) Menorrhagia

   (Hyper/hypo) Exophthalmos

2. You see a 38-year-old woman with hypothyroidism who is currently taking levothyroxine 75 mcg/d with excellent adherence, stating, "I take the medicine every morning on an empty stomach with a big glass of water." She is feeling well. Results of today's laboratory testing includes a TSH=4.5 mIU/mL. The next best step in her care is to:

   A. Continue on the same levothyroxine dose and obtain a repeat TSH in 1 year.

   B. Decrease the levothyroxine dose by 25 mcg/d and repeat a TSH in 1 month.

   C. Increase the levothyroxine dose by 25 mcg/d and repeat a TSH in 2 months.

   D. Provide counseling to take the medication with breakfast.

Primary Hypothyroidism Treatment Algorithm

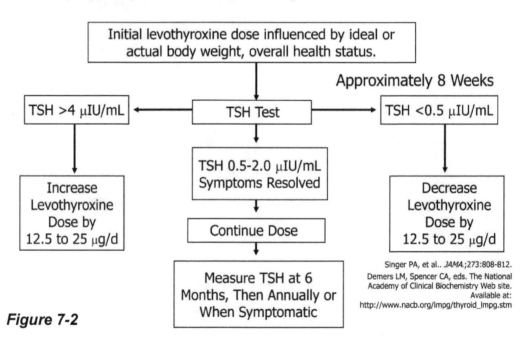

Figure 7-2

Singer PA, et al.. *JAMA*.;273:808-812.
Demers LM, Spencer CA, eds. The National
Academy of Clinical Biochemistry Web site.
Available at:
http://www.nacb.org/lmpg/thyroid_lmpg.stm

3. Mrs. Lange is a 79-year-old woman with a >20-year history of well-controlled hypertension and dyslipidemia, currently taking an ACE inhibitor, low-dose thiazide diuretic, and a statin. She presents today with a chief complaint of a 6-month history of progressive symptoms, including fatigue, difficulty initiating and maintaining sleep, increased difficulty with raising her arms above her head, and a sensation of "my heart not beating right, sometimes I feel like it's going to hop right out of my chest." She denies shortness of breath, chest pain, cough, or difficulty breathing when supine and admits to "losing weight without even trying." Cardiac examination reveals an irregularly irregular cardiac rhythm, without S_3, S_4, or murmur and no neck vein distention. Electrocardiogram is as shown.

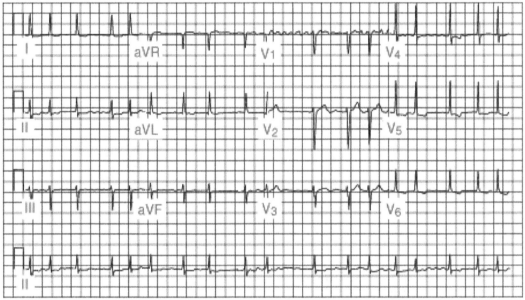

The result of Mrs. Lange's electrocardiogram is consistent with:

   A. Sinus tachycardia.

   B. Multifocal atrial tachycardia.

   C. First-degree heart block.

   D. Atrial fibrillation.

Figure 7-3

4. The remainder of her physical examination reveals flat affect, fine tremor, 3–4+ DTR response, mild proximal muscle weakness, symmetric thyroid enlargement without tenderness or mass and a 10-lb (4.5-kg) weight loss since her last visit 8 months ago. The remainder of Mrs. Lange's examination is at her baseline. Which of the following is the most likely diagnosis?

   A. Thyrotoxicosis

   B. Statin-induced myopathy

   C. Heart failure

   D. Hypothyroidism

5. Choose the two most important tests to help support Mrs. Lange's diagnosis.

    A. Serum creatine kinase

    B. Serum electrolytes

    C. Serum thyroid stimulating hormone

    D. B-type natriuretic peptide

    E. Free thyroxine (FT$_4$)

Table 7-7: Evaluation of a Solitary Thyroid Nodule	
What is a thyroid nodule?	Palpable thyroid mass, not a term specific to any diagnosis, typically >1 cm in diameter.
What is the risk of a palpable thyroid nodule being a malignant lesion?	Presentation of benign and malignant thyroid lesions typically the same. Risk that any thyroid nodule is malignant=about 5%.
What are the findings most consistent with a malignant thyroid nodule?	History of head or neck irradiation Size larger than 4 cm Firmness, nontender on palpation Relatively fixed position (nonmobile) Persistent nontender cervical lymphadenopathy Dysphonia Hemoptysis

Source: https://www.aace.com/files/thyroid-guidelines.pdf

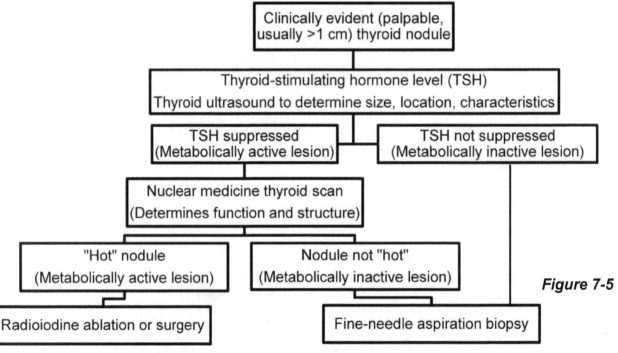

Figure 7-5

6. One of the most common causes of asymptomatic hypercalcemia in an otherwise well adult is:

    A. Excessive use of calcium supplements.

    B. Primary hyperparathyroidism.

    C. Renal insufficiency.

    D. Intestinal malabsorption.

Table 7-8: Primary and Secondary Hyperparathyroidism

Disease	Etiology	Clinical presentation and diagnosis	Intervention
Primary hyperparathyroidism	Elevated level of parathyroid hormone (PTH). (PTH role=Appropriate body calcium levels) Excess PTH production= Hypercalcemia Etiology= Overactivity of ≥1 of four parathyroid glands, by enlargement (hyperplasia), adenoma (benign), or malignant tumor.	Variable, characterized by "moans, groans, stones, and bones…with psychic overtones." Common signs and symptoms include loss of energy, poor concentration and/or memory, depression, osteoporosis/ osteopenia, insomnia, GERD, decreased libido, hair loss, and bone and joint aches. Other signs include kidney stones, hypertension, arrhythmias, atrial fibrillation, liver dysfunction, and abnormal blood protein levels. Diagnosis typically by elevated serum calcium without other obvious cause, confirmed elevated parathyroid hormone. Additional test includes 24-h urine calcium to determine disease severity. Special consultation advised	• Surgery to remove problematic gland(s) or lesion. Approximately 95% curative. • Cinacalcet (Sensipar®, calcimimetic), use to treat hyperparathyroidism in chronic kidney disease or parathyroid cancer. Use results in less parathyroid hormone release. • To prevent bone loss, bisphosphonates and/or hormone replacement therapy (for post-menopausal women) should be considered. • In mild or asymptomatic cases, avoid use of thiazide diuretics and lithium, as these can elevate levels of both PTH and calcium, thus exacerbating the condition. If these medications are being taken, PTH and calcium levels should be reassessed after a medication-free period to confirm the diagnosis.
Secondary hyperparathyroidism	Result of another condition that lowers serum calcium levels, therefore causing the parathyroid glands to overproduce PTH. Causes include severe calcium or vitamin D deficiency and/or chronic kidney disease	Presentation is similar as primary hyperparathyroidism. Diagnosis most commonly made with findings of low-normal serum calcium, elevated PTH, and presence of severe renal dysfunction (often on dialysis and/or significant kidney problems over several years).	• Vitamin D analogues, phosphate binders, and calcimimetics (cinacalcet [Sensipar®]) • Surgery only considered if medical therapy fails • Ensure adequate amount of calcium and vitamin D intake. • See comment above on use of lithium or thiazide diuretics

Sources: Michels TC, Kelly KM. Parathyroid disorders. *Am Fam Physician*. 2013;88:249-57.
Kim L. Hyperparathyroidism. Medscape, July 2016. Available at:
http://emedicine.medscape.com/article/127351-overview#a3.
Norman Parathyroid Center. Symptoms of hyperparathyroidism. Available at:
http://parathyroid.com/parathyroid-symptoms.htm.

Table 7-9: Screening for Thyroid Dysfunction: Recommendations for Asymptomatic Adults	
Organization	**Recommendation**
American Thyroid Association	Women and men >35 years of age should be screened every 5 years.
American Association of Clinical Endocrinologists	Older patients, especially women, should be screened periodically.
American Academy of Family Physicians	Patients age 60 or older should be screened.
American College of Physicians	Women age 50 or older with an incidental finding suggestive of symptomatic thyroid disease should be evaluated
US Preventive Services Task Force	Evidence is insufficient to recommend for or against routine screening for thyroid disease in adults.

Source: Garber JR, Cobin RH, Gharib H, et al. Clinical Practice Guidelines for Hypothyroidism in Adults: Cosponsored by the American Association of Clinical Endocrinologists and the American Thyroid Association (2012). Available at http://journals.aace.com/doi/abs/10.4158/EP12280.GL

Bonus questions for this chapter available through your Fitzgerald Health learning portal at fhea.com/npexpert.

Resources for Additional Study

Books:

Desai, S. (2009) <u>Clinician's Guide to Laboratory Medicine: Pocket</u>, Houston, TX: MD2B.

Ferri, F. (2014) <u>Ferri's Best Test: A Practical Guide to Clinical Laboratory Medicine and Diagnostic Imaging</u>, 3rd Edition, St. Louis, MO: Elsevier Health Sciences.

Fitzgerald, M. A. (2017) Endocrine Disorders, <u>Nurse Practitioner Certification Examination and Practice Preparation</u>, 5th Edition, Philadelphia, PA: F.A. Davis.

Audio programs:

Fitzgerald, M. A. <u>Laboratory Data Interpretation: A Case Study Approach</u>, North Andover, MA: Fitzgerald Health Education Associates.

CD-ROM programs:

Miller, S. K. <u>12-Lead ECG Interpretation: A Primary Care Perspective</u>, North Andover, MA: Fitzgerald Health Education Associates.

Miller, S. K. <u>Beyond the Basics in 12-Lead ECG Interpretation</u>, North Andover, MA: Fitzgerald Health Education Associates.

Miller, S. K. <u>Cardiac Rhythms: The Clinician's Approach to Accurate Interpretation</u>, North Andover, MA: Fitzgerald Health Education Associates.

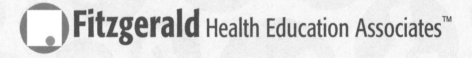
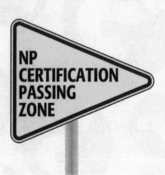

Chapter 8: Differential Diagnosis and Treatment of Headache

Table 8-1: Primary vs. Secondary Headache	
Primary headache	**Secondary headache**
Not associated with other diseases, likely complex interplay of genetic, developmental, and environmental risk factors	Associated with or caused by other conditions, generally will not resolve until the specific cause is diagnosed and addressed
Migraine, tension-type, cluster	Tumor, intracranial bleeding, increased intracranial pressure, use of select medications (such as nitrates), meningitis, accelerated hypertension, giant cell arteritis, viremia, others

Table 8-2: Consider diagnosis other than primary headache if headache "red flags" present. SNOOP mnemonic	
Presence of **s**ystemic symptoms, **s**econdary headache risk factors	Systemic symptoms, including fever, unintended weight loss, others
	Secondary headache risk factors, including HIV, malignancy, pregnancy, anticoagulation, hypertension, others
Neurologic signs, symptoms	Any newly-acquired neurological finding, including confusion, impaired alertness or consciousness, nuchal rigidity, hypertension, papilledema, cranial nerve dysfunction, abnormal motor function, others
Onset	Sudden, abrupt, or split-second, the "thunderclap" headache is suggestive of subarachnoid hemorrhage.
	Onset of headache with exertion, sexual activity, coughing, and sneezing is suggestive of increased intracranial pressure.
Onset (age at onset of headache)	Older (>50 years) and younger (<5 years)
	Serious-origin secondary headache is more likely to be found in individuals at either end of the lifespan.
Previous headache history	Primary HA pattern usually established in youth-young adult years. More worrisome if first headache report in adult ≥30 years.
	New onset of different headache, change in attack frequency, severity or clinical features, including progressive headache without headache-free period

Sources: Dodick DW. *Adv Stud Med*. 2003;3:87-92.
Merck Manual: Approach to the Patient with Headache, available at
www.merckmanuals.com/professional/neurologic_disorders/headache/approach_to_the_p
atient_with_headache.html

Table 8-3: Primary Headache: Clinical Presentation and Diagnosis

Headache type	Headache characteristics
Tension-type headache	Lasts 30 min to 7 d (usually 1–24 h) with ≥2 of the following characteristics: • Pressing, nonpulsatile pain • Mild to moderate in intensity • Usually bilateral location • Notation of 0–1 of the following (>1 suggests migraine) ○ Nausea, photophobia, or phonophobia Female:Male ratio=5:4
Migraine without aura	Lasts 4 to 72 h with ≥2 of the following characteristics: • Usually unilateral location, though occasionally bilateral • Pulsating quality, moderate to severe in intensity • Aggravation by normal activity, such as walking, or causes avoidance of these activities During headache, notation of ≥1 of the following characteristics: • Nausea and/or vomiting, photophobia, phonophobia Female:Male ratio=3:1 Positive family history in 70–90%
Migraine with aura	Migraine-type HA occurs with or after aura. • Focal dysfunction of cerebral cortex or brain stem causes ≥1 aura symptoms developing over 4 min, or ≥2 sx occurs in succession. • Symptoms can include feeling of dread or anxiety, unusual fatigue, nervousness, or excitement, GI upset, visual or olfactory alteration. • No aura symptom should last >1 h. If this occurs, an alternate diagnosis should be considered. Positive family history in 70–90%
Cluster headache	Tendency of headache to occur daily in groups or clusters, hence the name cluster headache Clusters usually last several weeks to months, then disappear for months to years. • Usually occurs at characteristic times of year, such as vernal and autumnal equinox with 1–8 episodes/d, at the same time of day. Common time is ~1 h into sleep, hence the term "alarm clock" headache, as the pain awakens the person. • Headache is often located behind 1 eye with a steady, intense ("hot poker in the eye") sensation, severe pain in a crescendo pattern lasting 15 min to 3 h, with most in the range of 30–45 minutes. Pain intensity has helped earn the condition the term, "suicide headache." Most often with ipsilateral autonomic signs, such as lacrimation, conjunctival injection, ptosis, and nasal stuffiness Female:Male ratio=~1:3 to 1:8 (depending on information source) Family history of cluster headache present in ~20%

Sources: National Headache Foundation: Advances in Preventive Therapies for Migraine;
National Headache Foundation: Comorbidities of Migraine; Migraine and Associated
Symptoms: Meeting the Treatment Challenge, available at www.headaches.org

Tension-type? Migraine? Both? Cluster?	
Pattern and patient description typical of which primary headache?	**Headache type**
Figure 8-1 "During a headache, I have constant pressure and pain on both sides of my head."	Tense
Figure 8-2 "During a headache, I have a throbbing feeling on one side of my head that is worse above my eye and at the base of my skull."	Migraine.
Figure 8-3 "During a headache, I have really strong constant pain behind one eye along with runny nose and watery eyes."	

Table 8-4: Primary Headache Treatment Options

Important terms:
Abortive or acute therapies- Used to control headache symptoms, best effect when taken at headache onset
Prophylactic or preventing therapies- Used to minimize risk of headache

Headache therapy	Intervention	Comment
Lifestyle modification	Recognize and avoid triggers (chocolate, alcohol, certain cheeses, monosodium glutamate [MSG], artificial sweeteners, perfume, stress, too much or too little sleep, altered routine, hunger, others). Encourage regular exercise, attend to posture at workstation as appropriate, use tinted lens to minimize glare and bright lights.	Highly effective and infrequently used
Analgesics	NSAIDs, acetaminophen, others. Best effect if taken at headache onset.	Limit use to 2 treatment-days per week to avoid analgesic rebound headache. Use with triptan therapy to enhance headache relief.
Migraine-specific medications	Triptans (selective serotonin receptor agonists, [sumatriptan, almotriptan, rizatriptan, others]), select ergot derivatives (dihydroergotamine [Migranal®], available as nasal spray or injection). Best effect if taken at headache onset.	Caution about use in pregnancy, cardiovascular disease, uncontrolled HTN due to potential vascular effect Helpful in tension-type headache that does not respond to analgesic therapy Also used in treatment of cluster headache, as is high-flow oxygen
Prophylactic (prevention) medications	Best evidence for migraine prophylaxis • Beta blockers- Metoprolol, propranolol • Tricyclic antidepressants- Amitriptyline, nortriptyline • Antiepileptic drugs (AEDs)- Divalproex sodium, sodium valproate, topiramate • Nutritional supplements: Butterbur, feverfew, coenzyme Q10, magnesium, and riboflavin • Lithium (specific to cluster headache) Calcium channel blockers, including verapamil, considered ineffective, not recommended.	Indication for prophylaxis (controller therapy), any or all of the following: Use of any product more than 3 times per week, ≥2 migraines per month that produce disabling symptoms ≥3 days, poor symptom relief from various abortive therapies, presence of select concomitant health condition, including hypertension, hemiplegic or basilar migraine. Goal of prophylaxis (controller therapy): Reduce headache frequency and severity; allow headache medications to be more effective in controlling headache symptoms.
Rescue therapy	Opioids, antiemetics, short course of systemic corticosteroids	When standard therapy ineffective or with severe or specific symptoms

Sources: Silberstein SD, Holland S, Freitag F, et al. Evidence-based guideline update: pharmacologic treatment for episodic migraine prevention in adults. Report of the Quality Standards Subcommittee of the American Academy of Neurology and the American Headache Society. *Neurology.* 2012;78:1337-1345.
National Headache Foundation: Comorbidities of Migraine; Migraine and Associated Symptoms: Meeting the Treatment Challenge, available at www.headaches.org

1. Katie is a 33-year-old woman who reports a 10-year history of unilateral, pulsing headache that lasts about 6–10 hours, occurring 3–4 times per month. The headache is typically preceded by a gradual onset of paresthesia affecting the ipsilateral face and arm, which lasts about 20 minutes. She reports severe photophobia and phonophobia as well as left-sided cephalgia during the 6–10 h headache duration. She states the headaches appear randomly. As a result of her headaches, Katie typically needs to either call in sick or leave work early at least once a month due to headache. Katie has used OTC medications with partial relief of pain but continued photo- and phonophobia. She is currently headache-free and neurological exam is within normal limits. Katie's presentation is consistent with:

    A. Migraine with aura.

    B. Tension-type headache.

    C. Cluster headache.

    D. Intracranial lesion.

2. Katie asks if she needs "any tests to see what causes my headaches." You respond that she should:

    A. Have head CT conducted.

    B. Keep a headache diary for the next month.

    C. Be promptly referred to a neurologist.

    D. Have head MRI conducted.

Table 8-5: Referral to Specialist is Warranted When the Patient:
Requires a healthcare service that the NP cannot provide or is beyond the scope of the NP's practice.   o   Example: Referring a patient who needs a cholecystectomy to a surgeon
Likely has a diagnosis that needs to be supported or clarified by a specialist.   o   Examples: Referring a patient with suspected immunologic condition, such as rheumatoid arthritis or systemic lupus erythematosus, to a rheumatology specialist
Has a diagnosed complex health condition for which input into ongoing care from a specialist is warranted.   o   Example: Referring a patient with significant cardiovascular disease, such as heart failure or angina pectoris, to a cardiology specialist
Fails to respond to standard, evidence-based care.   o   Examples: Referring a patient with chronic low back pain who has failed to respond to standard therapies to pain management

Source: The Fitzgerald Health Education Associates, Nurse Practitioner Certification Exam Review and Advanced Practice Update Faculty.

Table 8-6: Head MRI vs. CT: When neuroimaging in headache is indicated	
Neuroimaging usually not warranted in any primary headache type but usually indicated in secondary headaches.	
Imaging modality	**Capable of revealing**
CT without contrast (Most common test performed in acute severe headache with abnormality on neurological examination when neuroimaging indicated)	Acute or chronic hemorrhage, regardless of etiology
	Stroke
CT with contrast	Tumor, abscess
MRI	Tumor

Source: Evidence-Based Guidelines in the Primary Care Setting: Neuroimaging in Patients with Nonacute Headache, available at
http://tools.aan.com/professionals/practice/pdfs/gl0088.pdf

3. Given Katie's clinical presentation, you prescribe which of the following. More than 1 can apply.

   A. An oral triptan

   B. Migraine prophylactic therapy

   C. An oral NSAID

   D. A short course of a systemic corticosteroid

4. Katie requests advice on family planning. She has not been pregnant in the past. Given her history, which of the following is the least desirable contraceptive form for Katie?

   A. Levonorgestrel IUD (Skyla®, Lilleta®, Mirena®)

   B. Copper IUD (ParaGard®)

   C. Combined estrogen-progestin oral contraceptive

   D. A progestin-only implant (Nexplanon®)

5. When considering evidence-based practice (EBP) recommendations for the use of prophylactic migraine treatment, which of the following is the preferred agent?

   A. Propranolol

   B. Ergotamine

   C. Rizatriptan

   D. Verapamil

6. Which of the following represents the best choice of abortive migraine therapy for a 55-year-old woman with poorly-controlled hypertension?

   A. Verapamil

   B. Ergotamine

   C. Ibuprofen

   D. Almotriptan

7. According to the EBP recommendations, nutraceutical options for the prevention of recurrent migraine include the use of all of the following except:

   A. Butterbur.

   B. Feverfew.

   C. Magnesium.

   D. Vitamin C.

8. Mrs. Jensen is an 82-year-old woman with generalized osteoarthritis and systolic hypertension who presents with a 3-day history of right-sided headache with accompanying right-sided jaw pain on chewing. OTC analgesics have provided little relief. She states she is eating little due to the pain on chewing but is taking liquids without difficulty. Mrs. Jensen reports, "I can hardly wash my hair, my scalp is so sore." Physical examination reveals the following: BP=168/88 mm Hg bilateral, P=88 regular, RR=18, alert, appears uncomfortable with poorly-groomed hair on the right only, PERLA, cranial nerve function II–XII intact, remaining neurological exam WNL, carotid upstroke within normal limits without bruit. There is a tender, palpable, pulseless structure in the right temple area. Mrs. Jensen's clinical presentation is most consistent with:

   A. Postherpetic neuralgia.

   B. Transiet ischemic attack.

   C. Giant cell arteritis.

   D. Acute venous occlusion.

9. Which of the following represents the best choice of initial test to support Mrs. Jensen's presumptive diagnosis?

   A. Erythrocyte sedimentation rate

   B. Enhanced contrast brain MRI

   C. Head CT without contrast

   D. Arterial biopsy

10. As you develop a treatment plan for Mrs. Jensen, you consider that likely:

    A. NSAIDs will be helpful.

    B. Reducing her blood pressure is important.

    C. Long-term, high-dose systemic corticosteroid therapy will be needed.

    D. Opioid use is contraindicated.

11. Which of the following is a potential serious complication of Mrs. Jensen's presumptive diagnosis?

    A. Hemiparesis

    B. Arthritis

    C. Blindness

    D. Anterior uveitis

Table 8-7: Giant Cell Arteritis		
Etiology	**Clinical presentation and diagnosis**	**Intervention**
Autoimmune vasculitis that affects medium- and large-sized vessels as well as the temporal artery. Inflammation and swelling of the arteries leads to decreased blood flow and its associated symptoms. Disease occurs most commonly in individuals 50 to 85 years old, more common in females	Tender or nodular pulseless vessel (usually the temporal artery) accompanied by severe unilateral headache. Approximately 50% will experience visual impairment, including transient visual blurring, diplopia, eye pain, or sudden loss of vision. CRP and ESR are usually markedly elevated; usually first test done with high index of suspicion. Definitive diagnosis involves superficial temporal artery biopsy. Color duplex ultrasonography can be used as an alternative or complement to biopsy.	Treatment is aimed to reduce pain and minimize risk of blindness. Treatment includes high-dose systemic corticosteroid therapy (1–2 mg/kg per day prednisone until disease is stabilized) followed by careful reduction in the dose and continued for 6 months to 2 years. Aspirin can be used to reduce risk of stroke. GI cytoprotection (e.g., PPI or misoprostol) and bone protection (e.g., bisphosphonate) should be provided to minimize adverse effects of long-term corticosteroid therapy.

Sources: Fitzgerald, M. A. (2017) <u>Nurse Practitioner Certification Examination and Practice Preparation</u>, 5th Edition, Philadelphia, PA: F. A. Davis.

Seetharaman M. Giant cell arteritis (temporal arteritis). Available at: http://emedicine.medscape.com/article/332483-overview

Table 8-8: Potential Dietary Triggers Influencing the Onset or Severity of Migraine or Other Primary Headache Symptoms

Patients with headache should be advised to avoid eating the following. With certain foods, small amounts eaten infrequently will be tolerated.

- Sour cream
- Ripened cheeses (cheddar, Stilton, Brie, Camembert)
- Sausage, bologna, salami, pepperoni, summer sausage, hot dogs
- Pizza
- Chicken liver, pâté
- Herring (pickled or dried)
- Any pickled, fermented, or marinated food
- MSG (found in soy sauce, meat tenderizers, seasoned salt)
- Freshly baked yeast products, sourdough bread
- Chocolate
- Nuts or nut butters including peanut butter
- Broad beans, lima beans, fava beans, snow peas
- Onions
- Figs, raisins, papayas, avocados, red plums
- Citrus fruits
- Bananas
- Caffeinated beverages (tea, coffee, cola, "energy" drinks, etc.)
- Alcoholic beverages (wine, beer, whiskey, etc.)
- Aspartame/phenylalanine-containing foods or beverages

Source: Diagnosis and treatment of primary headache in adults, available at
http://www.guideline.gov/content.aspx?id=47060

Table 8-9: Potential Lifestyle Triggers Influencing the Onset or Severity of Migraine or Other Primary Headache Symptoms

Patients with migraine or other primary headache should be advised that these issues can be a headache trigger. Avoidance when possible is an important part of migraine care. In general, people with primary headache have less headache-related issues when maintaining a regular schedule of adequate sleep, nutrition, hydration and exercise.

- Menses, ovulation, or pregnancy
- Illness of any kind
- Intense or strenuous activity/exercise, particularly in a normally sedentary person
- Altered sleep patterns: Too much, too little, jet lag, others
- Altered eating pattern: Fasting, missing meals
- Bright or flickering lights
- Excessive or repetitive noises
- Odors, fragrances, tobacco smoke
- Weather, seasonal changes
- High altitudes
- Medications including SSRI, SNRI, other mental health medications, analgesic overuse, hormonal contraception (progestin with or without estrogen), postmenopausal hormone therapy
- Stress or stress letdown

Source: Diagnosis and treatment of primary headache in adults, available at
http://www.guideline.gov/content.aspx?id=47060

Bonus questions for this chapter available through your Fitzgerald Health learning portal at fhea.com/npexpert.

Resources for Additional Study

Audio programs:

Fitzgerald, M. A. <u>Laboratory Data Interpretation: A Case Study Approach</u>, North Andover, MA: Fitzgerald Health Education Associates.

Fitzgerald, M. A. <u>Migraine and Tension Headache: The Latest Treatment Options</u>, North Andover, MA: Fitzgerald Health Education Associates.

Miller, S. K. <u>Prescribing for the Relief of Symptoms Update</u>, North Andover, MA: Fitzgerald Health Education Associates.

Video programs:

Wright, W. L. <u>Expert Exam: The Primary Care Neurologic Exam</u>, North Andover, MA: Fitzgerald Health Education Associates.

Chapter 9: Evaluation and Intervention in Select Gastrointestinal and Hepatic Disorders

Table 9-1: Diagnosis and Management of Gastroesophageal Reflux Disease (GERD)
Establishing the diagnosis of GERD
A presumptive diagnosis of GERD can be established in the setting of typical symptoms of heartburn and regurgitation. Diagnostics (upper endoscopy, barium radiograph, *H. pylori* testing) should not be performed as part of GERD evaluation.
Endoscopy is recommended in the presence of alarming findings (dysphagia [difficulty swallowing], odynophagia [painful swallowing], unintended weight loss, hematemesis [vomiting blood], melena [black or bloody stools], chest pain, or choking) and for screening of patients at high risk for complications.
Management of GERD
Empiric therapy with a proton pump inhibitor (PPI) is recommended with the presumptive GERD diagnosis. PPI therapy should be initiated at once-a-day dosing, before the first meal of the day for maximum pH control.
Protracted PPI use is associated with vitamin B_{12}, calcium, magnesium, iron malabsorption and possible increased fracture and *Clostridium difficile*-associated diarrhea risk. Patients who do not respond to PPIs should be referred for evaluation.
Weight loss is recommended for GERD patients who are overweight or obese. Head-of-bed elevation and avoidance of meals 2–3 h before bedtime should be recommended for patients with nocturnal GERD.
Foods that are known to trigger symptoms should be eliminated or minimized. Routine global elimination of food that can trigger reflux (including chocolate, caffeine, alcohol, acidic foods) is not recommended in the treatment of GERD.

Source: American College of Gastroenterology: Diagnosis and Management of Gastroesophageal Reflux Disease, available at http://gi.org/guideline/diagnosis-and-managemen-of-gastroesophageal-reflux-disease

1. Which of the following is unlikely to be reported by Mr. Kane, a 45-year-old man with a BMI=41 kg/m^2 who presents with typical GERD symptoms?

    A. Unintended weight loss

    B. Hoarseness

    C. A recurrent cough

    D. Chronic pharyngitis

2. Mr. Lam, a 78-year-old man with longstanding GERD, presents with a 1-month history of "feeling like the food gets stuck way down in my throat." This sensation occurs with meats and other solid food types and less likely with softer or liquid foods. He denies nausea, vomiting, constipation, diarrhea, aspiration, or melena. His physical examination is unremarkable. A hemogram today reveals a microcytic hypochromic anemia with an elevated RDW. The most likely etiology of this anemia is:

    A. Anemia of chronic disease.

    B. Vitamin B_{12} deficiency.

    C. Iron deficiency.

    D. Acute blood loss.

3. All of the following diagnostic studies are available as part of Mr. Lam's evaluation. Rank from 1 (most helpful) to 3 (least helpful) as these tests pertain to the evaluation of Mr. Lam's symptoms.

_②_ Barium swallow

_①_ Upper endoscopy

_③_ Abdominal ultrasound

4. When choosing pharmacologic intervention to prevent recurrence of duodenal ulcer, you prescribe:

A. A proton pump inhibitor.

B. Timed antacid use.

C. Antimicrobial therapy.

D. A H_2-receptor antagonist.

Table 9-2: WBC Cell Line (Total WBC [TWBC] = 6,000–10,000/mm^3 in health)

Leukocytosis (WBC>10,000/mm^3) = Anticipated response in significant bacterial infection such as appendicitis, pyelonephritis, bacterial pneumonia, noninfectious reasons such as stress, pain, environmental extremes.

Mnemonic to help recall cell lines and order of reporting	WBC cell line	Point of action	In health, % of differential	When cell line elevated
Nobody	Neutrophil (AKA poly or segs) Bands–Young neutrophil form	Bacteria	~60%	Neutrophilia
Likes	Lymphocyte	Virus	~30%	Lymphocytosis
My	Monocyte	Debris	~6%	Monocytosis
Educational	Eosinophil	Allergens, parasites (worms, wheezes, and weird diseases)	~3%	Eosinophilia
Background	Basophil	Anaphylaxis, not fully understood	~1%	Basophilia

Table 9-3: Most likely with WBC response in serious bacterial infection? In significant viral infection?

Case A	Case B
TWBC: 5,500/mm^3 • Neutrophils (polys, segs): 40% • Bands: 3% • Lymphs: 55% w/reactive forms	TWBC: 16,500/mm^3 • Neutrophils (polys, segs): 71% w/toxic granulation • Bands: 6% • Lymphs: 20%

5. Anticipated clinical findings in acute appendicitis for Jordan, an otherwise well 24-year-old man with a BMI=32 kg/m^2 include all of the following except:

   A. Leukocytosis with neutrophilia and bandemia.

   B. Positive obturator and psoas signs.

   C. A 2-hour history of sudden onset of vomiting and generalized abdominal pain accompanied by fever.

   D. A 12-hour history of epigastric discomfort and anorexia that gradually shifts to nausea and right lower quadrant abdominal pain.

6. The most helpful imaging study in the evaluation of appendicitis for Jordan is an abdominal:

   A. Flat plate.

   B. CT with contrast.

   C. MRI.

   D. Radionuclide scan.

7. Of the following imaging studies, place in rank order from greatest to least amount of ionizing radiation burden to the patient.

   ___3___ Abdominal ultrasound

   ___1___ Abdominal CT

   ___2___ Abdominal flat plate

8. Match each clinical presentation with one of the following conditions.

A. Erosive gastritis

B. Acute pancreatitis

C. Duodenal ulcer

D. Cholecystitis

E. Diverticulitis

Clinical presentation	Condition
A 45-year-old man who drinks 8–10 beers/day with a 12-hour history of acute-onset epigastric pain radiating into the back with bloating, nausea, vomiting Objective: Epigastric tenderness, hypoactive bowel sounds, abdomen distended and hypertympanic. Laboratory evaluation reveals elevated lipase and amylase.	B
A 64-year-old woman with a 3-day history of intermittent left lower quadrant (LLQ) abdominal pain accompanied by fever, cramping, nausea, and 4–5 loose stools per day Objective: Abdomen soft, +bowel sounds, tenderness to LLQ abdominal palpation, negative Blumberg's sign. Laboratory evaluation reveals leukocytosis with neutrophilia.	E
A 34-year-old man w/3-month history of intermittent upper abdominal pain described as epigastric burning, gnawing pain about 2–3 h PC. Relief with foods, antacids. Awakening at 1–2 AM with symptoms Objective: Tender at the epigastrium, LUQ, slightly hyperactive bowel sounds	C
A 52-year-old woman who was recently laid off from her job, taking 3–4 doses of ibuprofen/day for the past 2–3 months to help with headaches; 1-month history of intermittent nausea, burning, and pain, limited to upper abdomen, often worse with eating Objective: Tender at the epigastrium, LUQ, hyperactive bowel sounds	A
A 54-year-old woman who presents with a 24-h history of significant epigastric and RUQ abdominal pain that is constant with 2–3-minute periods of increased pain, accompanied by nausea, 2 episodes of vomiting, and intermittent fever. Objective: Tenderness at the epigastrium and abdominal RUQ, positive Murphy's sign, moderately elevated AST, ALT, and ALP.	D

9. Risk factors for pancreatic cancer include all of the following except:

A. Hypertension.

B. History of chronic pancreatitis.

C. Tobacco use.

D. Diabetes mellitus.

10. Match the viral hepatitis type with the **most common** method of acquisition. *An option can only be used once.*

A. Hepatitis A

B. Hepatitis B

C. Hepatitis C

Acquisition method	Hepatitis type
Fecal-contaminated food or water	A
Injection drug use	C
Sexual contact	B

11. Janet, a 47-year-old well woman who is 64" (163 cm) tall with BMI=25 kg/m^2, presents for a periodic health evaluation and to establish care in your practice. She reports drinking approximately 1 to 2 mixed drinks containing 1.5 oz (44.4 mL) 80-proof liquor per week and takes approximately 1 to 2 doses of acetaminophen per month. Her last visit with a healthcare provider was more than 5 years ago; she was told that her "liver tests were a bit higher than normal." She felt well and decided not to return for follow-up. She denies history of injection drug use and has no tattoos. Her last vaccines were administered more than 10 years ago. She is without complaint. Abdominal examination is within normal limits.

Janet's laboratory results are as follows.

   HBsAg=positive (evidence HBV onboard)

   Anti-HAV=positive (immune to HAV)

   Anti-HCV=negative (no evidence of past or present HCV infection)

   AST=56 unit/L (0–40) (modest elevation, with ALT>AST)

   ALT=98 unit/L (0–40) (modest elevation, with ALT>AST)

These findings are most consistent with which of the following? Chose two that apply.

A. Chronic hepatitis B

B. Evidence of hepatitis B infection immunity

C. Evidence of hepatitis A immunity

D. Acute hepatitis B infection

E. Evidence of hepatitis C infection

12. Choosing all that apply, you offer Janet the following immunizations against:

    A. Hepatitis B.

    B. Hepatitis A.

    C. Seasonal influenza.

    D. Tetanus, diphtheria, and acellular pertussis.

13. Thomas is a 45-year-old man who has a past history of injection drug use, currently with 5 years of sobriety. He is unsure about his vaccine history but believes he had "some when I was a child." Results of recent laboratory tests reveal the following.

    HCV RNA=positive (evidence of current HCV infection)

    Anti-HBs=positive (evidence of HBV immunity)

    Anti-HAV=negative (no evidence of HAV infection or immunity)

    AST=45 unit/L (0–40) (modest elevation, with ALT>AST)

    ALT=72 unit/L (0–40) (modest elevation, with ALT>AST)

You offer the following immunization(s) against:

    A. Hepatitis B.

    B. Hepatitis A.

    C. Hepatitis A and B.

    D. Seasonal influenza, tetanus, diphtheria, and acellular pertussis.

14. True or false?

    (T/F) Adults born from 1945 through 1965 should be encouraged to be screened for HCV regardless of HCV risk factors.

Table 9-4: Infectious Hepatitis: Key Features to Transmission and Diagnosis

Type	Route of transmission	IZ available? Post-exposure prophylaxis?	Next steps if positive for infection	Sequelae	Disease marker
Hepatitis A	Fecal-oral	IZ=Yes Post-exposure prophylaxis with immune globulin (Gammagard®) and/or immunization for close contacts that are not immune to HAV.	Liver function tests (e.g., ALT, AST, bilirubin); notify local public health authorities Treatment: Generally supportive care; liver transplantation an option in select cases of fulminant hepatic failure, rare occurrence, typically when HAV contracted in presence of preexisting liver disease	None, survive or die (low mortality rate)	*Acute disease markers* • HAV IgM (M=Miserable) • Elevated hepatic enzymes ≥10 x ULN *Chronic disease markers* • None, as chronic hepatitis A does not exist. *Disease in past, Hx IZ=* • Anti-HAV (total of HAV IgM and HAV Ig**G** [G=Gone]) present • Hepatic enzymes normalize *Still susceptible to hepatitis A infection* • Anti-HAV negative (Negative="Never had")

Hepatitis B	Blood, body fluids	IZ=Yes
		
		Post-exposure prophylaxis with hepatitis B immune globulin (HBIG) and HBV immunization for blood, body fluid contacts in nonimmune individuals.
			Liver function tests; screen for coinfection with hepatitis A, C, HIV, and other STIs. Immunize against HAV if required.
			
			Refer for expert consultation for antiviral therapy consideration
				Chronic hepatitis B, hepatocellular carcinoma (HCC, primary liver cancer, hepatoma), hepatic failure, in absence of successful treatment for chronic HBV.	*Acute disease markers*
					• HBV core IgM ab=Earliest marker to become positive post–HBV exposure, denotes acute infection
					• HBs**A**g=**A**lways **g**rowing, surrogate marker for HBV
					• HB**e**Ag=Notes a time when HBV is **e**xtra contagious, **e**xtra growing
					• Elevated hepatic enzymes ≥10 x ULN
					Chronic disease markers
					• Patient without symptoms
					• NL or slightly elevated hepatic enzymes
					• HBs**A**g (**A**g=Always growing)
					  ○ Only present if HBV on board
					  ○ Surrogate marker for HBV
					Hepatitis B in past, Hx IZ
					• HBsA**b** (Anti-HBs)
					  ○ **B**=Bye, as no HBV on board
					  ○ A protective antibody, unable to get HBV in the future
					• Hepatic enzyme normalized
					Still susceptible to hepatitis B infection
					• HBsAg negative
					• Anti-HBc negative
					• HBsAb (Anti-HBs) negative
					See CDC table for additional clarification.

Continued...

Table 9-4 (cont.): Infectious Hepatitis: Key Features to Transmission and Diagnosis					
Type	Route of transmission	IZ available? Post-exposure prophylaxis?	Next steps if positive for infection	Sequelae	Disease marker
Hepatitis C	Blood, body fluids	No No	Liver function tests; screen for coinfection with hepatitis A, B, HIV, and other STIs Refer for expert consultation for antiviral therapy consideration	Chronic hepatitis C, hepatocellular carcinoma (HCC, primary liver cancer, hepatoma), hepatic failure	*Acute disease markers* • Anti-HCV present • HCV viral RNA • Elevated hepatic enzymes *Chronic disease markers* • Anti-HCV present • HCV viral RNA • Normal to slightly elevated hepatic enzymes *Disease in the past* • Anti-HCV present (non-protective antibody) • HCV RNA absent • Normalized hepatic enzymes
Hepatitis D	Blood, body fluids	No, but prevent B and you can prevent D	See hepatitis B recommendations	Severe infection, hepatic failure, death	*Acute or chronic* hepatitis B (HBsAg) markers *plus* hepatitis D IgM, usually with markedly elevated hepatic enzymes.

NB: The content of this table is not meant to be a comprehensive guide for the diagnosis of infectious hepatitis but rather an overview. See Ferri, F. (2014) Ferri's Best Test: A Practical Guide to Clinical Laboratory Medicine and Diagnostic Imaging, 3rd Ed. St. Louis, MO: Elsevier Health Sciences and Desai, S. (2009) Clinician's Guide to Laboratory Medicine: Pocket, Houston, TX: MD2B for additional information.

Source: Fitzgerald, M. A. (2017) Abdominal Disorders, Nurse Practitioner Certification Examination and Practice Preparation, (5th Ed). Philadelphia, PA: F. A. Davis.
Gilroy RK. Hepatitis A Workup. Available at: http://emedicine.medscape.com/article/177484-overview
Dhawan VK. Hepatitis C Workup. Available at: http://emedicine.medscape.com/article/177792-workup
Centers for Disease Control and Prevention. Viral Hepatitis. Available at: www.cdc.gov/hepatitis/

The ABCs of Hepatitis

	HEPATITIS A is caused by the Hepatitis A virus (HAV)	HEPATITIS B is caused by the Hepatitis B virus (HBV)	HEPATITIS C is caused by the Hepatitis C virus (HCV)
U.S. Statistics	• Estimated 17,000 new infections in 2010	• Estimated 38,000 new infections in 2010 • Estimated 1.2 million people with chronic HBV infection	• Estimated 17,000 new infections in 2010 • Estimated 3.2 million people with chronic HCV infection
Routes of Transmission	Ingestion of fecal matter, even in microscopic amounts, from: • Close person-to-person contact with an infected person • Sexual contact with an infected person • Ingestion of contaminated food or drinks	Contact with infectious blood, semen, and other body fluids, primarily through: • Birth to an infected mother • Sexual contact with an infected person • Sharing of contaminated needles, syringes or other injection drug equipment • Needlesticks or other sharp instrument injuries	Contact with blood of an infected person, primarily through: • Sharing of contaminated needles, syringes, or other injection drug equipment Less commonly through: • Sexual contact with an infected person • Birth to an infected mother • Needlestick or other sharp instrument injuries
Persons at Risk	• Travelers to regions with intermediate or high rates of Hepatitis A • Sex contacts of infected persons • Household members or caregivers of infected persons • Men who have sex with men • Users of certain illegal drugs (injection and non-injection) • Persons with clotting-factor disorders	• Infants born to infected mothers • Sex partners of infected persons • Persons with multiple sex partners • Persons with a sexually transmitted disease (STD) • Men who have sex with men • Injection drug users • Household contacts of infected persons • Healthcare and public safety workers exposed to blood on the job • Hemodialysis patients • Residents and staff of facilities for developmentally disabled persons • Travelers to regions with intermediate or high rates of Hepatitis B (HBsAg prevalence of ≥2%)	• Current or former injection drug users • Recipients of clotting factor concentrates before 1987 • Recipients of blood transfusions or donated organs before July 1992 • Long-term hemodialysis patients • Persons with known exposures to HCV (e.g., healthcare workers after needlesticks, recipients of blood or organs from a donor who later tested positive for HCV) • HIV-infected persons • Infants born to infected mothers
Incubation Period	15 to 50 days (average: 28 days)	45 to 160 days (average: 120 days)	14 to 180 days (average: 45 days)
Symptoms of Acute Infection	**Symptoms of all types of viral hepatitis are similar and can include one or more of the following:** • Fever • Fatigue • Loss of appetite • Nausea • Vomiting • Abdominal pain • Gray-colored bowel movements • Joint pain • Jaundice		
Likelihood of Symptomatic Acute infection	• < 10% of children < 6 years have jaundice • 40%–50% of children age 6–14 years have jaundice • 70%–80% of persons > 14 years have jaundice	• < 1% of infants < 1 year develop symptoms • 5%–15% of children age 1-5 years develop symptoms • 30%–50% of persons > 5 years develop symptoms **Note:** Symptoms appear in 5%–15% of newly infected adults who are immunosuppressed	• 20%–30% of newly infected persons develop symptoms of acute disease
Potential for Chronic Infection	None	• Among unimmunized persons, chronic infection occurs in >90% of infants, 25%–50% of children aged 1–5 years, and 6%–10% of older children and adults	• 75%–85% of newly infected persons develop chronic infection • 15%–25% of newly infected persons clear the virus
Severity	Most persons with acute disease recover with no lasting liver damage; rarely fatal	• Most persons with acute disease recover with no lasting liver damage; acute illness is rarely fatal • 15%–25% of chronically infected persons develop chronic liver disease, including cirrhosis, liver failure, or liver cancer • Estimated 3,000 persons in the United States die from HBV-related illness per year	• Acute illness is uncommon. Those who do develop acute illness recover with no lasting liver damage. • 60%–70% of chronically infected persons develop chronic liver disease • 5%–20% develop cirrhosis over a period of 20–30 years • 1%–5% will die from cirrhosis or liver cancer • Estimated 12,000 persons in the United States die from HCV-related illness per year
Serologic Tests for Acute Infection	• IgM anti-HAV	• HBsAg in acute and chronic infection • IgM anti-HBc is positive in acute infection only	• No serologic marker for acute infection

	HEPATITIS A	**HEPATITIS B**	**HEPATITIS C**
Serologic Tests for Chronic Infection	• Not applicable—no chronic infection	• HBsAg (and additional markers as needed)	• Screening assay (EIA or CIA) for anti-HCV • Verification by an additional, more specific assay (e.g., nucleic acid testing (NAT) for HCV RNA)
Screening Recommendations for Chronic Infection	• Not applicable—no chronic infection Note: Screening for past acute infection is generally not recommended	Testing is recommended for: • All pregnant women • Persons born in regions with intermediate or high rates of Hepatitis B (HBsAg prevalence of ≥2%) • U.S.–born persons not vaccinated as infants whose parents were born in regions with high rates of Hepatitis B (HBsAg prevalence of ≥8%) • Infants born to HBsAg-positive mothers • Household, needle-sharing, or sex contacts of HBsAg-positive persons • Men who have sex with men • Injection drug users • Patients with elevated liver enzymes (ALT/AST) of unknown etiology • Hemodialysis patients • Persons needing immunosuppressive or cytotoxic therapy • HIV-infected persons • Donors of blood, plasma, organs, tissues, or semen	Testing is recommended for: • Persons born from 1945–1965 • Persons who currently inject drugs or who have injected drugs in the past, even if once or many years ago • Recipients of clotting factor concentrates before 1987 • Recipients of blood transfusions or donated organs before July 1992 • Long-term hemodialysis patients • Persons with known exposures to HCV (e.g., healthcare workers after needlesticks, recipients of blood or organs from a donor who later tested positive for HCV) • HIV-infected persons • Children born to infected mothers (do not test before age 18 mos.) • Patients with signs or symptoms of liver disease (e.g., abnormal liver enzyme tests) • Donors of blood, plasma, organs, tissues, or semen
Treatment	• No medication available • Best addressed through supportive treatment	• Acute: No medication available; best addressed through supportive treatment • Chronic: Regular monitoring for signs of liver disease progression; some patients are treated with antiviral drugs	• Acute: Antivirals and supportive treatment • Chronic: Regular monitoring for signs of liver disease progression; some patients are treated with antiviral drugs
Vaccination Recommendations	Hepatitis A vaccine is recommended for: • All children at age 1 year • Travelers to regions with intermediate or high rates of Hepatitis A • Men who have sex with men • Users of certain illegal drugs (injection and non-injection) • Persons with clotting-factor disorders • Persons who work with HAV-infected primates or with HAV in a research laboratory • Persons with chronic liver disease, including HBV- and HCV-infected persons with chronic liver disease • Family and care givers of recent adoptees from countries where Hepatitis A is common • Anyone else seeking long-term protection	Hepatitis B vaccine is recommended for: • All infants at birth • Older children who have not previously been vaccinated • Susceptible sex partners of infected persons • Persons with multiple sex partners • Persons seeking evaluation or treatment for an STD • Men who have sex with men • Injection drug users • Susceptible household contacts of infected persons • Healthcare and public safety workers exposed to blood on the job • Persons with chronic liver disease, including HCV-infected persons with chronic liver disease • Persons with HIV infection • Persons with end-stage renal disease, including predialysis, hemodialysis, peritoneal dialysis, and home dialysis patients • Residents and staff of facilities for developmentally disabled persons • Travelers to regions with intermediate or high rates of Hepatitis B (HBsAg prevalence of ≥2%) • Unvaccinated adults with diabetes mellitus 19–59 (for those aged ≥60 years, at the discretion of clinician) • Anyone else seeking long-term protection	There is no Hepatitis C vaccine.
Vaccination Schedule	2 doses given 6 months apart	• Infants and children: 3 to 4 doses given over a 6- to 18-month period depending on vaccine type and schedule • Adults: 3 doses given over a 6-month period (most common schedule)	No vaccine available

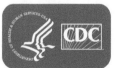

U.S. Department of Health and Human Services
Centers for Disease Control and Prevention

Publication No. 21-1076

August 2012

Important additional study resources available through your Fitzgerald Health online learning portal at fhea.com/npexpert

- Resource 9-1: Irritable Bowel Syndrome (IBS) vs. Inflammatory Bowel Disease (IBD)
- Resource 9-2: Evaluation and Treatment Options in Diverticulitis
- Resource 9-3: Diagnostic Testing and Treatment Options for *H. pylori*

Bonus questions for this chapter available through your Fitzgerald Health learning portal at fhea.com/npexpert.

Resources for Additional Study

Books:

Desai, S. (2009) <u>Clinician's Guide to Laboratory Medicine: Pocket</u>, Houston, TX: MD2B.

Ferri, F. (2014) <u>Ferri's Best Test: A Practical Guide to Clinical Laboratory Medicine and Diagnostic Imaging,</u> 3rd Edition, St. Louis, MO: Elsevier Health Sciences.

Fitzgerald, M. A. (2017) Abdominal Disorders, <u>Nurse Practitioner Certification Examination and Practice Preparation</u>, 5th Edition, Philadelphia, PA: F. A. Davis.

Audio programs:

Fitzgerald, M. A. <u>Laboratory Data Interpretation: A Case Study Approach</u>, North Andover, MA: Fitzgerald Health Education Associates.

Miller, S. K. <u>Assessment and Intervention in Common GI Disorders: PUD, Gastritis, GERD, IBS, and IBD</u>, North Andover, MA: Fitzgerald Health Education Associates.

Video programs:

Fitzgerald, M. A. <u>Expert Exam: Abdomen</u>, North Andover, MA: Fitzgerald Health Education Associates.

Chapter 10: Lower Respiratory Tract Disease

Table 10-1: Community-acquired Pneumonia Defined:
Infection of lungs and bronchi, caused by select pathogens, acquired while residing in the community, not while in hospital or long-term care facility

Suitable for treatment as an outpatient	***Likely causative pathogens*** S. pneumoniae (Gram-positive) M. pneumoniae (Atypical pathogen) C. pneumoniae (Atypical pathogen) Respiratory viruses, including influenza A/B, respiratory syncytial virus (RSV), adenovirus, parainfluenza
Requiring inpatient treatment but not in the ICU	***Likely causative pathogens*** S. pneumoniae (Gram-positive) M. pneumoniae (Atypical pathogen) C. pneumoniae (Atypical pathogen) Legionella spp. (Atypical pathogen) H. influenzae (Gram-negative) Respiratory viruses, including influenza A/B, RSV, adenovirus, parainfluenza

Source: Mandell, L. et al. Infectious Diseases Society of America/American Thoracic Society Consensus Guidelines on the Management of Community-acquired Pneumonia in Adults. *Clin Infect Dis.*;44:S21-S72. Available at https://www.thoracic.org/statements/resources/mtpi/idsaats-cap.pdf

Table 10-2: Causative Pathogens in Community-acquired Pneumonia (CAP)

Pathogen Description	Antimicrobial resistance mechanism Preferred antimicrobials	Comment
S. pneumoniae Gram-positive diplococci Most common cause of fatal CAP	Resistance via altered protein-binding sites in bacterial cell (~25% nationwide) Drug-resistant *S. pneumoniae* (DRSP) factors: Recent systemic antimicrobial use (within past 3 months), age ≥65 years, exposure to or being a child in daycare, alcohol abuse, medical comorbidities, immunosuppressive therapy or illness Preferred antimicrobials for non-resistant *S. pneumoniae*: Doxycycline, macrolides (azithro-, clarithro-, erythromycin), standard-dose amoxicillin (1.5–2.5 g/d), select cephalosporins Preferred antimicrobials with risk for DRSP: High-dose (HD) amoxicillin (3–4 g/d), respiratory fluoroquinolones (moxi-, levo-, gemifloxacin)	Macrolide use: Associated with potential QT prolongation and increased risk of CV death during use, particularly in those with highest cardiovascular risk. Fluoroquinolone use associated with tendon rupture risk, particularly in older adults, with concomitant systemic corticosteroid use, and/or select organ transplant. See previous advisory on FQ use. In CAP with DRSP risk, benefit likely outweighs risk.
H. influenzae Gram-negative bacillus	Resistance via beta-lactamase production (~30% nationwide) Effective antimicrobials: Those with activity against Gram-negative organisms and stable in presence of or active against beta-lactamase: Cephalosporins, amoxicillin-clavulanate, macrolides, respiratory fluoroquinolones, doxycycline	Common respiratory pathogen with tobacco-related lung disease
M. pneumoniae *C. pneumoniae* Not revealed by Gram stain	Effective antimicrobials: Macrolides, respiratory fluoroquinolones, doxycycline Ineffective antimicrobials: Beta-lactams (cephalosporins, penicillins)	Largely cough-transmitted, often seen in people who have recently spent extended time in close proximity (closed communities, such as correctional facilities, college dormitories, long-term care facilities, others)
Legionella spp. Not revealed by Gram stain	Effective antimicrobials: Macrolides, respiratory fluoroquinolones, doxycycline Ineffective antimicrobials: Beta-lactams (cephalosporins, penicillins)	Usually contracted by inhaling mist or aspirating liquid that comes from a water source contaminated with *Legionella* No evidence for person-to-person spread of the disease.

Table 10-3: Infectious Diseases Society of America/American Thoracic Society: Community-acquired Pneumonia Classification for Outpatient Treatment
Minimum diagnostic evaluation in CAP includes CBC with WBC differential, chest x-ray.
Additional testing based on patient presentation and comorbidity.
Recommended length of CAP therapy=Minimum of 5 days with evidence of increasing stability, afebrile for 48–72 h prior to antimicrobial discontinuation

IDSA/ATS classification	Likely causative pathogens	Recommended treatment	Comment
Previously healthy No recent (within 3 months) systemic antimicrobial use	*S. pneumoniae* (Gram-positive) with low DRSP risk, little risk of *H. influenzae* Atypical pathogens (*M. pneumoniae, C. pneumoniae*) Respiratory virus, including influenza A/B, RSV, adenovirus, parainfluenza	Doxycycline **Or** Azithromycin, clarithromycin, or erythromycin, taking into consideration local *S. pneumoniae* macrolide resistance rates	Erythromycin, clarithromycin: CYP3A4 inhibitors with significant drug-interaction and GI upset potential
Comorbidities including: COPD, diabetes, renal or heart failure, asplenia, alcoholism, immunosuppressing conditions or use of immunosuppressing medications, malignancy or use of a systemic antimicrobial in past 3 months	*S. pneumoniae* (Gram-positive) with DRSP risk *H. influenzae* (Gram-negative) Atypical pathogens (*M. pneumoniae, C. pneumoniae, Legionella*) Respiratory virus as mentioned above	Respiratory fluoroquinolone (moxi-, gemi-, levofloxacin*) **Or** Doxycycline, azithromycin or clarithromycin **plus** beta-lactam, such as HD amoxicillin (3–4 g/d), HD amoxicillin-clavulanate (4 g/d), ceftriaxone (Rocephin®), cefpodoxime (Vantin®), cefuroxime (Ceftin®)	Recent antimicrobial use increases risk of infection with DRSP. Given comorbidity, risk of poor outcome if treatment failure Recent use of a fluoroquinolone should dictate selection of a non-fluoroquinolone regimen, and vice versa

*For information about FDA fluoroquinolone warning, please see
http://www.fda.gov/Drugs/DrugSafety/ucm511530.htm
Source: Mandell, L. et al., Infectious Diseases Society of America/American Thoracic
Society Consensus Guidelines on the Management of Community-acquired Pneumonia in
Adults. *Clin Infect Dis.* 2007;44:S21-S72. Available at
https://www.thoracic.org/statements/resources/mtpi/idsaats-cap.pdf

Table 10-4: The CURB-65
Used to calculate location of appropriate treatment for a person with CAP. Each item carries a weight of 1 point. The higher the score, the greater risk of CAP-associated mortality.

- **C**onfusion of new onset
- Blood **u**rea nitrogen greater than 19 mg/dL (7 mmol/L)
- **R**espiratory rate of 30 breaths per minute or greater
- **B**lood pressure less than 90 mm Hg systolic or diastolic blood pressure 60 mm Hg or less
- Age **65** or older

CURB-65 results
- 0–1: Treat as an outpatient.
- 2: Consider a short stay in hospital or watch very closely as an outpatient.
- 3–5: Requires hospitalization with consideration as to whether patient needs to be in the intensive care unit.

Source: http://www.mdcalc.com/curb-65-severity-score-community-acquired-pneumonia/

1. Likely causative organisms in community-acquired pneumonia include:

   A. *S. pneumoniae* and select respiratory viruses.

   B. *H. influenzae* and *S. aureus.*

   C. *M. catarrhalis* and atypical pathogens.

   D. *K. pneumoniae* and *Legionella* species. _

2. Teresa, a 38-year-old woman with no chronic health problems, presents with a chief complaint of "A cold I cannot shake for the past three weeks." She also reports an intermittent frontal headache and has taken acetaminophen with relief, as well as general malaise and a dry cough that is particularly problematic at night. She denies nausea, vomiting, chills, fever, or dyspnea. She has not taken an antimicrobial within the past year, underwent a bilateral tubal ligation approximately 10 years ago, and is allergic to penicillin with a hive-form reaction. Examination reveals the following: SaO_2=97%, BP=114/70 mm Hg, T=98°F (36.7°C), HR=88, RR=20, bilateral coarse late inspiratory crackles without wheeze. She is in no acute distress. Chest x-ray demonstrates bilateral interstitial infiltrates. Which of the following describes the recommended additional diagnostic testing for Teresa?

   A. No further testing is required.

   B. CBC with WBC differential

   C. Blood culture

   D. Sputum culture

3. In treating Teresa, you prescribe the following.

   A. A 7-day course of oral doxycycline

   B. A 10-day course of oral moxifloxacin

   C. A 3-day course of parenteral ceftriaxone

   D. Timed inhaled short-acting beta$_2$-agonist use

4. Teresa's CURB-65 score=_____

5. Teresa's location of treatment= outpatient

6. Mr. Spaulding is a 70-year-old man with a 50 pack-year cigarette smoking history, chronic obstructive pulmonary disease, and hypertension, who presents with a 24-hour history of increasing dyspnea and productive cough with white-yellow sputum. He is alert, oriented, and answers questions with ease. Physical examination reveals the following: Alert, breathing slightly labored at rest, BP=130/78 mm Hg, T=99.8°F (37.7°C), HR=96, RR=22, dullness to percussion over the left base with increased tactile fremitus and tubular breath sounds as well as crackles in the right base. Cardiac examination reveals no S_3, no S_4, no murmur, with nondistended neck veins. His physical examination findings are suggestive of:

A. A left lower lobe consolidation.

B. Diffuse hyperinflation.

C. Heart failure.

D. Compromised pulmonary vascular perfusion.

7. Which of the numbered areas on the chest x-ray best correlates with Mr. Spaulding's physical examination findings?

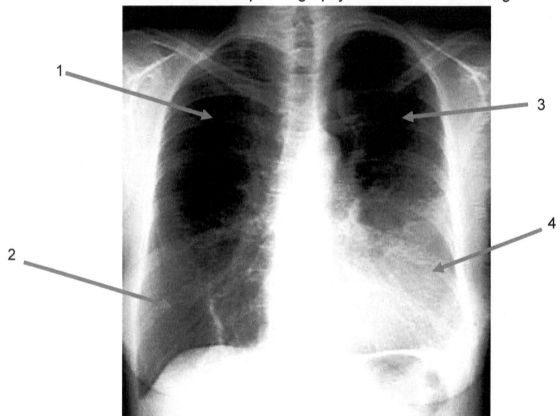

Figure 10-9

| Table 10-5: Common Physical Examination Findings in Pneumonia ||
Condition	Physical exam findings
Consolidation (Caused most often by pneumonia, less commonly by hemorrhage)	Dullness to percussion —— • Dense tissue when percussed sounds dull *(Dense=Dull)* Increased tactile fremitus • *Increases* with *increased* tissue density · Bronchial or tubular breath sounds, often with late inspiratory crackles that do not clear with cough
Pleural inflammation (pleurisy) (Associated with pneumonia, less commonly with pulmonary embolism)	Patient report of sharp, localized pain, worse with deep breath, movement, cough Audible pleural friction rub, from movement of inflamed pleura layers • Sound similar to stepping into fresh snow

8. Mr. Spaulding's current medications include an inhaled corticosteroid, a long-acting beta$_2$-agonist, an ACE inhibitor with a thiazide diuretic, a statin, and low-dose aspirin, as well as a short-acting beta$_2$-agonist as needed. Laboratory testing reveals BUN and hematocrit=WNL. The preferred choice of antimicrobial therapy for Mr. Spaulding is a:

A. 7-day course of clarithromycin.

B. 5-day course of levofloxacin.

C. 10-day course of amoxicillin-clavulanate.

D. 14-day course of cefpodoxime.

9. Mr. Spaulding's CURB-65 score= ___2___

10. Location of treatment= *out ptnl*

Table 10-4: The CURB-65
Used to calculate location of appropriate treatment for a person with CAP. Each item carries a weight of 1 point. The higher the score, the greater risk of CAP-associated mortality.
• Confusion of new onset • Blood **u**rea nitrogen greater than 9 mg/dL (7 mmol/L) • **R**espiratory rate of 30 breaths per minute or greater • **B**lood pressure less than 90 mm Hg systolic or diastolic blood pressure 60 mm Hg or less • Age **65** or older
CURB-65 results • 0–1: Treat as an outpatient • 2: Consider a short stay in hospital or watch very closely as an outpatient • 3–5: Requires hospitalization with consideration as to whether patient needs to be in the intensive care unit

Source: http://www.mdcalc.com/curb-65-severity-score-community-acquired-pneumonia/

11. Mr. Spaulding returns in 3 days. He states that he is feeling somewhat better, with less shortness of breath but with continued fatigue and production of small amounts of white-yellow sputum. He states he has taken his antimicrobial therapy as advised without difficulty. Physical examination reveals the following: Alert, BP=130/78 mm Hg, T=97.8°F (36.6°C), HR=88, RR=18, dullness to percussion over the left base with increased tactile fremitus and tubular breath sounds. Cardiac examination reveals no S_3, no S_4, no murmur, with nondistended neck veins. At this point, you consider the following two best options:

   A. A repeat chest x-ray should be obtained today.

   B. His antimicrobial needs to be changed to an agent with wider spectrum of activity.

   C. Mr. Spaulding should be advised to complete his current course of therapy.

   D. Pneumococcal and seasonal influenza vaccines should be updated today as needed.

12. Which of the following is the most common pathogen implicated in acute bronchitis?

   A. *S. pneumoniae*

   B. *H. influenzae*

   C. *M. pneumoniae*

   D. Respiratory virus

Table 10-6: Acute Bronchitis: Inflammation of the lower airways found in the absence of other airway disease, including asthma and COPD Likely Causative Pathogens		
Organism	**% of total**	**Comment**
Respiratory tract viruses		Consider using muscarinic antagonist bronchodilator, such as ipratropium bromide (Atrovent®), inhaled beta$_2$-agonist, such as albuterol, or short course of oral corticosteroid (for example, prednisone 40 mg PO daily dose for 3–5 days) with protracted, problematic cough
Bacterial pathogens, such as *M. pneumoniae, C. pneumoniae, B. pertussis*		Consider use of macrolide or doxycycline when antimicrobial therapy indicated.

Sources: Irwin, R. et al. , American College of Chest Physicians (ACCP) Evidence-Based Clinical Practice Guidelines: Diagnosis and Management of Cough. *Chest.* 2006;129:1S-23S.

Gilbert, D., Chambers, H., Eliopoulos, G., Saag, M., Pavia, A. (2016) The Sanford Guide to Antimicrobial Therapy (46th ed.). Sperryville, VA: Antimicrobial Therapy, Inc.

13. A 63-year-old man who resides at the homeless shelter is brought to the ED with a chief complaint of chronic cough and chest pain. His temperature is 102.3°F (39.1FC), respiratory rate of 45 bpm, and blood pressure of 135/85 mm Hg. Which of the following findings would best support a diagnosis of active tuberculosis infection?

    A. Erythematous plaques over the torso

    B. Hemoptysis

    C. Absent or clear sputum

    D. Unexplained weight gain

Table 10-7: Active Tuberculosis	
Risk factors	**Clinical presentation**
HIV infection	Cough
History of positive PPD result	Unexplained weight loss/anorexia
History of prior TB treatment	Fever
TB exposure	Night sweats
Travel to or emigration from an area where TB is endemic	Hemoptysis
	Chest pain
Homelessness, shelter-dwelling, incarceration	Fatigue

Source: Herchline TE. Tuberculosis. Available at:
http://emedicine.medscape.com/article/230802-overview.

14. The chest x-ray of a 47-year-old man with suspected tuberculosis reveals the following:

The radiograph likely shows:

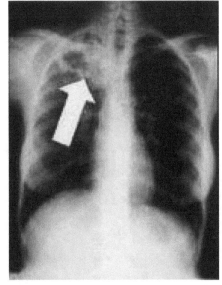

    A. Infiltrate in the left upper lobe.

    B. Infiltrate in the right upper lobe.

    C. Pleural effusion in the left upper lobe.

    D. Pleural effusion in the right upper lobe.

Table 10-8: Making the diagnosis: Is it asthma?	
Asthma defined	A common chronic disorder that is complex and characterized by underlying airway inflammation that leads to variable airflow obstruction and bronchial hyperresponsiveness. ***Airway inflammation first, bronchospasm follows.***
Symptoms consistent with asthma	Recurrent cough, wheeze, shortness of breath and/or chest tightness due to variable airflow obstruction and bronchial hyperresponsiveness triggered by underlying airway inflammation. Symptoms occur or worsen at night, or with exercise, viral respiratory infections, aeroallergens and/or pulmonary irritants (such as first- or second-hand smoke)
Airflow obstruction that is at least partially reversible	Increase in $FEV_1 \geq 12\%$ from baseline post-short-acting beta$_2$-agonist use
Consider the diagnosis of asthma and perform spirometry if any of these indicators are present.	These indicators are not diagnostic by themselves, but the presence of multiple key indicators increases the probability of the diagnosis of asthma. Spirometry is needed to make the diagnosis of asthma. Peak flow meter is used for monitoring, not for diagnosing, asthma. ***Objective evaluation for airflow obstruction should be conducted with every asthma-related visit.***

Source: Expert Panel Report 3: Guidelines for the Diagnosis and Management of Asthma, EPR-3, available at www.nhlbi.nih.gov/guidelines/asthma/asthgdln.pdf, p. S42.

Table 10-9: Key Points for EPR-3 Asthma Guideline Implementation	
Goals of therapy	Reduce impairment Reduce risk of exacerbation or other complication Optimize health and function
Assessment	Classify asthma severity (initial visit) and asthma control (follow-up visits). Identify precipitating and exacerbating factors, including comorbid conditions that aggravate asthma. Identify patients at high risk for exacerbations and death from asthma Regularly assess patient's and family's knowledge and skills for self-management, including medication device technique
Visit frequency	Well-controlled: 3–6 months Not well-controlled: 2–6 weeks
Treatment	Short-acting beta$_2$-agonist as acute reliever Controller for persistent asthma (inhaled corticosteroid preferred) Step-up therapy if not well-controlled Written asthma action plan Education

Table 10-10: Asthma Controller Medications

Inhaled corticosteroids (ICS) • Mometasone (Asmanex®) • Fluticasone (Flovent®) • Budesonide (Pulmicort®) • Beclomethasone (QVAR®) • Ciclesonide (Alvesco®) • Others	Preferred controller treatment for persistent asthma. Less than 20% of ICS dose absorbed systemically. ***Requires consistent, daily use for optimal effect***
Inhaled corticosteroids/long-acting beta₂-agonists (ICS/LABA) • Budesonide + formoterol (Symbicort®) • Fluticasone + salmeterol (Advair®) • Mometasone + formoterol (Dulera®) • Others	Preferred treatment for moderate to severe persistent asthma. FDA boxed warning: Increased death in asthma patients using LABAs; ICS with LABA should not be used in patients whose asthma is well-controlled with an ICS alone. **(Boxed warning does not extend into LABA use in COPD.)** ***Requires consistent, daily use for optimal effect***
Leukotriene modifiers (LTM) • Montelukast (Singulair®)	Additional benefit with allergic rhinitis, most often used in conjunction with ICS. Approx. 50% as potent as ICS in inflammation control. ***Requires consistent, daily use for optimal effect***

Source: Expert Panel Report 3: Guidelines for the Diagnosis and Management of Asthma (EPR-3), available at www.nhlbi.nih.gov/guidelines/asthma/asthgdln.pdf

Table 10-11: Estimated Comparative Daily Dosages for ICS in Patients Age ≥12 Years

ICS	Low daily dose	Medium daily dose	High daily dose
Beclomethasone HFA (QVAR®) 40 or 80 mcg/puff	80–240 mcg	>240–480 mcg	>480 mcg
Budesonide DPI (Pulmicort®) 180 mcg/inhalation	180–540 mcg	>540–1080 mcg	>1080 mcg
Fluticasone HFA MDI (Flovent®) 44, 110, or 220 mcg/puff	88–264 mcg	264–440 mcg	>440 mcg
Fluticasone DPI (Flovent®) 50, 100, or 250 mcg/puff	100–300 mcg	300–500 mcg	>500 mcg
Mometasone DPI (Asmanex®) 200 mcg/puff	200 mcg	400 mcg	>400 mcg

Source: www.nhlbi.nih.gov/guidelines/asthma/asthgdln.pdf

Table 10-12: Asthma Reliever Medications

Clinical condition	Medication	Comment
Acute reliever (rescue) medications for intervention in acute bronchospasm	Short-acting beta$_2$-agonists (SABA), such as albuterol (Proventil®), pirbuterol (Maxair®), levalbuterol (Xopenex®) *(Beta$_2$-agonists=Activates beta$_2$ receptors in airways going to the two lungs.)*	Regardless of classification, all individuals with asthma should have ready access to a SABA. Use >2 days/week (except for exercise) suggests a need for better control. Prudent practice dictates that the prescriber and patient monitor frequency and amount of use. Drug of choice for preventing exercise-induced bronchospasm (EIB). Use 15–30 mins prior to activity.
Aggressive treatment of inflammation during asthma flare	Systemic corticosteroids	Example: Prednisone 40–60 mg/d × 3–10 d (average 5–7 d). No therapeutic benefit to using an injectable corticosteroid when compared with oral product. Taper usually not needed with the aforementioned dosing and duration of therapy. During asthma flare, increase use of rescue drug.

Table 10-13: Additional Medications Used in the Treatment of Asthma

Medication	Indication	Comment
Inhaled muscarinic antagonists (AKA inhaled anticholinergics)	Bronchodilator via blockage of cholinergic/muscarinic receptors. Emerging role in asthma treatment. Well-established role in COPD therapy. Use primarily for prevention, not treatment, of bronchospasm	Ipratropium bromide [Atrovent®]= Example of short-acting muscarinic antagonist (SAMA) Tiotropium bromide [Spiriva®])= Example of a long-acting muscarinic antagonist (LAMA)
Theophylline	Mild to moderate bronchodilator	Use requires periodic monitoring of theophylline levels, multiple drug-drug interaction potential limits its clinical utility. See EPR-3 for full details on its use.

Table 10-14: Classifying Asthma Severity in Youths ≥12 Years of Age and Adults Initial Diagnosis: Determine Severity and Treatment Needed					
Components of Severity		**Classification of Asthma Severity (Youths ≥12 years of age and adults)**			
			Persistent		
		Intermittent	**Mild**	**Moderate (most commonly encountered)**	**Severe**
Impairment **Normal FEV₁/FVC:** **8–19 y 85%** **20–39 y 80%** **40–59 y 75%** **60–80 y 70%**	**Symptoms**	≤2 days/week	>2 days/week but not daily	Daily	Throughout the day
	Nighttime awakenings	≤2×/month	3–4×/month	>1×/week but not nightly	Often 7×/week
	Short-acting beta$_2$-agonist use for symptom control (not prevention of EIB)	≤2 days/week	>2 days/week but not >1×/day	Daily	Several times per day
	Interference with normal activity	None	Minor limitation	Some limitation	Extreme limitation
	Lung function	Normal FEV₁ between exacerbations			
		FEV₁>80% predicted	FEV₁>80% predicted	FEV₁>60% but <80% predicted	FEV₁<60% predicted
		FEV₁/FVC normal	FEV₁/FVC normal	FEV₁/FVC reduced 5%	FEV₁/FVC reduced >5%
Risk	Exacerbations requiring oral systemic corticosteroids	0–1/year (see note)		≥2/year (see note)	
		Consider severity and interval since last exacerbation. Frequency and severity may fluctuate over time for patients in any severity category.			
		Relative annual risk of exacerbations may be related to FEV₁			
Recommended Step for Initiating Treatment		Step 1	Step 2	Step 3	Step 4
					and consider short course of oral systemic corticosteroids
		In 2 to 6 weeks, evaluate level of asthma control that is achieved and adjust therapy accordingly.			

Level of severity is determined by assessment of both impairment and risk. Assess impairment domain by patient's/caregiver's recall of previous 2–4 weeks and spirometry. Assign severity to the most severe category in which any feature occurs.
At present, there are inadequate data to correspond frequencies of exacerbations with different levels of asthma severity. In general, more frequent and intense exacerbations (e.g., requiring urgent, unscheduled care, hospitalization, or ICU admission) indicate greater underlying disease severity. For treatment purposes, patients who had ≥2 exacerbations requiring oral systemic corticosteroids in the past year may be considered the same patients who have persistent asthma, even in the absence of impairment levels consistent with persistent asthma.

Table 10-15: Stepwise Approach for Managing Asthma in Patients Age≥12 Years

Intermittent Asthma	Persistent Asthma: Daily Medication Consult with asthma specialist if Step 4 care or higher is required. Consider consultation at Step 3.	

Step 6
Preferred:
High-dose ICS + LABA + Oral Corticosteroid
AND
Consider Omalizumab for Patients Who Have Allergies

Step 5
Preferred:
High-dose ICS + LABA
AND
Consider Omalizumab for Patients Who Have Allergies

Step 4
Preferred:
Medium-dose ICS + LABA
Alternative:
Medium-dose ICS + either LTM or theophylline

Step 3
Preferred:
Low-dose ICS + LABA
OR
Medium-dose ICS
Alternative:
Low-dose ICS + either LTM or theophylline

Step 2
Preferred:
Low-dose ICS
Alternative:
LTM (montelukast) or theophylline

Step 1
Preferred:
SABA PRN

↑ **Needed**
(first, check adherence, environmental control, and comorbid conditions)

Assess Control

Step Down if Possible
(and asthma is well controlled at least 3 months)

↓

Steps 2-4: Consider subcutaneous allergen immunotherapy for patients who have allergic asthma

Quick-relief medication for all patients

- SABA as needed for symptoms. Intensity of treatment depends on severity of symptoms: up to 3 treatments at 20-minute intervals as needed. Short course of systemic oral corticosteroids may be needed
- Use of SABA >2 days a week for symptom relief (not prevention of EIB) generally indicates inadequate control and the need to step up treatment

www.nhlbi.nih.gov/guidelines/asthma/asthgdln.pdf

Table 10-16: Assessing Asthma Control in Youths ≥12 Years of Age and Adults Follow-up Visits: Determine Level of Control and Treatment Needed				
Components of Control		**Classification of Asthma Control** **(Youths ≥12 years of age and adults)**		
	Symptoms	Well-controlled (therapeutic goal)	Not well-controlled	Very poorly controlled
		≤2 days/week	>2 days/week	Throughout the day
Impairment	Nighttime awakenings	≤2×/month	1–3×/week	≥4×/week
	Interference with normal activity	None	Some limitation	Extreme limitation
	Short-acting beta$_2$-agonist use for symptom control (not prevention of EIB)	≤2 days/week	>2 days/week	Several times per day
	FEV$_1$ or peak flow	>80% predicted/personal best	60–80% predicted/personal best	<60% predicted/personal best
	Validated Questionnaires ATAQ ACQ ACT	0 ≤0.75* ≥20	1–2 ≥1.5 16–19	3–4 N/A ≤15
Risk	Exacerbations	0–1/year	≥2/year (see note)	
		Consider severity and interval since last exacerbation		
	Progressive loss of lung function	Evaluation requires long-term follow-up care.		
	Treatment-related adverse effects	Medication adverse effects can vary in intensity from none to very troublesome and worrisome. The level of intensity does not correlate to specific levels of control but should be considered in the overall assessment of risk.		
Recommended action for treatment		• Maintain current step. • Regular follow-ups every 1–6 months to maintain control • Consider step down if well-controlled for at least 3 months.	• Step up 1 step and reevaluate in 2–6 weeks. • For adverse effects, consider alternative treatment options.	• Consider short course of oral systemic corticosteroids. • Step up 1–2 steps and reevaluate in 2 weeks. • For adverse effects, consider alternative treatment options.

*ACQ values of 0.76–1.4 are indeterminate regarding well-controlled asthma.
Key: EIB, exercise-induced bronchospasm; FEV$_1$, forced expiratory volume in 1 second.

15. You anticipate finding the following on physical examination during an acute asthma or chronic obstructive pulmonary disease (COPD) flare:

A. Intercostal retraction.

B. Inspiratory crackles.

C. Increased tactile fremitus.

D. Hyperresonance.

| Table 10-17: Physical Examination Findings in Select Lower Airway Disease ||
Condition	Objective findings
Air trapping • COPD, consistently present, worsens with exacerbation • Asthma, present during exacerbation	Hyperresonance Decreased tactile fremitus Wheeze (expiratory first, inspiratory later) Low diaphragms Increased anteroposterior (AP) diameter ("barrel chest," most often in COPD or with longstanding, poorly-controlled asthma)

Chest x-ray in COPD with hyperinflation findings

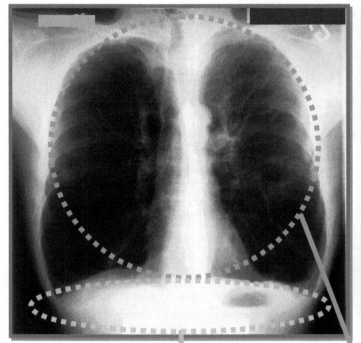

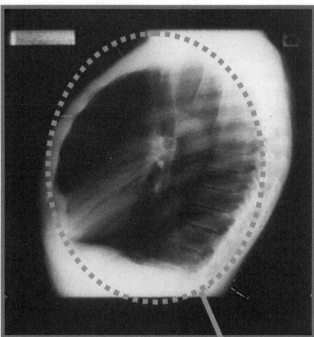

Low, Flattened Diaphragm

Air Trapping

Figure 10-17

Increased A-P Diameter

Figure 10-18

16. You see Michelle, a 38-year-old woman with moderate persistent asthma who is using medium-dose inhaled fluticasone daily and albuterol via MDI as needed. In a typical month, she uses albuterol 2 puffs "about 2 times, when I feel my chest getting a little tight, and it works right away." In an average month, she has no episodes of nocturnal awakening with cough or wheeze, typically has excellent activity tolerance. Which of the following is the most important additional clinical parameter to obtain today in evaluating Michelle's baseline asthma control?

A. SaO_2

B. Peak expiratory flow

C. Auscultation of breath sounds

D. Resting respiratory rate

17. Michelle returns for an urgent care visit three weeks later with a 2-day history of URI symptoms with a dry cough and reports, "The albuterol is not working as well as usual. I was up all night coughing." She denies fever, productive cough, nausea, or vomiting. Which of the following is the most important clinical parameter in assessing Michelle's asthma flare?

A. $SaO_2=97\%$

B. Peak expiratory flow=55% of personal best

C. Presence of bilateral expiratory wheezes

D. Patient report of reduced response to $beta_2$-agonist use

18. In managing Michelle's asthma flare, her medication regimen should be adjusted to include which of the following?

A. An oral systemic bronchodilator titrated to therapeutic level

B. A short course of an oral corticosteroid

C. An oral macrolide antimicrobial

D. A single dose of injectable corticosteroid

Global Initiative for Chronic Obstructive Lung Disease:
Guide to COPD Diagnosis, Management and Treatment
Source: www.goldcopd.org

Table 10-18: COPD Overview	
What is COPD?	COPD is a preventable and treatable disease with some significant extrapulmonary effects that may contribute to its severity in individual patients. Its pulmonary component is characterized by airflow limitation that is not fully reversible. Exacerbations and comorbidities contribute to the overall severity in individual patients.
Goals of COPD treatment	Relieve symptoms and reduce the impact of symptoms, reduce risk of future adverse health events, including exacerbations
What are the most common COPD symptoms?	Chronic cough, chronic sputum production, activity intolerance, symptoms typically progressive over time.
What are the most common COPD risk factors?	Exposure to irritants including tobacco use, occupational exposure to irritants, indoor/outdoor air pollution. Also family history of COPD, advancing age. Consider COPD diagnosis in individuals with risk factors and age >40 years.
Who is at highest risk for COPD exacerbation and COPD death?	Individuals with COPD with a history of ≥2 exacerbations within the last year, FEV_1<50% of predicted value and/or hospitalization for COPD exacerbation in the past year.

Table 10-19: Assessment in COPD	
Degree of airflow limitation	Spirometry is required for diagnosis. When possible, use age-related values to avoid over-diagnosis in elders. FEV_1:FVC<0.70 post-bronchodilator confirms persistent airflow limitation/COPD. Classification of severity determined by FEV_1
CAT or CCQ Questionnaire	Validated questionnaires such as the COPD Assessment Test (CAT) or the Clinical COPD Questionnaire (CCQ) are recommended for a comprehensive assessment of symptoms.
Alpha-1 Antitrypsin Deficiency Screening	Perform when COPD develops in patients of European ancestry under 45 years or with a strong family history of COPD.

Table 10-20: Classification of Severity of Airflow Limitation in COPD Based on Post-bronchodilator FEV_1 Comprehensive COPD evaluation includes applying the Combined Assessment of COPD recommendations from GOLDCOPD.ORG		
In patients with FEV_1/FVC<0.70:		
GOLD 1	Mild	FEV_1≥80% predicted
GOLD 2	Moderate	50%≤FEV_1<80% predicted
GOLD 3	Severe	30%≤FEV_1<50% predicted
GOLD 4	Very severe	FEV_1<30% predicted

Source: Global Initiative for Chronic Obstructive Lung Disease, Pocket Guide to COPD Diagnosis, Management and Prevention, www.goldcopd.org/guidelines-pocket-guide-to-copd-diagnosis.html

Table 10-21: Medications Used in the Treatment of COPD: A Focus on Therapeutic Goals

For all groups, smoking cessation, physical activity, and appropriate influenza and pneumococcal vaccine recommended.

Pulmonary rehabilitation recommended for improvement in overall health and respiratory function

Medications mentioned represent examples of the given drug class, not a comprehensive list of all options.

Medication	Therapeutic goal
Short-acting beta$_2$-agonist (SABA) (albuterol), short-acting anticholinergic/muscarinic antagonist (SAMA) (ipratropium bromide) (inhaled)	Relief of bronchospasm ***Usually used PRN***
Long-acting beta$_2$-agonist (LABA) (salmeterol) (inhaled)	Protracted duration bronchodilation ***Used on a daily set schedule***
Long-acting muscarinic antagonist (LAMA) (tiotropium bromide) (inhaled)	Protracted duration bronchodilation Minimizes risk of COPD exacerbation ***Used on a daily set schedule***
Inhaled corticosteroid (ICS)	Antiinflammatory Minimizes risk of COPD exacerbation ***Used on a daily set schedule***
Theophylline (oral)	Bronchodilator ***Used on a daily set schedule***
PDE-4 inhibitor (roflumilast) (oral)	Minimizes risk of COPD exacerbation ***Used on a daily set schedule***

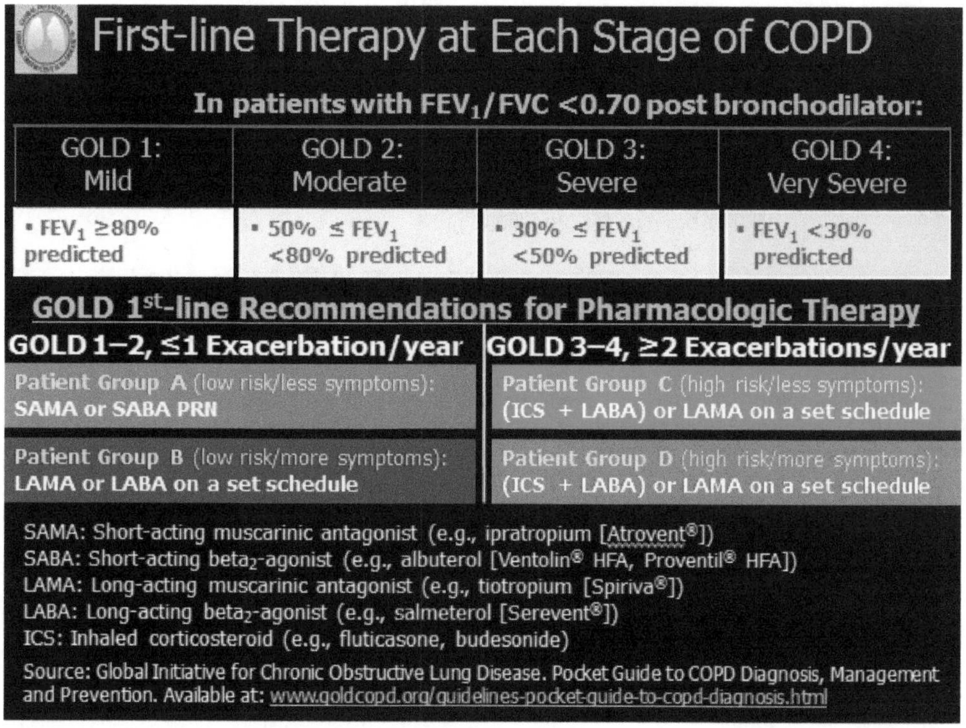

First-line Therapy at Each Stage of COPD

In patients with FEV$_1$/FVC <0.70 post bronchodilator:

GOLD 1: Mild	GOLD 2: Moderate	GOLD 3: Severe	GOLD 4: Very Severe
• FEV$_1$ ≥80% predicted	• 50% ≤ FEV$_1$ <80% predicted	• 30% ≤ FEV$_1$ <50% predicted	• FEV$_1$ <30% predicted

GOLD 1st-line Recommendations for Pharmacologic Therapy

GOLD 1–2, ≤1 Exacerbation/year	GOLD 3–4, ≥2 Exacerbations/year
Patient Group A (low risk/less symptoms): **SAMA or SABA PRN**	**Patient Group C** (high risk/less symptoms): (ICS + LABA) or LAMA on a set schedule
Patient Group B (low risk/more symptoms): **LAMA or LABA on a set schedule**	**Patient Group D** (high risk/more symptoms): (ICS + LABA) or LAMA on a set schedule

SAMA: Short-acting muscarinic antagonist (e.g., ipratropium [Atrovent®])
SABA: Short-acting beta$_2$-agonist (e.g., albuterol [Ventolin® HFA, Proventil® HFA])
LAMA: Long-acting muscarinic antagonist (e.g., tiotropium [Spiriva®])
LABA: Long-acting beta$_2$-agonist (e.g., salmeterol [Serevent®])
ICS: Inhaled corticosteroid (e.g., fluticasone, budesonide)

Source: Global Initiative for Chronic Obstructive Lung Disease. Pocket Guide to COPD Diagnosis, Management and Prevention. Available at: www.goldcopd.org/guidelines-pocket-guide-to-copd-diagnosis.html

Figure 10-19

Table 10-22: Comprehensive Pharmacologic Therapy for Stable COPD: 1st, 2nd, and Alternative Options*

Patient group	First-choice	Second-choice	Alternative choice**
A Low Risk Less Symptoms **GOLD 1–2** 1 or fewer exacerbations per year	SA muscarinic antagonist (ipratropium [Atrovent®]) PRN *or* SA beta$_2$-agonist (albuterol [Ventolin® HFA, Proventil® HFA]) PRN	LA muscarinic antagonist (tiotropium [Spiriva®]) *or* LA beta$_2$-agonist (salmeterol [Serevent®]) *or* SA beta$_2$-agonist *and* SA muscarinic antagonist (ipratropium bromide with albuterol [Combivent Respimat®])	Oral theophylline
B Low Risk More Symptoms **GOLD 1–2** 1 or fewer exacerbations per year	LA muscarinic antagonist (tiotropium [Spiriva®]) *or* LA beta$_2$-agonist (salmeterol [Serevent®])	LA muscarinic antagonist (tiotropium [Spiriva®]) *with* LA beta$_2$-agonist (salmeterol [Serevent®])	SA beta$_2$-agonist (albuterol [Ventolin® HFA, Proventil® HFA]) *and/or* SA muscarinic antagonist (ipratropium [Atrovent®]) (ipratropium bromide with albuterol [Combivent Respimat®])
C High Risk Less Symptoms **GOLD 3–4** 2 or more exacerbations per year	ICS (fluticasone, budesonide) + LA beta$_2$-agonist (salmeterol, formoterol [Advair®, Symbicort®]) *or* LA muscarinic antagonist (tiotropium [Spiriva®])	LA muscarinic antagonist (tiotropium [Spiriva®]) *with* LA beta$_2$-agonist (salmeterol [Serevent®]) (vilanterol with umeclidinium bromide [Anoro Ellipta®]=LAMA with LABA)	PDE-4 inhibitor (roflumilast [Daliresp®***]) SA beta$_2$-agonist (albuterol [Ventolin® HFA, Proventil® HFA]) *and/or* SA muscarinic antagonist (ipratropium [Atrovent®]) Theophylline (do not use w/roflumilast)
D High Risk More Symptoms **GOLD 3–4** 2 or more exacerbations per year	ICS (fluticasone, budesonide) + LA beta$_2$-agonist (salmeterol, formoterol [Advair®, Symbicort®]) *or* LA muscarinic antagonist (tiotropium [Spiriva®])	ICS (fluticasone [Flovent® HFA], budesonide [Pulmicort Flexhaler®]) and LA muscarinic antagonist (tiotropium [Spiriva®]) *or* ICS (fluticasone, budesonide) + LA beta$_2$-agonist (salmeterol, formoterol [Advair®, Symbicort®]) *with* LA muscarinic antagonist (tiotropium [Spiriva®]) *or* ICS + LA beta$_2$-agonist (Advair®, Symbicort®) *with* PDE-4 inhibitor (roflumilast [Daliresp®***]) *or* LA muscarinic antagonist *and* LA beta$_2$-agonist (vilanterol with umeclidinium bromide [Anoro Ellipta®]) *with* LA muscarinic antagonist (tiotropium [Spiriva®]) *with* PDE-4 inhibitor (roflumilast [Daliresp®***])	Carbocysteine (mucolytic) SA beta$_2$-agonist (albuterol [Ventolin® HFA, Proventil® HFA]) *and/or* SA muscarinic antagonist (ipratropium [Atrovent®]) Theophylline

*Medications in each box are mentioned in alphabetical order and therefore not necessarily in order of preference.
**Medications in this column can be used alone or in combination with other options in the First- and Second-choice columns.
***Roflumilast (Daliresp®) (phosphodiesterase 4 [PDE-4] inhibitor), therapeutic option to reduce the risk of COPD exacerbations in patients with severe and very severe COPD associated with chronic bronchitis who have a history of exacerbations. Not a bronchodilator and not indicated for relief of acute bronchospasm. Adverse effects include unintended weight loss, changes in mood, thinking, and behavior. Not to be used with theophylline.

Source: Global Initiative for Chronic Obstructive Lung Disease. Pocket Guide to COPD Diagnosis, Management and Prevention, available at www.goldcopd.org

Table 10-23: Treatment of COPD Exacerbation

COPD Exacerbation: Definition, evaluation, and treatment: An event in the natural course of the disease characterized by a change in the patient's baseline dyspnea, cough, and/or sputum beyond day-to-day variability sufficient to warrant a change in management.

Source: www.goldcopd.org

Use of bronchodilators	Short-acting beta$_2$-agonist and/or muscarinic antagonist (ipratropium bromide) PRN
	Consider adding long-acting bronchodilator (LABA, [salmeterol], LAMA [tiotropium bromide]) if patient currently not using one.
Systemic corticosteroids to shorten recovery time, hypoxemia and minimize relapse risk	Example- Prednisone 40 mg/d for 5–10 days. Study supports shorter (5-day) course equally effective with fewer adverse effects than longer (10-day) course. Consider adding inhaled corticosteroid if not currently using.
Encourage smoking cessation	Smoking cessation is associated with COPD exacerbation reduction and reduction in rate of loss of lung function.
Antimicrobial therapy in COPD exacerbation	Likely indicated in the presence of 3 cardinal symptoms: Increased dyspnea, increased sputum volume, and increased sputum purulence, though evidence varies.

Source: www.goldcopd.org

Table 10-24: Antimicrobial Therapy in COPD Exacerbation

Aside from bacterial infection, tobacco use, air pollution, and viruses common contributing factors to COPD flare.

Causative bacterial pathogens (contributing to 30–50% of exacerbations) include select Gram-negative (*Haemophilus influenzae, Haemophilus parainfluenzae, Moraxella catarrhalis*) and Gram-positive (*Streptococcus pneumoniae*) pathogens. Less common pathogens include atypical pathogens, other Gram-positive and -negative organisms.

Consider chest x-ray only with fever and/or low SaO$_2$ to help rule out concomitant pneumonia.

Mild to moderate COPD exacerbation/ acute exacerbation of chronic bronchitis *Antimicrobial therapy usually not indicated. If prescribed, consider spectrum of antimicrobial activity and risks associated with the use of each product.*	If prescribed, consider using the following agents: — Amoxicillin — TMP-SMX — Doxycycline

More severe COPD exacerbation/acute exacerbation of chronic bronchitis *Role of antimicrobial therapy debated even for severe disease. If prescribed, consider spectrum of antimicrobial activity and benefit vs. risk ratio with each product.* Consider severity of COPD and comorbidities in decision-making process.	Use one of the following agents:
	— Beta-lactam
	  • Amoxicillin-clavulanate
	  • Cephalosporin (cefdinir, cefpodoxime, others)
	— Macrolide
	  • Azithromycin
	  • Clarithromycin
	— Respiratory fluoroquinolone
	  • Moxi-, levofloxacin

Source: Gilbert, D., Chambers, H., Eliopoulos, G., Saag, M., Pavia, A. (2016) <u>The Sanford Guide to Antimicrobial Therapy</u> (46th ed.). Sperryville, VA: Antimicrobial Therapy, Inc.

19. Which of the following is consistent with the diagnosis of all stages of chronic obstructive pulmonary disease?

    A. FEV_1:FVC ratio <0.70 post-bronchodilator

    B. Dyspnea on exertion

    C. Hypoxemia

    D. Orthopnea

20. Ms. Matthews is a 78-year-old woman with severe COPD, who is currently using tiotropium bromide via inhaler and medium-dose inhaled fluticasone with salmeterol via MDI, and who presents for an acute care visit. Her current medications include enalapril, hydrochlorothiazide, lovastatin, and low-dose aspirin. She reports increasing dyspnea and a productive cough with small amounts of yellow-green sputum for the past 24 hours. She states, "I hardly slept at all last night. I kept waking up coughing." She denies nausea, vomiting, or fever. Physical examination reveals bilateral expiratory wheezes and rhonchi with hyperresonance to percussion without increased tactile fremitus or dullness to percussion. SaO_2=98%, T=97.6°F (36.4°C), BP=136/84 mm Hg, P=92, regular, RR=20. When considering pharmacologic therapy to treat Ms. Matthews, the NP prescribes:

    A. Cefpodoxime and a single dose of an injectable, sustained-release corticosteroid.

    B. Clarithromycin with an increase of her inhaled corticosteroid/LABA via MDI by 2 puffs per day.

    C. Amoxicillin-clavulanate and an opioid-containing cough suppressant.

    D. Doxycycline with a short-course of an oral corticosteroid.

Table 10-25: Long-term Oxygen Therapy in COPD	
Goal	To ensure adequate oxygen delivery to the vital organs by increasing the baseline PaO_2 at rest to ≥60 mm Hg at sea level and/or producing a SaO_2≥90%
Indications to initiate long-term (>15 hours/day) oxygen therapy	PaO_2<55 mm Hg *or* SaO_2<88% with or without hypercapnia
	PaO_2=55–59 mm Hg *or* SaO_2=89% in the presence of cor pulmonale, right heart failure, or polycythemia (Hct>56% [0.56 proportion])

Source: www.goldcopd.org/guidelines-pocket-guide-to-copd-diagnosis.html

Important additional study resources available through your Fitzgerald Health online learning portal at fhea.com/npexpert

- Resource 10-1: Biological Attack: Human Pathogens, Biotoxins, and Agricultural Threats

- Resource 10-2: Hantavirus Pulmonary Syndrome: What You Need To Know

- Resource 10-3: American College of Chest Physicians: Diagnosis and Management of Cough

- Resource 10-4: Monitoring Control in Clinical Practice: Asthma Control Test™ for Patients Age≥12 Years

- Resource 10-5: The COPD Assessment Test™ (CAT)

- Resource 10-6: Inhalation and Cutaneous Anthrax

Bonus questions for this chapter available through your Fitzgerald Health learning portal at fhea.com/npexpert.

Resources for Additional Study

Books:

Fitzgerald, M. A. (2017) Chest Disorders, <u>Nurse Practitioner Certification Examination and Practice Preparation</u>, 5th Edition, Philadelphia, PA: F. A. Davis

Audio programs:

Fitzgerald, M. A. <u>Antibiotic Update: A Focus on Treatment Options in Community-acquired Pneumonia</u>, North Andover, MA: Fitzgerald Health Education Associates.

Yates, C. M. <u>Acute Asthma Exacerbations and Acute Uncomplicated Bronchitis: An Evidence-based Approach to Management</u>, North Andover, MA: Fitzgerald Health Education Associates.

Yates, C. M. <u>Asthma in Adults and Adolescents: Are They at Risk for an Exacerbation?</u>, North Andover, MA: Fitzgerald Health Education Associates.

Yates, C. M. <u>Asthma Update: An Evidence-based Approach to Management Throughout the Lifespan</u>, North Andover, MA: Fitzgerald Health Education Associates.

Video programs:

Campo, T. M. <u>Chest Pain Evaluation: From Differential Diagnosis to Diagnostic Imaging</u>, North Andover, MA: Fitzgerald Health Education Associates.

Campo, T. M. <u>Chest X-ray Interpretation: A Systematic Approach</u>, North Andover, MA: Fitzgerald Health Education Associates.

Kaminsky, D. <u>Demystifying Pulmonary Function Testing</u>, North Andover, MA: Fitzgerald Health Education Associates.

Chapter 11: Diabetes Mellitus

Type 1 or type 2 diabetes mellitus?	
An autoimmune process involving beta cell destruction resulting in insulin deficiency	
Insulin resistance with eventual insulin deficiency	
Short history of significant symptoms, including recent unexplained weight loss, ketonuria, and the classic "polys," polydipsia, polyphagia, and polyuria, usually diagnosed in the acutely ill child or younger adult	
Few if any symptoms Usually diagnosed during routine screening	

Table 11-1: Criteria for Diabetes Testing in Asymptomatic Adults T2DM Secondary Prevention
Testing should be considered in all adults who are overweight (BMI≥25 kg/m^2*) and have additional risk factors. <ul><li>Physical inactivity</li><li>First-degree relative with type 2 diabetes</li><li>Members of a high-risk ethnic population (e.g., African American, Latino, Native American, Asian American, Pacific Islander)</li><li>Women who have given birth to a baby weighing >9 lbs (4.08 kg) or were diagnosed with gestational diabetes mellitus (GDM; screen women with recent dx of GDM at 6–12 weeks postpartum)</li><li>Hypertension (≥140/90 mm Hg or on therapy for hypertension)</li><li>HDL cholesterol level <35 mg/dL (0.90 mmol/L) and/or a triglyceride level >250 mg/dL (2.82 mmol/L)</li><li>Women with polycystic ovary syndrome</li><li>A1C≥5.7% (0.057 proportion), impaired glucose tolerance (IGT), or impaired fasting glucose (IFG) on previous testing</li><li>Other clinical conditions associated with insulin resistance (e.g., severe obesity, acanthosis nigricans)</li><li>History of CVD</li></ul>
In the absence of the above criteria, screening for diabetes should begin at age 45 years.
If results are normal, testing should be repeated at least at 3-year intervals, with consideration of more frequent testing, depending on initial results and risk status.
*At-risk BMI can be lower in some ethnic groups.

Source:
American Diabetes Association Standards of Medical Care in Diabetes, available at http://care.diabetesjournals.org/content/39/Supplement_1

Criteria for Diabetes Testing in Children can be found in "The Primary Care of the Well and Sick Infant, Child, and Teen" chapter of this workbook.

Table 11-2: Diagnosis of Diabetes Mellitus, Categories of Increased Risk for Diabetes			
	Plasma glucose	**Oral glucose tolerance test (OGTT)**	**A1C**
Diabetes mellitus	Fasting (no caloric intake for ≥8 h)≥126 mg/dL (≥7.0 mmol/L) Random≥200 mg/dL (≥11.1 mmol/L) with symptoms including polyphagia, polyuria, polydipsia, and unexplained weight loss or hyperglycemic crisis. Most common method of diagnosing T1DM.	2-h plasma glucose ≥200 mg/dL (≥11.1 mmol/L) after a 75-g glucose load	A1C≥6.5% (0.065 proportion) No special patient preparation, can be done non-fasting, no protracted time needed to test like OGTT, improved standardization of A1C measurement. Provides a 3-month look-back at overall glycemic control. A1C repeat recommended in asymptomatic adult with glucose≤200 mg/dL (≤11.1 mmol/L). Repeat not needed in presence of DM symptoms and/or random or fasting glucose levels greater than 200 mg/dL (11.1 mmol/L)
Categories of increased risk for diabetes (impaired fasting glucose [IFG], impaired glucose tolerance [IGT], prediabetes)	IFG=100 mg/dL (5.6 mmol/L) to 125 mg/dL (6.9 mmol/L)	IGT=140 to 199 mg/dL (7.8 to 11 mmol/L) on the 75-g OGTT	A1C=5.7–6.4% (0.057–0.064 proportion)

Sources:
American Diabetes Association Standards of Medical Care in Diabetes, available at
http://care.diabetesjournals.org/content/39/Supplement_1

Table 11-3: Targets for Glycemic Control

Obtain A1C at least two times a year in patients who are meeting treatment goals and who have stable glycemic control; quarterly in patients whose therapy has changed or who are not meeting glycemic goals.

Biochemical index	NL	ADA
		Goal
Hemoglobin A1C (proportion of hemoglobin)	<5.6% (0.056)	<7% (0.07) for most < 6% (0.06 proportion) with low hypoglycemia risk, long life expectancy, anticipated long life expectancy and no CVD. For older adults, esp. frail or limited life expectancy, ≤8% (0.08 proportion), due to risks of hypoglycemia outweigh benefits of stringent glycemic control.
Fasting (preprandial) plasma glucose	<100 mg/dL (5.6 mmol/L)	80–130 mg/dL (3.9–7.2 mmol/L)
Peak postprandial (1–2 h post meal) plasma glucose	<140 mg/dL (7.8 mmol/L)	<180 mg/dL (10 mmol/L)
Bedtime	<120 mg/dL (6.7 mmol/L)	90–150 mg/dL (5–8.3 mmol/L)

Sources: American Diabetes Association Standards of Medical Care in Diabetes, available at http://care.diabetesjournals.org/content/39/Supplement_1

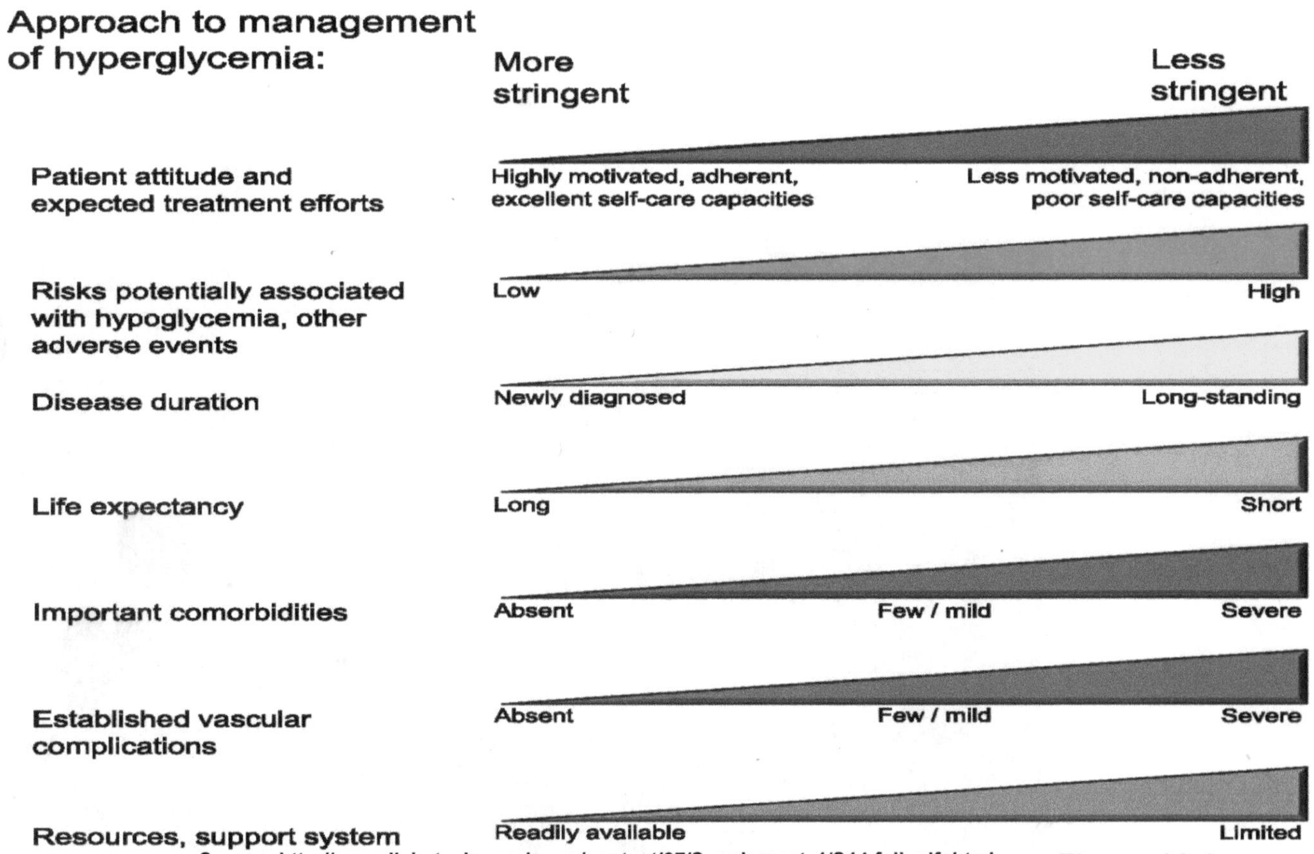

Approach to management of hyperglycemia:

	More stringent		Less stringent
Patient attitude and expected treatment efforts	Highly motivated, adherent, excellent self-care capacities		Less motivated, non-adherent, poor self-care capacities
Risks potentially associated with hypoglycemia, other adverse events	Low		High
Disease duration	Newly diagnosed		Long-standing
Life expectancy	Long		Short
Important comorbidities	Absent	Few / mild	Severe
Established vascular complications	Absent	Few / mild	Severe
Resources, support system	Readily available		Limited

Source: http://care.diabetesjournals.org/content/37/Supplement_1/S14.full.pdf+html

Figure 11-1

Table 11-4: Relationship Between Estimated Average Glucose (eAG) and A1C

A1C		Estimated average plasma glucose	
%	Proportion	mg/dL	mmol/L
5	0.05	97	5.4
5.5	0.055	111	6.2
6	0.06	126	7
6.5	0.065	140	7.8
7	0.07	154	8.5
7.5	0.075	169	9.4
8	0.08	183	10.2
8.5	0.085	197	10.9
9	0.09	212	11.8
9.5	0.095	226	12.5
10	0.10	240	13.3
10.5	0.105	255	14.2
11	0.11	269	14.9
11.5	0.115	283	15.7
12	0.12	298	16.5

Sources: American Diabetes Association, available at www.diabetes.org/living-with-diabetes/treatment-and-care/blood-glucose-control/a1c/?keymatch=eag, Online Calculator of Estimated Average Glucose (eAG), available at http://www.globalrph.com/hba1c.htm

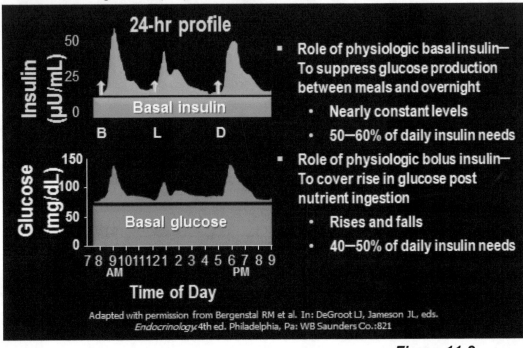

Figure 11-2

Table 11-5: Pharmacologic Intervention in T2DM		
Consider what therapeutic goal is. Correction of fasting glucose, postprandial glucose, action on insulin resistance, increasing insulin availability, offloading of glucose? Hypoglycemia risk? Cost? Adverse effects? Medication(s) that help with these issues?		
Medication **Anticipated A1C reduction**	**Mechanism of action**	**Comment**
Biguanide Example- Metformin (Glucophage®) A1C reduction with intensified use=1–2% (0.01–0.02 proportion) **First-line medication unless contraindicated**	*Insulin sensitizer, reduces hepatic glucose production and intestinal glucose absorption* *Action on fasting and postprandial glucose, minimal to no inherent hypoglycemic risk when used as a solo product*	Lactic acidosis risk (rare) usually with identified risk factors including impaired renal or hepatic function, hypovolemia, low perfusion state including heart failure, and/or advanced age (>80 years). National Institutes of Health- eGFR below 45 mL/min per 1.73 m^2 for metformin discontinuation. With condition that can potentially alter hydration status (radiocontrast use, surgery, other), omit metformin for the day of and ≥48 h post condition resolution and reinitiate once baseline hydration and renal function have been reestablished. Metformin for DM prevention at 1500–2000 mg daily for prevention of type 2 diabetes can be considered in those at highest risk for developing T2DM. Metformin use increases risk of vitamin B_{12} deficiency due to B_{12} malabsorption, risk appears dose- and length of therapy-dependent.
Thiazolidinedione (TZD, glitazones) Examples- Pioglitazone (Actos®), rosiglitazone (Avandia®) A1C reduction with intensified use=1–2% (0.01–0.02 proportion)	*Insulin sensitizer* *Action on fasting and postprandial glucose, minimal to no inherent hypoglycemic risk when used as a solo product*	Edema risk, particularly when used with insulin or SU. Do not initiate with risk or in presence of heart failure. In consideration of cardiovascular risk, use with insulin or nitrates not recommended. Rare risk (<0.5%) of hepatic toxicity with use. Monitor ALT periodically.
Sulfonylurea (SU) Examples- Glipizide (Glucotrol®), glyburide (DiaBeta®), glimepiride (Amaryl®) A1C reduction with intensified use=1–2% (0.01–0.02 proportion) **Often considered, in addition to metformin, when a 2nd medication is needed.**	*Increases insulin release* from pancreatic beta cells *Action on fasting and postprandial glucose, hypoglycemia risk, especially in elders, presence of impaired renal function*	Due to failing beta cell function, typically less effective after many years T2DM Dx, older adults, in the presence of severe hyperglycemia.

Continued...

Table 11-5 (cont.): Pharmacologic Intervention in T2DM		
Medication **A1C reduction**	**Mechanism of action**	**Comment**
Dipeptidyl peptidase-4 (DPP-4) inhibitor Examples- Sitagliptin (Januvia®), saxagliptin (Onglyza®), linagliptin (Tradjenta®), alogliptin (Nesina®) A1C reduction with intensified use=0.6–1.4% (0.006–0.014 proportion)	*Increases insulin release, largely in response to increased blood glucose post meal.* *Action largely on postprandial blood glucose, minimal to no inherent hypoglycemia risk*	Per FDA advisory, pancreatitis risk with use, also unexplained joint aches with DPP-4 inhibitor use.
GLP-1 agonist **Injection only** Examples- Exenatide (Bydureon®, Byetta®), liraglutide (Victoza®, Saxenda®), albiglutide (Tanzeum®) A1C reduction with intensified use=1–2% (0.01–0.02 proportion)	*Increases insulin release, largely in response to increased blood glucose post meal.* *Action largely on postprandial blood glucose, little inherent hypoglycemia risk* Slows gastric emptying, often leading to appetite suppression and weight loss.	Major adverse effect=N/V, usually better with dose adjustment, continued use, contraindicated in gastroparesis Rare pancreatitis risk with GLP-1 agonist use. Discontinue GLP-1 agonist use if pancreatitis symptoms or with history of pancreatitis. **Source:** **http://www.fda.gov/Safety/MedWatch/SafetyInformation/ucm194556.htm** Do not prescribe with severe renal impairment or ESRD.
Sodium glucose cotransporter-2 (SGLT2) inhibitor Examples- Canagliflozin (Invokana®), dapagliflozin (Farxiga®), empagliflozin (Jardiance®) A1C reduction with intensified used=0.7–1% (0.007–0.01 proportion)	*Action largely by lowering plasma glucose levels by increasing the amount of glucose excreted in urine.* *Primarily postprandial glucose effect.* *Hypoglycemic risk related to glucose offload, increased when used with insulin and insulin secretagogues.*	Adverse effects=Genital mycotic infection (~10% female, ~5% male), UTI, increased urination. Modest weight loss (4–7 lbs [1.8–3.2 kg]), greater with higher dose Adjust dose or discontinue in renal impairment due to increased risk of adverse effects, electrolyte disturbances, less therapeutic effect. FDA advisory about diabetic ketoacidosis and urosepsis risk with SGLT2 inhibitor use. See http://www.fda.gov/downloads/Drugs/DrugSafety/UCM446954.pdf for details.

Source: http://care.diabetesjournals.org/content/33/Supplement_1/S3.full

Location of action for type 2 diabetes medications

Figure 11-3

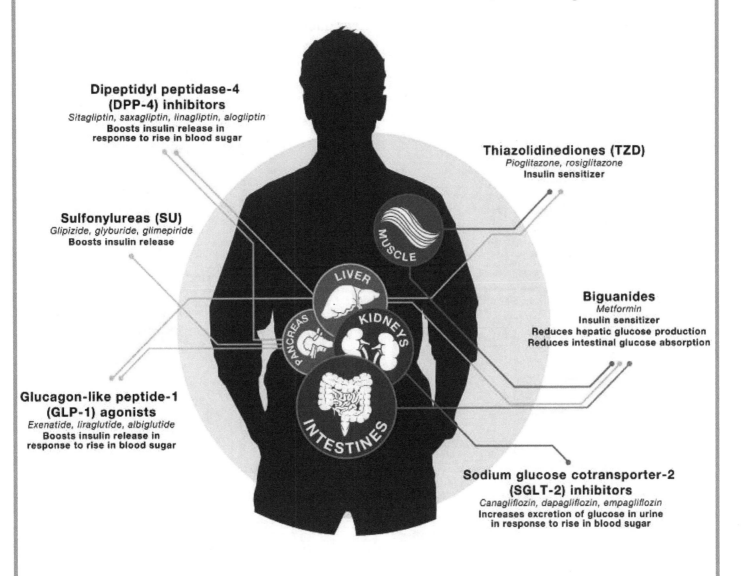

Dipeptidyl peptidase-4 (DPP-4) inhibitors
Sitagliptin, saxagliptin, linagliptin, alogliptin
Boosts insulin release in response to rise in blood sugar

Thiazolidinediones (TZD)
Pioglitazone, rosiglitazone
Insulin sensitizer

Sulfonylureas (SU)
Glipizide, glyburide, glimepiride
Boosts insulin release

Biguanides
Metformin
Insulin sensitizer
Reduces hepatic glucose production
Reduces intestinal glucose absorption

Glucagon-like peptide-1 (GLP-1) agonists
Exenatide, liraglutide, albiglutide
Boosts insulin release in response to rise in blood sugar

Sodium glucose cotransporter-2 (SGLT-2) inhibitors
Canagliflozin, dapagliflozin, empagliflozin
Increases excretion of glucose in urine in response to rise in blood sugar

ADA Clinical Practice Recommendations in T2DM
Keep in mind action and anticipated clinical effect of each medication.

Figure 11-4

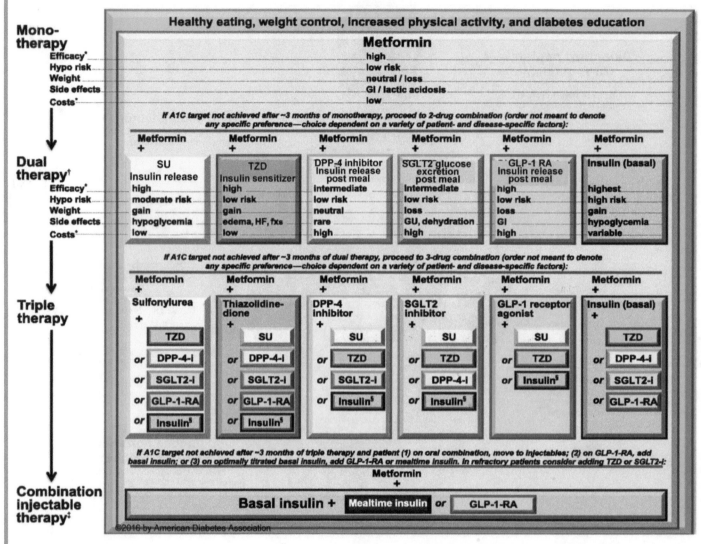

Table 11-6: When to Use Insulin in DM Treatment

Type 1 DM	Type 2 DM
All patients Basal insulin with adjustments for meals via multiple injections or pump • Basal (long-acting) =40–50% total daily insulin • Bolus (rapid-acting) =50–60% total daily insulin, given in response to carbohydrate intake post meals and with snacks	At time of diagnosis to help achieve initial glycemic control, particularly when A1C at time of diagnosis ≥9% with symptoms (classic polys, visual changes, others). • Impaired insulin release and action is a consequence of hyperglycemia. Hyperglycemia itself induces insulin resistance and impairs pancreatic β cell function. A short course (2–3 weeks) of insulin to help achieve normoglycemia When ≥2 standard agents at optimized doses are inadequate to maintain glycemic control When acutely ill • In critically ill surgical and nonsurgical patients with type 1 or type 2 DM, blood glucose levels should be kept generally 140–180 mg/dL (7.8–10 mmol/L). Overtreatment and undertreatment of hyperglycemia represent major safety concerns.

Source: American Diabetes Association. Standards of Medical Care in Diabetes, available at
http://care.diabetesjournals.org/content/27/5/1028.full.pdf

Table 11-7: Insulin: Type, Onset, Peak, and Duration of Action Is there a pharmacodynamic difference in insulins? Critical to consider onset of action, peak of action, duration of action when prescribing insulin.			
Insulin type	**Onset of action**	**Peak** (Most likely when hypoglycemic reaction can occur)	**Duration of action**
Short-acting, rapid-acting (preferred short-acting insulin form) Insulin glulisine (Apidra®), insulin lispro (Humalog®), and insulin aspart (NovoLog®)	Approximately 15 min	Approximately 1 h	Approximately 4 h
Short-acting (Regular, trade names Humulin R®, Novolin R®)	Approximately 30 min	Approximately 2–3 h	3–6 h
Long-acting (preferred basal insulin form) Insulin detemir (Levemir®) and insulin glargine (Basaglar KwikPen®, Lantus®, Lantus Solostar Pen®, Toujeo SoloStar®)	Approximately 1–2 h	None	Approximately 24 h
Intermediate-acting (NPH trade names Novolin N®, Humulin N®)	1–2 h	6–14 h	16–24 h

Source:
http://www.diabetes.org/living-with-diabetes/treatment-and-care/medication/insulin/insulin-basics.html

1. You see Kevin, a 25-year-old man with a BMI=38 kg/m^2 and hyperpigmented plaques with a velvet-like appearance at the nape of the neck and axillary region. He states his skin has had this appearance since he was approximately age 13 and it has not changed significantly over time. He denies itch or pain in these areas. This most likely represents:

    A. Acanthosis nigricans.

    B. Lichens planus.

    C. Actinic keratosis.

    D. Erythema migrans.

2. As part of Kevin's healthcare, consideration should be given for obtaining which of the following laboratory tests?

    A. Hemoglobin A1C

    B. Serum transaminases

    C. Rapid plasma reagent

    D. Erythrocyte sedimentation rate

3. With Kevin's skin condition, lesions are most often found in all of the following areas except:

 A. Groin folds.

 B. Over the knuckles.

 C. Elbows.

 D. Plantar surface of the feet.

4. You see an 81-year-old woman with type 2 DM. Today she presents for follow-up care. Results of recent laboratory assessment include the following: GFR=45 mL/min/1.73 m^2, A1C=7.2% (0.072 proportion), K$^+$=4.8 mEq/L (4.8 mmol/L). Her current medications include metformin, glyburide, lisinopril, and simvastatin. She is generally feeling well, is self-sufficient in ADL, and states, "I can get around in my home with my cane. I am a little less certain on my feet if I do not use the cane." As part of her ongoing healthcare, you consider all of the following except:

 A. Due to age and impaired renal function, her risk of adverse effects from metformin is increased.

 B. Glipizide is preferred over glyburide as a sulfonylurea in the older adult.

 C. With poor hydration, she is at risk for hyperkalemia.

 D. She should be treated to an A1C goal of <7% (0.07 proportion).

5. You see a 55-year-old woman with type 2 diabetes mellitus, hypertension, and dyslipidemia. Evaluation today reveals a BMI=36 kg/m^2. She states, "I just do not know where to start in trying to lose some weight." Which of the following is the most appropriate response to this statement?

 A. "How much weight do you want to lose?"

 B. "How do you feel about your weight?"

 C. "What barriers do you see to losing weight?"

 D. "Your blood sugar control will likely improve if you lose some weight."

Table 11-8: Motivational Interviewing (MI) – (William Miller)	
Evidence-based practice	Evidence to support use of MI with substance use disorders, chronic medical illnesses (e.g., diabetes, cardiovascular disease, obesity)
Guiding principles	Partnership with patient, work on self-efficacy. Provider doesn't have what the patient needs; the patient has what he/she needs. Struggles with ambivalence are expected and normal.
Goals	To support change in a person that is consistent with their own values and concerns

Techniques	Express empathy
	Develop a discrepancy
	Roll with resistance
	Support self-efficacy
	Reflective listening
	Change talk (examples)
	  • Explore pros and cons of behavior change
	  • Look back to a previous time—how were things different?
	  • Explore values
	  • Explore negative side of ambivalence
	Ask open-ended questions
	Affirming statements: Recognize patient's strengths
	Summarize: Review of session
	Provide information
	  • Ask-provide-ask

Sources: Miller W, Rose G. Toward a theory of motivational interviewing. *Am Psychol.* 2009;64(6):527-537.

Rollnick, S., Miller, W., & Butler, C. (2008). <u>Motivational interviewing in health care: Helping patients change behavior</u>. New York, NY: Guilford Press.

Table 11-9: DM Type 2: Additional Care Considerations

A	Aspirin 75–162 mg/d (use clopidogrel [Plavix®] 75 mg/d in aspirin allergy) in most, esp. men age>50 years, women age>60 years with DM and ≥1 additional CVD risk factor such as HTN, smoking, family history, others
B	Blood pressure control with T2DM and HTN, ≥2 agents including thiazide-type diuretic, ACEI, or ARB, usually required per ADA recommendations
C	Cholesterol: HMG-CoA reductase inhibitor (statin) therapy usually indicated, in particular for anyone age>40 years or with a history of ACS. Check fasting lipid profile annually, consider less often if evidence of stability. Creatinine (renal function): Check serum creatinine, calculated GFR, and urine microalbumin annually.
D	Diet: Limit trans and saturated fats, healthiest foods in appropriate amounts at every meal. Medical nutritional therapy (MNT) with a registered dietician advisable. Dental care: Reinforce ongoing dental care and treatment of dental disease.
E	Exercise, increase physical activity, if not contraindicated, to ≥150 min/wk of moderate activity, such as walking, best in the form of ≥30 min, ≥5 times/wk, resistance exercise ≥3 times/wk. Vigorous aerobic or resistance activity is potentially contraindicated in the presence of proliferative or severe nonproliferative retinopathy due to the possible risk of vitreous hemorrhage or retinal detachment. Eye exam (dilated) annually, increase frequency as dictated by developing retinopathy or other eye problems
F	Foot examination (visual) with every visit, teach protective foot behavior, comprehensive lower extremity sensory exam annually, using 10 g monofilament with ≥1 of the following: Vibration using a 128 Hz tuning fork, pinprick sensation, ankle reflexes, or vibration threshold
G	Goals: Periodically review overall goals of care with patient.

Sources: American Diabetes Association. Standards of Medical Care in Diabetes—2014,
available at http://care.diabetesjournals.org/content/37/Supplement_1/S14.extract

Massachusetts Guidelines for Adult Diabetes Care, available at
www.mass.gov/eohhs/docs/dph/com-health/diabetes/diabetes-guidelines-adult.pdf

Table 11-10: Metabolic Syndrome

Components	Pathophysiology	Treatment and goals
• Large waistline • Hypercholesterolemia • Low HDL cholesterol • High blood pressure • High glucose	Causes include overweight and obesity, an inactive lifestyle, and insulin resistance. Other factors include older age and genetics. Multiple mechanisms of metabolic syndrome lead to various target organ damage. Condition increases risk of heart disease, diabetes, renal dysfunction, and stroke.	Lifestyle changes to lose weight through healthy diet and increasing activity; smoking cessation. Treat each component to goal as determined by nationally-recognized guidelines: • Reduce LDL-cholesterol with statins • Increase HDL-cholesterol with lifestyle modification, possibly with use of fibrate or niacin • Reduce high blood pressure through various agents (diuretics, ACE inhibitors, ARBs, CCBs) • Reduce blood sugar with standard oral diabetes medication or insulin injection • Aspirin to reduce risk of blood clots and stroke

Sources: Wang SS. Metabolic syndrome. Available at:
http://emedicine.medscape.com/article/165124-overview

National Heart, Lung, and Blood Institute. Metabolic Syndrome. Available at:
http://www.nhlbi.nih.gov/health/health-topics/topics/ms/

Important additional study resources available through your Fitzgerald Health online learning portal at fhea.com/npexpert

- Resource 11-1: Diabetic Retinopathy, Including Visual Images, Assessment, and Intervention
- Resource 11-2: A Stepwise Approach to Prescribing Insulin

Texas Diabetes Council, available at http://www.tdctoolkit.org/algorithms-guidelines/

- Prevention and Delay of Type 2 Diabetes in Children and Adults
- Glycemic Control Algorithm for Type 2 Diabetes Mellitus in Adults
- Insulin Algorithm for Type 1 Diabetes Mellitus in Children and Adults

Bonus questions for this chapter available through your Fitzgerald Health learning portal at fhea.com/npexpert.

Insulin Algorithm for Type 2 Diabetes Mellitus in Children and Adults

TEXAS
Department of
State Health Services

Stock # 45-11647

TD
TEXAS DIABETES
COUNCIL

Revised 10/28/10

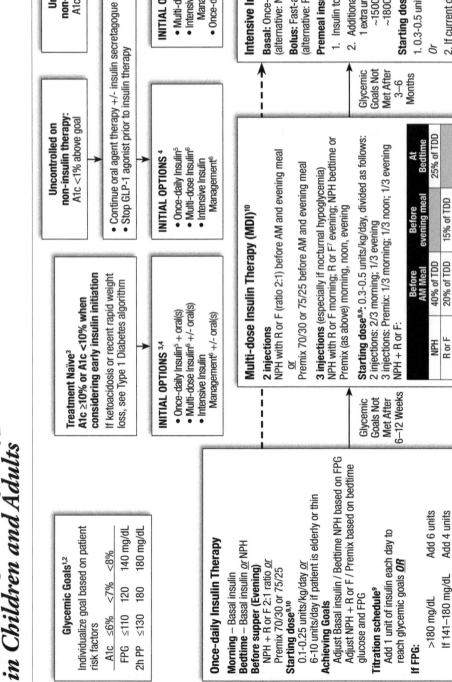

Glycemic Goals[1,2]

Individualize goal based on patient risk factors

A1c	≤6%	<7%	<8%
FPG	≤110	120	140 mg/dL
2h PP	≤130	180	180 mg/dL

Treatment Naïve[3]
A1c ≥10% or A1c <10% when considering early insulin initiation

If ketoacidosis or recent rapid weight loss, see Type 1 Diabetes algorithm

INITIAL OPTIONS[3,4]
- Once-daily Insulin[5] + oral(s)
- Multi-dose Insulin[6] +/- oral(s)
- Intensive Insulin Management[6] +/- oral(s)

Uncontrolled on non-insulin therapy:
A1c <1% above goal

- Continue oral agent therapy +/- insulin secretagogue
- Stop GLP-1 agonist prior to insulin therapy

INITIAL OPTIONS[4]
- Once-daily Insulin[5]
- Multi-dose Insulin[6]
- Intensive Insulin Management[6]

Uncontrolled on non-insulin therapy:
A1c ≥1% above goal

INITIAL OPTIONS[4]
- Multi-dose Insulin[6]
- Intensive Insulin Management[6]
- Once-daily Insulin[5]

Basal insulin: Glargine or Detemir
Bolus insulin: Aspart or Glulisine or Lispro
Fast-acting insulin: Aspart; Glulisine; Lispro
F: Fast-acting insulin
R: Regular insulin
FPG: Fasting plasma glucose
PP: Postprandial plasma glucose
SMBG: Self-monitored blood glucose
TDD: Total daily dose of insulin

Pramlintide
Consider as adjunct therapy to insulin in patients unable to stabilize post-prandial glucose

Once-daily Insulin Therapy

Morning – Basal insulin
Bedtime – Basal insulin or NPH
Before supper (Evening)
NPH + R or F 2:1 ratio or
Premix 70/30 or 75/25

Starting dose[9,10]
0.1–0.25 units/kg/day or
6-10 units/day if patient is elderly or thin

Achieving Goals
Adjust Basal insulin / Bedtime NPH based on FPG
Adjust NPH + R or F / Premix based on bedtime glucose and FPG

Titration schedule[9]
Add 1 unit of insulin each day to reach glycemic goals **OR**

If FPG:
>180 mg/dL	Add 6 units
If 141–180 mg/dL	Add 4 units
If 121–140 mg/dL	Add 2 units
If 100–120 mg/dL	Add 1 unit
If 80-99 mg/dL	No change
If <80 mg/dL	Subtract 2 units

Multi-dose Insulin Therapy (MDI)[10]

2 injections
NPH with R or F (ratio 2:1) before AM and evening meal
or
Premix 70/30 or 75/25 before AM and evening meal

3 injections (especially if nocturnal hypoglycemia)
NPH with R or F morning; R or F[7] evening; NPH bedtime or
Premix (as above) morning, noon, evening

Starting dose[8,9]: 0.3–0.5 units/kg/day, divided as follows:
2 injections: 2/3 morning; 1/3 evening
3 injections: Premix: 1/3 morning; 1/3 noon; 1/3 evening
NPH + R or F:

	Before AM Meal	Before evening meal	At Bedtime
NPH	40% of TDD		25% of TDD
R or F	20% of TDD	15% of TDD	

Intensive Insulin Management[10]

Basal: Once-daily, either morning or bedtime (alternative: NPH morning and bedtime)
Bolus: Fast-acting insulin before each meal; (alternative: R may be used)
Premeal insulin dose includes:
1. Insulin to cover carbohydrate ingested[11] &
2. Additional insulin to correct for high SMBG:
   1 extra unit premeal insulin ↓ glucose (mg/dL)
   ~1500/TDD for Regular;
   ~1800/TDD for Aspart/Glulisine/Lispro

Starting dose[8,9]:
1. 0.3-0.5 units/kg/day (1:1 basal:bolus ratio SQ)
Or
2. If current dose >0.5 units/kg/day
   Basal dose = 80% Total daily NPH *or*
   80% Total long-acting component of premix
   Bolus dose = 80% of basal dose divided between 3 meals

Glycemic Goals Not Met After 6–12 Weeks

Glycemic Goals Not Met After 3–6 Months

Follow A1c every 3-6 months and Adjust Regimen to Maintain Glycemic Goals

Footnotes

1. **Intensify management if:** Absent/stable cardiovascular disease, mild-moderate microvascular complications, intact hypoglycemia awareness, infrequent hypoglycemic episodes, recently diagnosed diabetes: **Less intensive management if:** Evidence of advanced or poorly controlled cardiovascular and/or microvascular complications, hypoglycemia unawareness, vulnerable patient (ie, impaired cognition, dementia, fall history). SEE "A1c Goal" treatment strategy for further explanation. A1c is referenced to a non-diabetic range of 4-6% using a DCCT-based assay. ADA Clinical Practice Recommendations Diabetes Care 2009;32(suppl 1):S19-20.

2. Current glucose meters give values corrected to plasma glucose.

3. May also begin combination oral agent therapy. See Glycemic Control Algorithm for Type 2 Diabetes Mellitus in Children and Adults.

4. Combining metformin with insulin therapy has been shown to result in less weight gain and better glycemic control with lower insulin requirements.

5. Continue combination oral agent therapy ± sulfonylurea.

6. Continue metformin (± 3rd oral agent); probably discontinue sulfonylurea.

7. Fast-acting insulin is given with the start of each meal. Regular insulin to be given 30-60 minutes before meals.

8. Dosage may differ in children and adolescents; consider referral to pediatric endocrinologist/comprehensive diabetes specialty team.

9. Start lower and increase slower for thin/elderly/complicated patients.

10. Consider referral to pediatric/adult endocrinologist/diabetes specialty team (option – insulin pump, Pramlintide).

11. Typical "carb" bolus = 1 unit bolus insulin covers 500/TDI x g carbohydrate from meal (~10-15 gm); **strongly recommend referral to Registered/Licensed Dietitian or Certified Diabetes Educator with experience in diabetes nutrition counseling (see Worksheet D).**

See disclaimer at www.tdctoolkit.org/algorithms_and_guidelines.asp

Initiation of Once Daily Insulin Therapy for Type 2 Diabetes Mellitus in Children and Adults

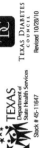
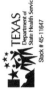

TEXAS
Department of
State Health Services

TEXAS DIABETES COUNCIL

Stock # 45-11647

Revised 10/28/10

Abbreviations:

FPG: Fasting plasma glucose

SMBG: Self-monitored blood glucose

PP: Postprandial plasma glucose

Glycemic Goals[2,3]

Individualize goal based on patient risk factors

A1c	≤6%	<7%	<8%
FPG	≤110	120	140 mg/dL
2h PP	≤130	180	180 mg/dL

Treatment Naïve[3]:

A1c ≥10% or A1c <10% when considering early insulin initiation

If ketoacidosis or recent rapid weight loss, see Type 1 Diabetes algorithm

→

Oral Agent Failure;
A1c above target

→

Initiate Insulin Therapy with daily Glargine or Detemir or bedtime NPH[5,6]

↓

Beginning Dosage: 10 units or 0.1–0.25 units/Kg

↓

Suggested Titration Schedule – Adjust Every 2-3 Days

If FPG:

>180 mg/dL	Add 6 units
If 141–180 mg/dL	Add 4 units
If 121–140 mg/dL	Add 2 units
If 100–120 mg/dL	Add 1 unit
If 80-99 mg/dL	No change
If <80 mg/dL	Subtract 2 units

OR

Add 1unit insulin each day until fasting SMBG is at goal

↓

If A1c remains >A1c goal over 3 months, discontinue oral secretagogue, continue oral insulin sensitizer(s) and initiate multi-dose insulin or intensive insulin therapy[1] or consult an endocrinologist

---

Footnotes

1   For the complete approach to insulin initiation in Type 2 Diabetes Mellitus, see Insulin Algorithm for Type 2 Diabetes Mellitus in Children and Adults.

2   **Intensify management if:** Absent/stable cardiovascular disease, mild-moderate microvascular complications, intact hypoglycemia awareness, infrequent hypoglycemic episodes, recently diagnosed diabetes. **Less intensive management if:** Evidence of advanced or poorly controlled cardiovascular and/or microvascular complications, hypoglycemia unawareness, vulnerable patient (ie, impaired cognition, dementia, fall history). See "A1c Goal" treatment strategy for further explanation. A1c is referenced to a non-diabetic range of 4-6% using a DCCT-based assay. ADA Clinical Practice Recommendations. *Diabetes Care* 2009;32(suppl 1):S19-20.

3   Current glucose meters give values corrected to plasma glucose.

4   Usually with an insulin secretagogue (sulfonylurea, repaglinide or nateglinide) and sensitizer (metformin or thiazolidinedione). See Glycemic Control Algorithm.

5   The pharmacokinetic profile of NPH compared to that of glargine or detemir is less predictable, therefore can result in blood sugar variations and increased nocturnal hypoglycemia. Cost of glargine or detemir is 1.5-2 times that of NPH. Lispro 75/25 or Aspart 70/30 can be considered at pre-supper adjusting dosage according to HS **and** fasting SMBG.

6   **IMPORTANT:** See package insert for dosing.

7   If daytime hypoglycemia develops, contact healthcare professional.

See disclaimer at www.tdctoolkit.org/algorithms_and_guidelines.asp

Worksheet: Advancing to Intensive/Physiologic Basal: Bolus Insulin Therapy

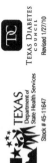

TEXAS
Department of
State Health Services
Stock #45-11647

TDC
TEXAS DIABETES
COUNCIL
Revised 1/27/10

Note: "Analog" = Rapid Acting (Bolus) Analog insulin throughout this document.

A. Conversion from once-daily insulin to intensive/physiologic insulin replacement:

Oral therapy failure: Once-daily glargine was added to the oral regimen and titrated to 30 units per day. How do you add analog insulin if the patient reports the following SMBG values?

	FPG	2-HR PP BRKFT	2-HR PP LUNCH	2-HR PP DINNER
Case 1	105	140	140	240
Case 2	105	140	190	240
Case 3	105	190	240	240

Case 1

a. Continue the oral agents (± sulfonylurea) and 30 units glargine or detemir (or NPH)

b. There are 2 approaches for adding analog (RAI) 10-15 minutes before a meal:

#1   Arbitrary start: 5 units
      Titrate: Add 2 units every 2 days to reach 2-hr pp goal

#2   Carb-counting   1 unit/50 mg/dL over 2-hr pp goal

            <u>PLUS</u>

            1 unit/15 grams carbohydrate

      Titrate: Add 1 unit/50 mg/dL >2-hr pp goal every 2 days

Cases 2 and 3

As above, but add and titrate analog before each meal where the postprandial glucose is above goal. Also, see part D below for more information on how to optimize the use of analog insulin. Re-evaluate each week to be certain that about half of the total daily dose is basal and half is bolus insulin.

B. Conversion from once-daily premix to intensive/physiologic insulin replacement:

Oral therapy failure: Once-daily 70/30 premixed insulin was added and titrated to 30 units per day. The fasting glucose is at goal, but daytime control is poor. How do you convert to physiologic insulin therapy?

a. **Basal insulin dose:** The first step in the conversion is based on the total dose of intermediate-acting insulin. In this case, the person is taking 21 units of NPH or aspart-protamine insulin (70% x 30 units=21 units). So, give 21 units basal glargine (use "unit-for-unit" conversion for once-daily intermediate regimens). *Remember, do not stop oral agents (+ sulfonylurea) at this time.*

b. **Bolus insulin dose:** There are several ways to start the analog.

  i. *See Case 1 (Arbitrary start or Carb-counting)*

  ii. Begin with the previous dose of fast-acting insulin, divide it before meals and titrate every 2 days. In this case, the person was using 30 units of 70/30 or about 9 units of fast-acting insulin (30% x 30 units=9 units). So give 3 units of analog before each meal and titrate every 2 days as per Case 1.

C. Conversion from twice-daily premix to intensive/physiologic insulin replacement:

Oral therapy failure in an 80 kg person: 70/30 premixed insulin was started and advanced to 60 units per day: 40 units before breakfast and 20 units before dinner. The fasting glucose was at goal, but wide glycemic excursions occurred at other times during the day and night. How do you convert this person to physiologic insulin therapy? There are several approaches. Use which ever method you want.

a. <u>Start over</u> and begin insulin at 0.5 units/kg. Give half as basal insulin and half as analog, divided before meals. In this case, the starting dose would be 40 units per day. Start giving 20 units glargine each morning and about 7 units analog before each meal. Titrate the basal and bolus insulins every 2 days to fasting and 2-hr postprandial goals.

b. Conversion based on current insulin usage:

  Basal dose: The first step in the conversion is based on the **80% of the total dose of intermediate-acting insulin.** In this case, the person is taking 42 units of NPH or aspart-protamine insulin (70% x 60 units = 42 units). When a person is taking multiple doses of intermediate-acting insulin, we give only 80% as glargine (80% x 42=~34). *Remember, do not stop oral agents (+ sulfonylurea) at this time.*

  Bolus insulin dose: There are several ways to start the analog.

  i. *See Case 1 (Arbitrary start or Carb-counting)*

  ii. Begin with the previous dose of fast-acting insulin, divide it before meals and titrate every 2 days. In this case, the person was using 60 units of 70/30 or 18 units of fast-acting insulin (30% x 60 units = 18 units). So, give 6 units of analog before each meal and titrate every 2 days as per Case 1.

c. The **"80%-80%" rule:** Similar to the above method, but yields an ideal ratio of basal:bolus insulin in one step. The dose of basal glargine will be 80% of the total intermediate insulin, and the analog will be 80% of the glargine dose, divided before meals.

Basal dose: = 80% of total intermediate insulin

= 80% x 42 units (70% x 60 = 42)

= 34 units glargine

Analog dose: = 80% of the glargine dose, divided TID

= 80% x 34 units = 27 units

= 27 units, divided TID = 9 units

= 9 units aspart, glulisine or lispro before meals

Note: Total dose of insulin is conserved and an ideal ratio between basal and bolus will always result with the "80%–80%" method.

D. Optimizing analog insulin use

Tight control of blood glucose requires that the patient participates in the management of their diabetes. This includes monitoring their blood glucose and learning to count carbohydrates or "carb count." The following material explains how to calculate the dose of analog required to cover a meal and how to add extra analog to correct a hyperglycemic event.

a. Determining the dose of analog insulin to use before a meal

The "**Rule of 500**" is used to determine how many grams of carbohydrate 1 unit of analog insulin will cover. When this number is known, then the person can easily give the correct dose of analog by simply counting the grams of carbohydrate they intend to eat at the meal.

Specifically, 500 divided by the total daily insulin dose (500/TDI) yields the number of grams of carbohydrate that 1 unit of analog will cover. For example, if a person has established that they require about 50 units of insulin per day, then it follows that 1 unit of analog will cover 10 grams of carbohydrate (500/50 = 10). If the person carb counts 140 grams in the dinner meal, then the dose of analog will be 14 units given 10 minutes before eating.

b. Correcting for hyperglycemia

The "**Rule of 1800**" is used to determine how much insulin to use to bring a high glucose reading back to goal. Even with tight control, hyperglycemia occurs and people need to be able to correct this situation.

Specifically, 1800 divided by the total daily insulin dose yields a value indicating how much 1 unit of analog insulin will lower the blood glucose. Thus, if a person uses 90 units of insulin per day, then 1 unit of analog will reduce the blood glucose by 20 mg/dL (1800/90 = 20). **This augment dose of insulin can be used by itself to correct hyperglycemia, or added to the bolus dose if glucose is high before a meal.**

References

1. Riddle MC, Rosenstock J, Gerich J. *Diabetes Care.* 2003; 26:3080-3086.

2. Spellman CW, Renda SM, Davis SN. *Realizing the Potential of Insulin Therapy in Type 2 Diabetes: A Case Presentation-Based Monograph.* presented at the American College of Osteopathic Internists 64th Annual Convention; Chicago, IL (September 30, 2004).

3. www.texasdiabetescouncil.org.

Reviews/Important Articles

- Abraira C, Colwell J, Nuttall F, et al. Cardiovascular events and correlates in the Veterans Affairs Diabetes Feasibility Trial. Veterans Affairs Cooperative Study on Glycemic Control and Complications in Type II Diabetes. *Arch Intern Med.* 1997;157(2):181-8.

- Anonymous. Intensive blood-glucose control with sulphonylureas or insulin compared with conventional treatment and risk of complications in patients with type 2 diabetes (UKPDS 33). UK Prospective Diabetes Study (UKPDS) Group. *Lancet.* 1998;352(9131):837-53.

- DeWitt DE, Dugdale DC. Using new insulin strategies in the outpatient treatment of diabetes: clinical applications. *JAMA.* 2003;289(17):2265-9.

- DeWitt DE, Hirsch IB. Outpatient insulin therapy in type 1 and type 2 diabetes mellitus: scientific review. *JAMA.* 2003;289(17):2254-64.

- Implementation Conference for ACE Outpatient Diabetes Mellitus Consensus Conference Recommendations: Position Statement, February 2, 2005. Available online at http://www.aace.com/pub/odimplementation/PositionStatement.pdf. Accessed on May 2, 2005.

- Hirsch IB. Insulin analogues. *N Engl J Med.* 2005;352(2):174-83.

Once Daily Insulin

Morning vs. Bedtime NPH

- Groop LC, Widen E, Ekstrand A, et al. Morning or bedtime NPH insulin combined with sulfonylurea in treatment of NIDDM. *Diabetes Care.* 1992;15(7):831-4.

Morning vs. Bedtime Glargine

- Fritsche A, Schweitzer MA, Haring HU. Glimepiride combined with morning insulin glargine, bedtime neutral protamine hagedorn insulin, or bedtime insulin glargine in patients with type 2 diabetes. A randomized, controlled trial. *Ann Intern Med.* 2003;138(12):952-9.

NPH vs. Glargine

- Riddle MC, Rosenstock J, Gerich J. The treat-to-target trial: randomized addition of glargine or human NPH insulin to oral therapy of type 2 diabetic patients. *Diabetes Care.* 2003;26(11):3080-6.

Once Daily vs. Twice Daily Regimen

- Raskin P, Allen E, Hollander P, et al. Initiating insulin therapy in type 2 diabetes: a comparison of biphasic and basal insulin analogs. *Diabetes Care.* 2005;28(2):260-5.

Multiple Dose Insulin Regimens (2-shot Regimens)

NPH/Regular vs. NPH/ short acting analogue therapy

- Vignati L, Anderson JH Jr, Iversen PW. Efficacy of insulin lispro in combination with NPH human insulin twice per day in patients with insulin-dependent or noninsulin-dependent diabetes mellitus. Multicenter Insulin Lispro Study Group. *Clin Ther.* 1997;19(6):1408-21.

70% NPH/ 30% Regular vs. Humalog Mix 75/25™ or Novolog Mix 70/30™

- Roach P, Yue L, Arora V. Improved postprandial glycemic control during treatment with Humalog Mix25, a novel protamine-based insulin lispro formulation. Humalog Mix25 Study Group. *Diabetes Care.* 1999;22(8):1258-61.

- Boehm BO, Home PD, Behrend C, et al. Premixed insulin aspart 30 vs. premixed human insulin 30/70 twice daily: a randomized trial in type 1 and type 2 diabetic patients. *Diabet Med.* 2002;19(5):393-9.

Multiple Dose Insulin Regimens (3-shot Regimens)

- Ohkubo Y, Kishikawa H, Araki E, et al. Intensive insulin therapy prevents the progression of diabetic microvascular complications in Japanese patients with non-insulin-dependent diabetes mellitus: a randomized prospective 6-year study. Diabetes Res Clin Pract. 1995;28(2):103-17.

Intensive Insulin Therapy

- Ohkubo Y, Kishikawa H, Araki E, et al. Intensive insulin therapy prevents the progression of diabetic microvascular complications in Japanese patients with non-insulin-dependent diabetes mellitus: a randomized prospective 6-year study. *Diabetes Res Clin Pract.* 1995;28(2):103-17.

- Saudek CD, Duckworth WC, Giobbie-Hurder A, et al. Implantable insulin pump vs multiple-dose insulin for non-insulin-dependent diabetes mellitus: a randomized clinical trial. Department of Veterans Affairs Implantable Insulin Pump Study Group. *JAMA.* 1996;276(16):1322-7.

- Raskin P, Bode BW, Marks JB, et al. Continuous subcutaneous insulin infusion and multiple daily injection therapy are equally effective in type 2 diabetes: a randomized, parallel-group, 24-week study. *Diabetes Care.* 2003;26(9):2598-603.

- Bretzel RG, Arnolds S, Medding J, et al. A direct efficacy and safety comparison of insulin aspart, human soluble insulin, and human premix insulin (70/30) in patients with type 2 diabetes. *Diabetes Care.* 2004;27(5):1023-7.

Resources for Additional Study

Books:

Fitzgerald, M. A. (2017) Endocrine Disorders, Nurse Practitioner Certification Examination and Practice Preparation, 5th Edition, Philadelphia, PA: F.A. Davis.

Audio programs:

Fitzgerald, M. A. Dyslipidemia: An Update on Treatment Goals and Options, North Andover, MA: Fitzgerald Health Education Associates.

Fitzgerald, M. A. Hypertension Update, North Andover, MA: Fitzgerald Health Education Associates.

Fitzgerald, M. A. Laboratory Data Interpretation: A Case Study Approach, North Andover, MA: Fitzgerald Health Education Associates.

Fitzgerald, M. A. Special Considerations in Geriatric Prescribing: Issues of Safety and Efficacy, North Andover, MA: Fitzgerald Health Education Associates.

Fitzgerald, M. A. Type 2 Diabetes Mellitus: Current Issues in Assessment and Intervention, North Andover, MA: Fitzgerald Health Education Associates.

Chapter 12: Cardiovascular Problems: Hypertension, Dyslipidemia, and Heart Failure

Learning activities are an integral part of the course available through your Fitzgerald Health learning portal at fhea.com/npexpert:

Online program for FNP and AGNPs: *Disorders Revealed by the Cardiac Exam: A Focus on Heart Sounds and Murmurs*

BP=HR (heart rate) × SV (stroke volume) × PVR (peripheral vascular resistance). Increase any part of the formula, BP rises; decrease any part of the formula, BP falls.

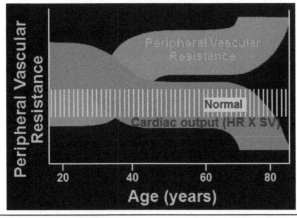

Figure 12-1

Table 12-1: Hypertension (HTN):	
A complex disease with a core defect of vascular dysfunction that leads to select target organ damage (TOD). Treating HTN minimizes risk for HTN TOD.	
Target organ	**Outcome**
Brain	Stroke, vascular (multi-infarct) dementia
Cardiovascular system	Atherosclerosis, myocardial infarction, left ventricular hypertrophy, heart failure
Kidney	Hypertensive nephropathy, renal failure
Eye	Hypertensive retinopathy with risk of blindness

Table 12-2: Hypertensive Retinopathy:		
Retinal Vascular Damage Caused by Poorly-controlled Hypertension *Is there only damage to the retinal vessels?*		
	Grade	**Findings**
Low grade	1 (Common in longstanding poorly-controlled HTN, reversible when HTN treated)	Narrowing of terminal arteriolar branches No vision change or permanent findings
Low grade	2 (Common in longstanding poorly-controlled HTN, reversible when HTN treated)	Narrowing of arterioles with severe local constriction No vision change or permanent findings
High grade	3 (Usually with DBP≥110 mm Hg)	Preceding signs with flame-shaped hemorrhages Potential for visual change and permanent findings
High grade	4 (Usually DBP≥130 mm Hg)	Papilledema with preceding signs Potential for visual change and permanent findings

Table 12-3: Lifestyle Modification Recommendations in HTN and Dyslipidemia

Modification	Recommendation	Average SBP reduction rate
Weight reduction for hypertension and dyslipidemia	Maintain normal body weight (BMI=18.5–24.9 kg/m^2)	5–20 mm Hg per 10 kg weight loss
DASH eating plan for hypertension and dyslipidemia	Adopt a diet rich in fruits, vegetables, and low-fat dairy products with reduced content of saturated and total fat	8–14 mm Hg
Dietary sodium reduction in hypertension	Reduce dietary sodium intake to <100 mmol/d (2.4 g sodium or 6 g sodium chloride)	2–8 mm Hg
Aerobic physical activity for hypertension and dyslipidemia	Moderate to vigorous aerobic physical activity (e.g., brisk walking) at least 40 min/d, 3–4 days of the week, no more than 48 hours without exercise	4–9 mm Hg
Moderation of alcohol consumption in hypertension	Men: Limit to <2 drinks* per day. Women and lighter-weight individuals: Limit to <1 drink* per day.	2–4 mm Hg

* 1 drink=12 oz (0.35 L) of beer, 5 oz (0.15 L) of wine, 1.5 oz (0.04 L) of 80-proof liquor

Source: Stone NJ, et al. 2013 ACC/AHA guideline on the treatment of blood cholesterol to reduce atherosclerotic cardiovascular risk in adults: a report of the American College of Cardiology/American Heart Association Task Force on Practice Guidelines. *Circulation*. 2014;129(25 Suppl 2):S1-45.

For additional information on DASH diet, www.nhlbi.nih.gov/health/public/heart/hbp/dash/new_dash.pdf

JNC-8 emphasizes the use of ACEI/ARB, thiazide diuretics and calcium channel blockers due to comparable clinical outcomes in cardiovascular, cerebrovascular, and renal outcomes, particularly in the general population without DM or CKD.

Table 12-4: Ethnic Differences in Cardiovascular Drug Response: Potential Contribution of Pharmacogenetics

Drug category	Mean BP reduction (SBP/DBP)		White-Black difference
	Whites	Blacks	
Diuretics	11.5/9.1	15/10.7	-3.5/-1.5
CCBs	15.3/12.6	16.9/13.3	-2.4/-0.6
β-blockers	11.7/11.3	5.9/9.5	6/2.9
ACEI/ARB	12.8/11.4	8.5/8	4.6/3

Source: www.ncbi.nlm.nih.gov/pmc/articles/PMC2730023/table/T2

Table 12-5: JNC-8 Blood Pressure Recommendations

For adults ≥18 years with hypertension:

- Implement lifestyle interventions (to be continued throughout management)
- Set blood pressure goal and initiate blood pressure-lowering medication based on age, diabetes mellitus, and chronic kidney disease (CKD)

Step 1: Set BP goal (SBP/DBP)

Any age with diabetes and/or CKD	<140/<90 mm Hg

No diabetes or CKD:
    Age<60 years
    Age≥60 years
	<140/<90 mm Hg
	    <150/<90 mm Hg

Step 2: Initiate therapy (for all ages)

Non-black race, no CKD, with or without DM	Initiate thiazide-type diuretic or ACEI or ARB or CCB, alone or in combination.
Black race, no CKD, with or without DM	Initiate thiazide-type diuretic or CCB, alone or in combination.
All races, with CKD, with or without DM	Initiate ACEI or ARB alone or in combination with other drug classes.

Step 3: Select a drug treatment titration strategy

A. Maximize dose of the first medication before adding second, *or*
B. Add second medication before reaching maximum dose of first medication, *or*
C. Start with 2 medication classes separately or as a fixed-dose combination

When blood pressure goal is met, continue the current treatment and monitoring.

Step 4: Get to Goal: Titrating therapy if needed after 1 month on initial therapy

If BP goal is not attained with initial treatment regimen:

- Reinforce medication and lifestyle adherence.
- For strategies A and B in **Step 3**, add and titrate thiazide-type diuretic or ACEI or ARB or CCB (use medication class not previously selected and avoid combined use of ACEI and ARB). Reevaluate effectiveness of regimen in 1 month.
- For strategy C, titrate initial medications to maximum advisable doses. Reevaluate effectiveness of regimen in 1 month.

If BP goal is still not attained after 1 month of titrated therapy as described above:

- Reinforce medication and lifestyle adherence.
- Add and titrate thiazide-type diuretic or ACEI or ARB or CCB (use medication class not previously selected and avoid combined use of ACEI and ARB). Reevaluate effectiveness of regimen in 1 month.

If BP goal is still not attained after 1 month of titrated therapy as described above:

- Reinforce medication and lifestyle adherence.
- Add additional medication class (e.g., beta-blocker, aldosterone antagonist, or others) and/or refer to healthcare provider with expertise in hypertension management. Reevaluate effectiveness of regimen in 1 month.

ACEI, angiotensin-converting enzyme inhibitor; ARB, angiotensin II receptor blocker; CCB, calcium channel blocker; CKD, chronic kidney disease. Do not prescribe ACEI with ARB.

Source: 2014 Evidence-based Guideline for the Management of High Blood Pressure in Adults: Report from the Panel Members Appointed to the Eighth Joint National Committee (JNC 8). *JAMA*. 2013 Dec 18. doi:10.1001/jama.2013.284427.

Table 12-6: Medications for Hypertension

Medication	Comment
Diuretic (thiazide) Examples: HCTZ (HydroDiuril®), chlorthalidone (Hygroton®) •MOA: Low-volume sodium depletion that leads to PVR reduction **BP=HR × SV × PVR↓**	W/HD (≥HCTZ 25 mg/d or its equivalent), potential for negative impact on dyslipidemia, glucose control Monitor for Na^+, K^+, Mg^{++} depletion. Calcium-sparing. Lower observed rate of fractures in women who are long-term thiazide diuretic users. Less effective with advancing renal impairment, in particular with GFR less than 30 mL/min/1.73 m². Loop diuretics such as furosemide (Lasix) remain effective with lower GFR.
Angiotensin-converting enzyme inhibitors (ACEI, -pril suffix) Lisinopril (Prinivil®, Zestril®), enalapril (Vasotec®), others **Angiotensin receptor blockers (ARB, -sartan suffix)** Losartan (Cozaar®), telmisartan (Micardis®), others •MOA: Minimize angiotensin II (AgII) effect (potent vasoconstrictor that also stimulates adrenal catecholamine release) by minimizing AgII production (ACEI) or blocking its action (ARB) **BP=HR × SV × PVR↓**	Adjust dose in renal insufficiency. Do not use in presence of bilateral renal artery stenosis. Modest hyperkalemia risk, especially with inadequate fluid intake, when used with aldosterone antagonist. ACEI-induced cough: Can use ARB as an alternative. Angioedema risk with ACEI use, less so with ARB use. Do not use during pregnancy (Category D).
Calcium channel blockers (CCB) Dihydropyridine (DHP) examples per JNC-8: Amlodipine (Norvasc®), all with -ipine suffix NonDHP CCB examples per JNC-8: Diltiazem (Cardizem LA®) •MOA: Causes vasodilatation **BP=HR × SV × PVR↓**	Ankle edema, particularly with DHP use, usually dose-dependent Avoid use or use with caution in presence of heart failure, renal or hepatic impairment.
Beta-adrenergic antagonists (beta blockers, -lol suffix) Atenolol (Tenoretic®), metoprolol (Toprol®, Lopressor®), propranolol (Inderal®, Inderal LA®), others •MOA: Block (antagonize) adrenergic beta$_1$-receptor sites (found in the heart), blunt catecholamine response; non-cardioselective (propranolol, nadolol, others) also block beta$_2$-receptor sites **BP=HR↓ × SV↓ × PVR**	Monitor for worsening airway obstruction when used with asthma, COPD. Lower-dose cardioselective beta-blocker therapy, usually acceptable in COPD, asthma. Small clinical effect in many populations leads to role as a 4th-line anti-HTN medication.
Aldosterone antagonist Spironolactone (Aldactone®), eplerenone (Inspra®) •MOA: Block effects of aldosterone, therefore better regulating of Na^+ and water homeostasis and maintenance of intravascular volume **BP=HR × SV × PVR↓**	Adverse effect profile leads to role as 4th-line anti-HTN medication. Gynecomastia risk with prolonged use. Hyperkalemia risk, particularly w/ACEI, ARB use or volume depletion, including excessive diuresis. Most often used in heart failure treatment.

1. Ms. Leonardo is a 68-year-old woman of Italian ancestry who presents with recently-diagnosed hypertension. Recent lab analysis reveals the following: A1C=5.3% (0.053 proportion), calculated GFR=98 mL/min/1.73 m^2. Physical examination findings include the following: BMI=26.4 kg/m^2, no S$_3$, S$_4$, or murmur, PMI at 5th ICS, MCL. Funduscopic examination is within normal limits. In the past 6 months, she has increased physical activity by walking for at least 40 minutes 5–6 days per week and has cut back on dietary sodium. Which of the following represent(s) the best advice? Choose all that apply.

   A. Advise adding a 3 oz (88.7 mL) glass of red wine with dinner nightly.

   B. Initiate therapy with hydrochlorothiazide.

   C. Encourage weight reduction.

   D. Advise Ms. Leonardo that drug therapy will be initiated when there is evidence of target organ damage.

2. Mr. Jones, a 52-year-old African-American man, presents for treatment of hypertension. He is currently taking a thiazide diuretic for the past 2 months. He is feeling well with no complaint and physical examination is within normal limits. His blood pressure today is 160/94 mm Hg bilaterally. The next best step is to:

   A. Add an ACEI and have the patient follow-up in 2 weeks.

   B. Discontinue the HCTZ and start an aldosterone antagonist.

   C. Advise Mr. Jones that his blood pressure is in an acceptable range and he should follow-up in approximately 2 months.

   D. Prescribe a calcium channel blocker and advise a 1-month follow-up.

3. Which of the following medications should be avoided in a 45-year-old man with poorly-controlled hypertension who asks, "What medications can I take when I have a cold?"

   A. Dextromethorphan

   B. Chlorpheniramine

   C. Pseudoephedrine

   D. Guaifenesin

ACC/AHA Guideline on the Treatment of Blood Cholesterol to Reduce Atherosclerotic Cardiovascular Risk in Adults: A Report of the American College of Cardiology/American Heart Association Task Force on Practice Guidelines

Source: http://circ.ahajournals.org/content/early/2013/11/11/01.cir.0000437738.63853.7a

Table 12-7: Dyslipidemia Screening and Detection

Recommendation	Comment
Lipoprotein profile, particularly in the person with significant cardiovascular risk (DM, HTN, strong family history of dyslipidemia, obesity, others)	Total cholesterol (TC), low-density lipoprotein cholesterol (LDL-C), high-density lipoprotein cholesterol (HDL-C), and triglycerides (TG) after 12-hour fast, non-caloric liquids allowed

Table 12-8: Dyslipidemia Intensive Therapeutic Lifestyle Changes

Intervention	Example	Comment
Dietary options to enhance ↓ LDL-C	Increase intake of plant sterols and stanols to 2 g/d, viscous or soluble fiber to 10–25 g/d	Viscous or soluble fiber found in oatmeal, oat bran, others. Plant stanols, sterols found in trace amounts in many foods, larger amounts as additive to Take Control® and Benecol® margarine, others
Reduce intake of saturated fat and cholesterol	Reduce saturated fat to <7% of total calories. Avoid *trans* fats. Reduce total cholesterol intake to <200 mg/d and dietary fat to 25–35% of total daily caloric intake.	Polyunsaturated fat intake (soybean, corn and safflower oil, fatty fish [salmon, mackerel, herring, trout, others], walnuts, sunflower seeds, others), monounsaturated fat intake (olive and canola oil, others) as part of the overall dietary fat intake Avoid tropical oils such as palm and coconut oil.
Increase intake of omega-3 fatty acids (eicosapentaenoic acid [EPA], docosahexaenoic acid [DHA])	For general population, AHA advises intake of a variety of (preferably oily) fish at least twice a week. Include oils and foods rich in α-linolenic acid (flaxseed, canola, and soybean oils, flaxseeds, walnuts).	With documented CHD, AHA advises intake of approximately 1 g of EPA + DHA per day, preferably from oily fish (approx. 4 oz [115 g] salmon). EPA + DHA (fish oil) supplement use could be considered in consultation with healthcare provider.

Table 12-9: High-, Moderate-, and Low-intensity Statin Therapy
LDL Reduction with Statin Therapy=
High-intensity≥1/2, Moderate-intensity≥1/3, Low-intensity≥1/4

High-intensity statin therapy (Avoid with higher risk for statin adverse effects, including age>80 y, impaired renal function, frailty, multiple comorbidities, with fibrate)	Moderate-intensity statin therapy (Preferred in select situations with high risk for adverse effects with high-intensity statin therapy.)	Low-intensity statin therapy (Not recommended as first-line therapy)
LDL-C reduction approx. ≥50%	LDL-C reduction approx. 30–49%	LDL-C reduction approx. <30%
Daily dose • Atorvastatin 40–80 mg • Rosuvastatin 20–40 mg	Daily dose • Atorvastatin 10–20 mg • Rosuvastatin 5–10 mg • Simvastatin 20–40 mg • Pravastatin 40–80 mg • Lovastatin 40 mg	Daily dose • Pravastatin 10–20 mg • Lovastatin 20 mg

Source: http://circ.ahajournals.org/content/early/2013/11/11/01.cir.0000437738.63853.7a

Major recommendations for statin therapy for ASCVD prevention

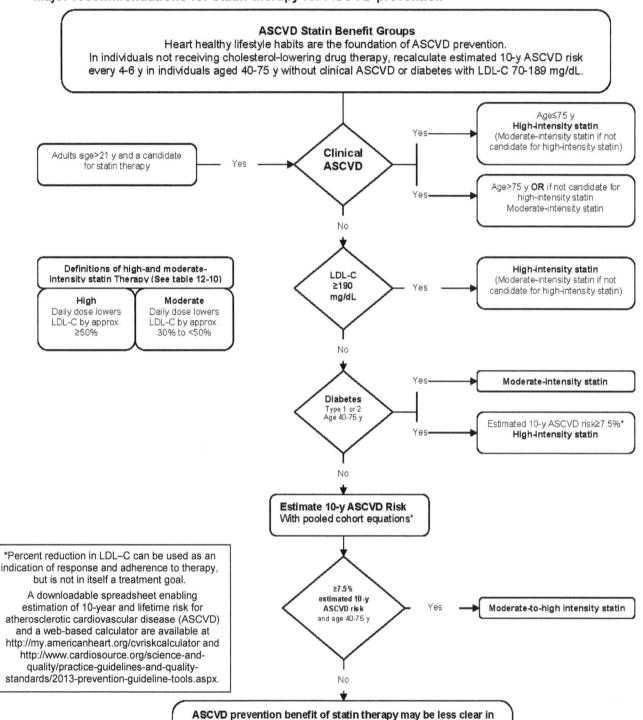

ASCVD Statin Benefit Groups
Heart healthy lifestyle habits are the foundation of ASCVD prevention.
In individuals not receiving cholesterol-lowering drug therapy, recalculate estimated 10-y ASCVD risk every 4-6 y in individuals aged 40-75 y without clinical ASCVD or diabetes with LDL-C 70-189 mg/dL.

Adults age>21 y and a candidate for statin therapy

Clinical ASCVD

Age≤75 y
High-intensity statin
(Moderate-intensity statin if not candidate for high-intensity statin)

Age>75 y **OR** if not candidate for high-intensity statin
Moderate-intensity statin

Definitions of high-and moderate-intensity statin Therapy (See table 12-10)

High	Moderate
Daily dose lowers LDL-C by approx. ≥50%	Daily dose lowers LDL-C by approx. 30% to <50%

LDL-C ≥190 mg/dL

High-intensity statin
(Moderate-intensity statin if not candidate for high-intensity statin)

Diabetes
Type 1 or 2
Age 40-75 y

Moderate-intensity statin

Estimated 10-y ASCVD risk≥7.5%*
High-intensity statin

Estimate 10-y ASCVD Risk
With pooled cohort equations*

*Percent reduction in LDL–C can be used as an indication of response and adherence to therapy, but is not in itself a treatment goal.

A downloadable spreadsheet enabling estimation of 10-year and lifetime risk for atherosclerotic cardiovascular disease (ASCVD) and a web-based calculator are available at http://my.americanheart.org/cvriskcalculator and http://www.cardiosource.org/science-and-quality/practice-guidelines-and-quality-standards/2013-prevention-guideline-tools.aspx.

≥7.5% estimated 10-y ASCVD risk and age 40-75 y

Moderate-to-high intensity statin

ASCVD prevention benefit of statin therapy may be less clear in other groups
In selected individuals, consider additional factors influencing ASCVD risk‡ and potential ASCVD risk benefits and adverse effects, drug-drug interactions, and patient preferences for statin treatment.

Figure 12-8

Source: Stone NJ, et al.
2013 ACC/AHA Blood Cholesterol Guideline
http://circ.ahajournals.org/

Notes:

Table 12-10: Medications for Dyslipidemia		
Medication	**Effect**	**Comment**
HMG-CoA reductase inhibitor (statin) Examples: Simvastatin (Zocor®), atorvastatin (Lipitor®), pravastatin (Pravachol®), pitavastatin (Livalo®), others ***Evidence-based dyslipidemia therapeutic leader***	↓ **LDL-C 18–55%** ↑ HDL-C 5–15% ↓ TG 7–30%	Check hepatic enzymes prior to initiation to establish baseline. No further routine hepatic enzyme monitoring warranted during statin use. T2DM risk slightly increased with higher potency statin use. Benefit outweighs risk. Caution with concomitant use of grapefruit juice (an intestinal CYP450 3A4 isoenzyme inhibitor) with the use of simvastatin, atorvastatin, lovastatin. Adverse effects: Rhabdomyolysis, myositis, rare but most often noted with higher statin dose with risk factors. See previous comments.
Bile acid resins (sequestrants) Examples: Cholestyramine (Questran®), colestipol (Colestid®), colesevelam (WelChol®)	↓ **LDL-C 15–30%** ↑ HDL-C 3–5% ↑ TG if ≥400 mg/dL (10.4 mmol/L)	Nonsystemic with no hepatic monitoring required. Adverse effects: GI distress, constipation, decreased absorption of other drugs if resin taken within 2 h of many medications
Selective cholesterol absorption inhibitor Example: Ezetimibe (Zetia®)	↓ **LDL-C 15–20%** ↑ HDL-C 3–5%	Adverse effects: Few due to limited systemic absorption No dose adjustment required for renal or hepatic dysfunction. When combined with simvastatin, drug combination known as Vytorin®
Niacin Examples: Generic niacin, Niaspan®, others	↑ **HDL-C 15–35%** ↓ **TG 20–50%** ↓ LDL-C 5–25%	Adverse effects: Flushing (potentially minimized by taking aspirin 1 h prior to niacin dose), hyperglycemia, hyperuricemia, upper GI distress, hepatotoxicity (rare)
Fibric acid derivatives (fibrates) Examples: Gemfibrozil (Lopid®), fenofibrate (TriCor®), fenofibric acid (Trilipix®)	↑ **HDL-C 10–20%** ↓ **TG 20–50%** ↓ LDL-C 5–20% (with normal TG) Can cause increase in LDL-C with very high TG	Adverse effects: Dyspepsia, gallstones, myopathy, including rhabdomyolysis, particularly if taken with a statin. Do not use in severe hepatic or renal disease.
Fish oil (omega-3 fatty acid) Example: Select prescription products, many OTC forms	At 4 g/d dose ↓ **TG 20–30%** ↑ HDL-C 1–5%	Adverse effects: Increased risk of bleeding due to modest antiplatelet effect, GI upset including "fishy" taste (can be minimized by freezing capsules, taking with food, avoiding hot beverages immediately post-ingestion).

Sources: http://circ.ahajournals.org/content/early/2013/11/11/01.cir.0000437738.63853.7a

Fitzgerald MA. Herbal facts, herbal fallacies. *American Nurse Today*. Volume 2, Number 12.

4. Mr. Kelly is a 66-year-old man with type 2 DM and HTN who presents with the following lipid profile:

  HDL=35 mg/dL (0.9 mmol/L)

  LDL=150 mg/dL (3.9 mmol/L)

  Triglycerides=210 mg/dL (2.4 mmol/L)

Which of the following represents the best choice of dyslipidemia therapy for Mr. Kelly?

  A. Low-intensity statin therapy

  B. Moderate-intensity statin therapy

  C. High-intensity niacin therapy

  D. Moderate-intensity fenofibrate therapy

5. A 45-year-old woman with hypertension and dyslipidemia is currently taking moderate-intensity statin therapy and she is at LDL-reduction goal. She is feeling well. As part of her ongoing healthcare, the NP considers that:

  A. Serum transaminases should be checked periodically.

  B. Evaluation of serum creatine kinase is needed.

  C. A CBC with WBC and platelet count is advised.

  D. In the absence of symptoms or concerns, no particular laboratory monitoring is recommended.

Diagnostic Algorithm in Heart Failure

Suspected heart failure?
- Dyspnea
- Fatigue
- Edema

↓

Seek Evidence of Underlying Heart Disease

1. Clinical history

- Previous MI/ACE
- Angina
- Hypertension
- Valvular disease/ rheumatic fever
- Palpitations

2. Clinical examination

- Tachycardia
- Increased jugular venous pressure (JVP)
- Displaced apex beat
- S_3 heart sound
- Murmur
- Pulmonary crackles
- Dependent edema

3. Investigation directed by clinical presentation

- Electrocardiogram (ECG)
- Chest x-ray (CXR)
- Echocardiogram
- Hemoglobin
- Blood chemistry
- Thyroid function tests

↓

Heart Failure Confirmed and Etiology Determined:

- Systolic left ventricular (LV) dysfunction (the most frequent cause for heart failure)
- Diastolic LV dysfunction
- Valvular disease
- Congenital heart disease
- Pericardial disease
- Endocardial disease
- Rhythm/conduction disturbance

Source: Concise Guide to the Management of Heart Failure, World Health Organization/Council on Geriatric Cardiology Task Force on Heart Failure Education

Figure 12-10

Heart Failure

At Risk for Heart Failure

STAGE A
At high risk for HF but without structural heart disease or symptoms of HF

STAGE B
Structural heart disease but without signs or symptoms of HF

STAGE C
Structural heart disease with prior or current symptoms of HF

STAGE D
Refractory HF

---

e.g., Patients with:
- HTN
- Atherosclerotic disease
- DM
- Obesity
- Metabolic syndrome

or

Patients:
- Using cardiotoxins
- With family history of cardiomyopathy

THERAPY

Goals
- Heart healthy lifestyle
- Prevent vascular, coronary disease
- Prevent LV structural abnormalities

Drugs
- ACEI or ARB in appropriate patients for vascular disease or DM
- Statins as appropriate

Structural heart disease

e.g., Patients with:
- Previous MI
- LV remodeling including LVH and low EF
- Asymptomatic valvular disease

THERAPY

Goals
- Prevent HF symptoms
- Prevent further cardiac remodeling

Drugs
- ACEI or ARB as appropriate
- Beta blockers as appropriate

In selected patients
- ICD
- Revascularization or valvular surgery as appropriate

Development of symptoms of HF

e.g., Patients with:
- Known structural heart disease and
- HF signs and symptoms

HFpEF

THERAPY

Goals
- Control symptoms
- Improve HRQOL
- Prevent hospitalization
- Prevent mortality

Strategies
- Identification of comorbidities

Treatment
- Diuresis to relieve symptoms of congestion
- Follow guideline driven indications for comorbidities, e.g., HTN, AF, CAD, DM

HFrEF

THERAPY

Goals
- Control symptoms
- Patient education
- Prevent hospitalization
- Prevent mortality

Drugs for routine use
- Diuretics for fluid retention
- ACEI or ARB
- Beta blockers
- Aldosterone antagonists

Drugs for use in selected patients
- Hydralazine /isosorbide dinitrate

In selected patients
- ACEI and ARB
- Digitalis
- CRT
- ICD
- Revascularization or valvular surgery as appropriate

Refractory symptoms of HF at rest, despite GDMT

e.g., Patients with:
- Marked HF symptoms at rest
- Recurrent hospitalizations despite GDMT

THERAPY

Goals
- Control symptoms
- Improve HRQOL
- Reduce hospital readmissions
- Establish patient's end - of-life goals

Options
- Advanced care measures
- Heart transplant
- Chronic inotropes
- Temporary or permanent MCS
- Experimental surgery or drugs
- Palliative care and hospice
- ICD deactivation

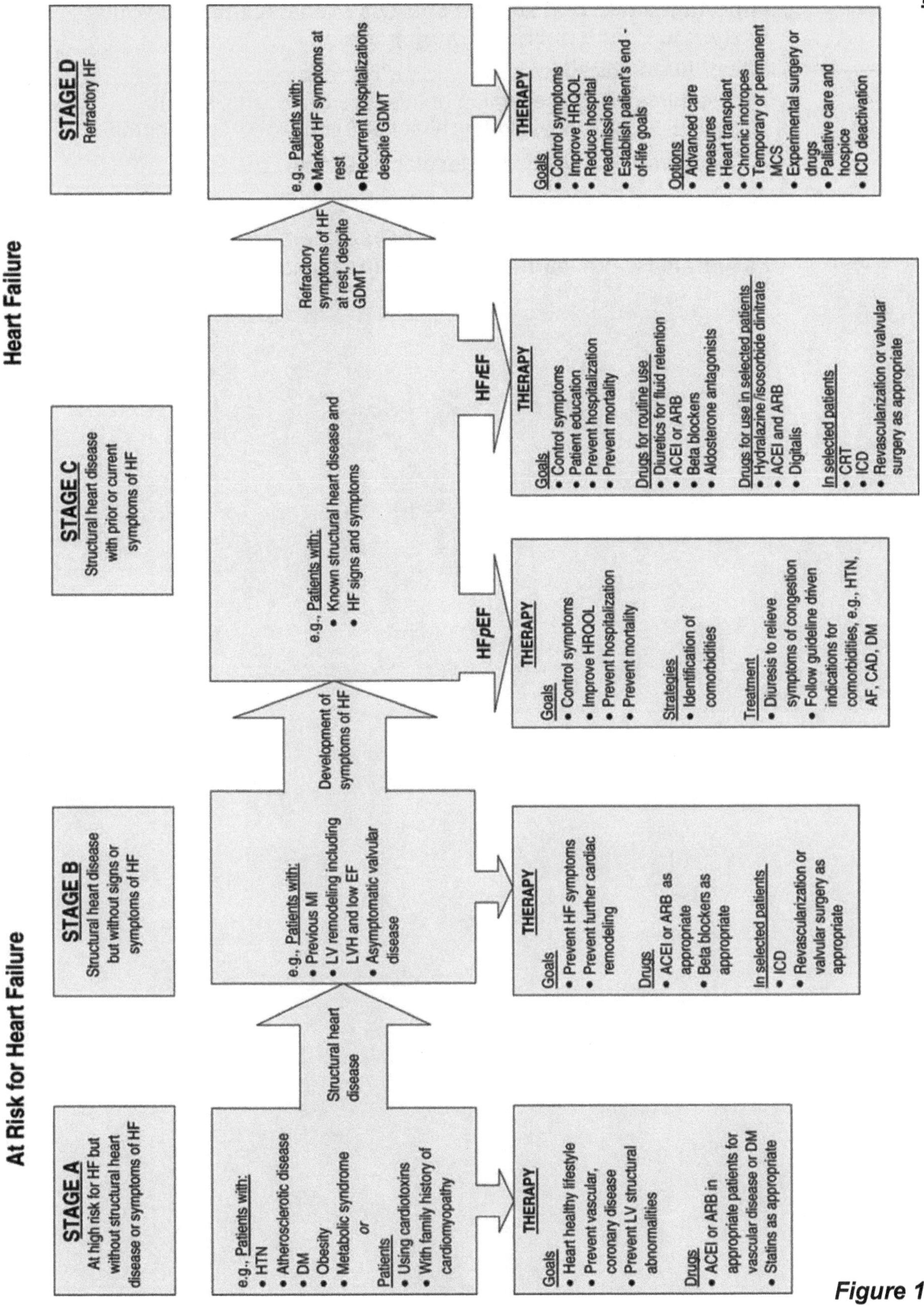

Figure 12-11

Source: http://circheartfailure.ahajournals.org

Important additional study resources available through your Fitzgerald Health online learning portal at fhea.com/npexpert

- Resource 12-1: Prevention of Infective Endocarditis (IE); Dental, Oral, or Respiratory Tract or Esophageal Procedures
- Resource 12-2: Retinal Arteriolar Sclerosis

Bonus questions for this chapter available through your Fitzgerald Health learning portal at fhea.com/npexpert.

Resources for Additional Study

Books:

Fitzgerald, M. A. (2017) Chest Disorders and Peripheral Vascular Disease, Nurse Practitioner Certification Examination and Practice Preparation, 5th Edition, Philadelphia, PA: F. A. Davis.

Audio programs:

Fitzgerald, M. A. Dyslipidemia: An Update on Treatment Goals and Options, North Andover, MA: Fitzgerald Health Education Associates.

Fitzgerald, M. A. Hypertension in the Elderly: The Latest Treatment Recommendations, North Andover, MA: Fitzgerald Health Education Associates.

Fitzgerald, M. A. Hypertension Update, North Andover, MA: Fitzgerald Health Education Associates.

CD-ROM programs:

Miller, S. K. 12-Lead ECG Interpretation: A Primary Care Perspective, North Andover, MA: Fitzgerald Health Education Associates.

Miller, S. K. Beyond the Basics in 12-Lead ECG Interpretation, North Andover, MA: Fitzgerald Health Education Associates.

Miller, S. K. Cardiac Rhythms: The Clinician's Approach to Accurate Interpretation, North Andover, MA: Fitzgerald Health Education Associates.

Video programs:

Tombasco, M., Wright, W. L. Expert Exam: Conducting a Pre-sports Physical Examination, North Andover, MA: Fitzgerald Health Education Associates.

161

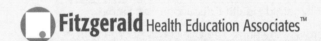
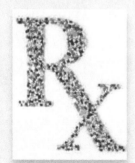
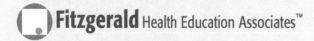

Chapter 13: Differential Diagnosis and Treatment in Commonly Encountered GU and GYN Problems

Learning activities are an integral part of the course available through your Fitzgerald Health learning portal at fhea.com/npexpert:
Online program for Family and Adult-Gerontology NPs:
Principles of Family Planning

Table 13-1: Vulvovaginitis Differential Diagnosis

Diagnostic criteria	Normal/healthy women of reproductive age	*Candida* vulvovaginitis Etiology: *Candida albicans* (80–90%)	Bacterial vaginosis Etiology: Unclear, likely polymicrobial, associated with *G. vaginalis*, *M. hominis*, others	Atrophic vaginitis Etiology: Estrogen deficiency
Discharge	White, clear, flocculent (physiologic leukorrhea)	White, curdy, "cottage cheese"–like, sometimes increased	Thin, homogeneous, white, gray, adherent, often increased	Scant, white-clear
Common patient complaints	None	Itching/burning, discharge	Discharge, foul odor, itching occasionally present	Itching/burning, discharge, but often without symptoms
Vaginal pH	3.8–4.2	<4.5 (usually)	5–7	>5
Amine odor (KOH "whiff" test)	Absent	Usually absent	Present (fishy)	Absent
Microscopic exam of vaginal discharge via saline wet mount	Lactobacilli	Mycelia, budding yeast, pseudohyphae w/KOH prep	>20 clue cells/HPF Few or no WBCs	Few or absent lactobacilli
Intervention	None	-azole antifungal, oral (fluconazole [Diflucan®]) or vaginal (miconazole [Monistat®], terconazole [Terazol®], others)	Metronidazole (topical [MetroGel®] or oral [Flagyl®]), clindamycin vaginal cream or ovules (Cleocin®), oral tinidazole (Tindamax®)	Topical and/or vaginal estrogen if symptomatic and/or recurrent UTI (Oral estrogen as solo intervention likely inadequate)

Source: Gilbert, D., Chambers, H., Eliopoulos, G., Saag, M., Pavia, A. (2016) The Sanford Guide to Antimicrobial Therapy (46th ed.). Sperryville, VA: Antimicrobial Therapy, Inc.
Centers for Disease Control and Prevention. STD treatment guidelines, available at www.cdc.gov/std/tg2015/

Table 13-2: Assessment and Treatment of Genitourinary Infection

In STI, especially *C. trachomatis*, expedited partner therapy (EPT), where patient is provided with prescription for partner, is encouraged.
See http://www.cdc.gov/Std/ept/default.htm for additional information.

Condition	Causative organism	Clinical findings	Treatment
Genital herpes	Human herpes virus 2 (HHV-2) (also known as herpes simplex type 2) less common by HHV-1 (also known as herpes simplex type 1)	Classic presentation of painful ulcerated lesions, marked lymphadenopathy with initial lesions. With recurrence, symptoms vary. Asymptomatic transmission common In women: Thin vaginal discharge if lesion located at vagina or introitus	Oral acyclovir (Zovirax®), famciclovir (Famvir®), valacyclovir (Valtrex®), dose and length of treatment dependent on medication choice, clinical presentation.
Nongonococcal urethritis and cervicitis	*Chlamydia trachomatis, Ureaplasma urealyticum, Mycoplasma genitalium* (obligate intracellular pathogen)	Irritative voiding symptoms, occasional mucopurulent discharge In women: Cervicitis common Often without symptoms in either gender Microscopic examination of discharge: Large number of WBCs	Azithromycin 1 g PO as a 1-time dose (preferred) Alternative options include PO doxycycline, erythromycin, ofloxacin, or levofloxacin (multiple days of therapy needed)
Gonococcal urethritis and vaginitis	*Neisseria gonorrhoeae* (Gram-negative bacteria)	Irritative voiding symptoms, occasional purulent discharge Often without symptoms in either gender Microscopic examination of discharge: Large number of WBCs	Ceftriaxone 250 mg IM as a one-time dose plus azithromycin 1 g PO × 1 dose Alternative option includes cefixime 400 mg (Suprax®) PO as 1-time dose only indicated if ceftriaxone IM unable to be used, with azithromycin 1 g PO × 1 dose. Data are limited for treatment options in face of severe beta-lactam allergy. One option is gemifloxacin (Factive®) 320 mg PO × 1 dose plus azithromycin 1 g PO as a single dose.
Trichomoniasis	*Trichomonas vaginalis* (Protozoan pathogen)	Dysuria, itching, vulvovaginal irritation, yellow-green vaginal discharge, occasionally frothy (~30%), cervical petechial hemorrhages ("strawberry spots") in about 30% Often without symptoms in either gender On microscopic exam: Motile organisms and large number of WBCs Alkaline pH	Metronidazole 2 g PO or tinidazole 2 g PO as a 1-time dose Patients should be advised to avoid consuming alcohol during treatment with oral metronidazole or tinidazole. Abstinence from alcohol use should continue for 24 hours after completion of metronidazole or 72 hours after completion of tinidazole. Alternative option is metronidazole 500 mg PO BID for 7 days.

Continued...

Table 13-2 (cont.): Assessment and Treatment of Genitourinary Infection

Condition	Causative organism	Clinical findings	Treatment
Syphilis	*Treponema pallidum* (Spirochete bacterium)	*Primary stage:* Chancre, firm, round, painless genital and/or anal ulcer(s) with clean base and indurated margins, accompanied by localized lymphadenopathy, ~3 weeks' duration, resolve without therapy *Secondary stage:* Nonpruritic skin rash, often involving palms and soles, as well as mucous membrane lesions Fever, lymphadenopathy, sore throat, patchy hair loss, headaches, weight loss, muscle aches, and fatigue commonly reported. Resolution without treatment possible. *Latent stage:* Presentation variable, occurs when primary and secondary symptoms have resolved.	Antimicrobial therapy, with dosage and length of therapy usually dictated by disease stage Options include injectable penicillin (preferred), PO doxycycline used in patients with beta-lactam allergy.
Genital warts (Condyloma acuminata)	Human papillomavirus, most commonly HPV-6, -11 causing genital warts (HPV-16, -18, -31, -33, -45, -52, -58, most commonly associated with GU malignancies. Infection with multiple HPV types common.) 9-Valent HPV vaccine (Gardasil® 9 protects against HPV-6, -11, -16, -18, -31, -33, -45, -52, -58) (For update on HPV-9 dosing, see https://www.cdc.gov/media/releases/2016/p1020-hpv-shots.html) Quadrivalent HPV vaccine (Gardasil® protects against HPV-6, -11, -16, -18)	Verruca-form lesions can be subclinical or unrecognized.	Prevent with immunization. Location of lesion can guide choice of treatment. Topical podofilox, liquid nitrogen, cryoprobe, trichloroacetic acid, bichloracetic acid, surgical removal, or topical imiquimod ([Aldara®]; imiquimod only indicated for external warts treatment) Podofilox, podophyllin, and sinecatechins should not be used during pregnancy; imiquimod use during pregnancy should be avoided until more data are available.

Table 13-2 (cont.): Assessment and Treatment of Genitourinary Infection			
Condition	**Causative organism**	**Clinical findings**	**Treatment**
Pelvic inflammatory disease (infectious, inflammatory disorder of the upper female reproductive tract, including uterus, fallopian tubes, adjacent pelvic structures)	*N. gonorrhoeae, C. trachomatis,* bacteroides, Enterobacteriaceae, streptococci	Irritative voiding symptoms, fever, abdominal pain, cervical motion tenderness, vaginal discharge Possible sequelae include tubal scarring with subsequent increased risk for ectopic pregnancy and/or infertility.	Recommended therapy for women with PID suitable for outpatient treatment: Ceftriaxone 250 mg IM as a single dose plus doxycycline 100 mg PO BID × 14 days with or without metronidazole 500 mg PO BID × 14 days. Alternative option includes cefoxitin 2 g IM as a single dose plus a single dose of probenecid 1 g PO plus doxycycline 100 mg PO BID × 14 days with or without metronidazole 500 mg PO BID × 14 days.

Sources: Gilbert, D., Chambers, H., Eliopoulos, G., Saag, M., Pavia, A. (2016) The Sanford Guide to Antimicrobial Therapy (46th ed.). Sperryville, VA: Antimicrobial Therapy, Inc.

Centers for Disease Control and Prevention. STD treatment guidelines, available at www.cdc.gov/std/tg2015/

1. Vulvovaginitis or STI diagnosis with the following findings on clinical or microscopic examination? Choose from the following:

   A. Bacterial vaginosis

   B. *Candida* vulvovaginitis

   C. Nongonococcal cervicitis/vaginitis

Microscopic finding	Diagnosis
Clue cells with alkaline pH	Bacterial vaginosis.
Pseudohyphae	B
Abundant WBCs	C /Nong..

2. Intervention in vulvovaginitis? Choose from the following (an option can be used more than once):

   A. *Candida* vulvovaginitis

   B. Trichomoniasis

   C. Bacterial vaginosis

Intervention	Diagnosis
Clotrimazole cream	A
Oral metronidazole	B–C
Metronidazole gel	C
Clindamycin cream	C

3. Treatment for which of the following STIs? Choose from the list below:

A. Genital warts

B. Gonococcal urethritis

C. *Chlamydia trachomatis* cervicitis

D. Syphilis

Intervention	Diagnosis
Ceftriaxone	B – Gonococcal urethritis
Injectable penicillin	D – Syphilis
Doxycycline	C – D – Chlamydia – Syphilis
Imiquimod	A – Genital warts

4. Genital *Candida albicans* infection in men typically presents with all of the following except:

A. Penile discharge.

B. Balanitis.

C. Groin-fold involvement.

D. Scrotal excoriation.

5. Considerations in caring for a 68-year-old man with a BMI=38 kg/m^2 who is otherwise well and presents with genital candidiasis includes which of two most helpful measures?

A. Advice on the use of antibacterial soap to the region.

B. Obtain an in-office blood glucose.

C. Prescribing topical miconazole.

D. Order a medium-potency topical corticosteroid to the affected region to help with symptom control.

Table 13-3: UTI Therapies

Information on antimicrobial resistance rates available in local antibiogram.

Type of infection	Usual pathogens	Regimens
Acute, uncomplicated urinary tract infection (cystitis, urethritis) in nonpregnant women	*E. coli (Gram-negative, most common pathogen), Klebsiella spp. (Gram-negative), S. saprophyticus (Gram-positive)* ***Growing concern about FQ resistance.***	***Primary*** If local *E. coli* resistance to TMP/SMX<20% and no allergy, then TMP/SMX-DS PO BID × 3 d If local *E. coli* resistance to TMP/SMX>20% or sulfa allergy, nitrofurantoin (Macrobid®) 100 mg PO BID × 5 d or fosfomycin (Monurol®) 3 g PO × 1 dose. Add phenazopyridine (Pyridium®) PO to help with symptom control. ***Alternative*** If local *E. coli* resistance to TMP/SMX>20% or sulfa allergy, ciprofloxacin 250 mg PO BID, ciprofloxacin ER 500 mg PO QD, levofloxacin 250 mg PO QD, or moxifloxacin 400 mg PO QD, all × 3 d. Add phenazopyridine (Pyridium®) PO to help with symptom control.

Source: Gilbert, D., Chambers, H., Eliopoulos, G., Saag, M., Pavia, A. (2016) The Sanford Guide to Antimicrobial Therapy (46th ed.). Sperryville, VA: Antimicrobial Therapy, Inc.

Table 13-4: Assessment and Treatment of Male GU Infection

Conditions	Causative organism	Clinical presentation	Treatment options
Epididymoorchitis (Upper reproductive tract infection with inflammation of epididymis/testis) Age≤35 y	*N. gonorrhoeae, C. trachomatis*	Irritative voiding symptoms, fever, and painful swelling of epididymis and scrotum Infertility potential post-infection	*Primary* Ceftriaxone 250 mg IM as a single dose plus doxycycline 100 mg PO BID × 10 d Advise scrotal elevation to help with symptom relief. (Prehn's sign=Relief of discomfort with scrotal elevation)
Epididymoorchitis Age>35 y or insertive partner in anal intercourse	Enterobacteriaceae (coliforms)	Irritative voiding symptoms, fever, and painful swelling of epididymis and scrotum Infertility potential post-infection	Levofloxacin 500 mg PO QD or ofloxacin 300 mg PO BID × 10 d
Acute bacterial prostatitis (Age≤35 y)	*N. gonorrhoeae, C. trachomatis*	Irritative voiding symptoms, suprapubic, perineal pain, fever, a tender, boggy prostate, leukocytosis	*Primary* Ceftriaxone 250 mg IM as 1-time dose with doxycycline 100 mg PO BID × 10 d
Acute bacterial prostatitis (Uncomplicated disease in men with low risk for STI)	Enterobacteriaceae (coliforms)	Irritative voiding symptoms, suprapubic, perineal pain, fever, a tender, boggy prostate, leukocytosis	Ciprofloxacin 500 mg PO BID or ofloxacin 200 mg PO daily × 14 d

Sources: Gilbert, D., Chambers, H., Eliopoulos, G., Saag, M., Pavia, A. (2016) The Sanford Guide to Antimicrobial Therapy (46th ed.). Sperryville, VA: Antimicrobial Therapy, Inc.

Centers for Disease Control and Prevention. STD treatment guidelines, available at www.cdc.gov/std/tg2015/

6. Which of the following is inconsistent with benign prostatic hyperplasia?

   A. Obliterated median sulcus

   B. Size ≥2.5 cm × 3 cm

   C. Symptoms improved with use of an alpha-1 receptor blockade such as tamsulosin.

   D. Surgical intervention should be offered early in the disease process.

Table 13-5: Conditions and Correlating Physical Examination Findings

Condition	Physical examination finding	Comment
Normal prostate	Firm, smooth, nontender	About as firm as pressing in on the tip of your nose
Acute prostatitis	Tender, boggy, indurated	About as firm as pressing in over your cheekbone
Prostate cancer	Nodular, firm, nontender	Usually malignant lesions not palpable until disease is advanced

7. Which of the following is least likely to be noted in the 55-year-old man who presents with bladder cancer?

    A. Textile worker for the past 25 years

    B. 60 pack-year cigarette smoking history

    C. Report of intermittent painless gross hematuria

    (D.) Report of recent-onset intermittent acute urinary retention

8. Which of the following is a worrisome finding noted during pelvic examination on a 62-year-old woman?

    A. Flattening of the vaginal rugae

    B. Vaginal pH=5.6

    (C.) Ovary palpable on bimanual examination

    D. Scant white vaginal discharge

9. Match the following urinary incontinence types:	
A. Urge incontinence B. Stress incontinence C. Functional incontinence D. Transient incontinence	
Associated with lifting	*B - Stress*
Occurs during an acute illness	*D - Transient*
Reports of strong sensation of needing to void	*A - Urge*
Often occurs in presence of mobility problems	*C - Functional*

Treatable causes of urinary incontinence

- *D*elirium
- *I*nfection (urinary)
- *A*trophic urethritis and vaginitis
- *P*harmaceuticals (diuretics, others)
- *P*sychologic disorders (depression)
- *E*xcessive urine output (heart failure, hyperglycemia due to undetected or poorly-controlled DM)
- *R*estricted mobility
- *S*tool impaction

Source: Resnick NM. Urinary incontinence in the elderly. *Medical Grand Rounds.* 1984;3:281-290.

Table 13-6: Assessment and Intervention in Urinary Incontinence

Type of urinary incontinence	Population most often affected	Clinical presentation	Treatment options
Urge incontinence	Most common form of incontinence in older adults	Strong sensation of needing to empty the bladder that cannot be suppressed, often coupled with involuntary loss of urine.	Behavioral therapy. Pharmacotherapy can include antimuscarinics (anticholinergics), such as tolterodine (Detrol®) oxybutynin (Ditropan®), solifenacin succinate (VESIcare®), darifenacin (Enablex®), fesoterodine fumarate (Toviaz®). Adverse effects= Dry mouth, sedation, mental status change, particularly in higher doses. Alternatives to anticholinergics include β3-agonist, mirabegron (Myrbetriq®), and botulinum toxin injections.
Stress incontinence	Most common form of incontinence in women; rare in men, occasionally noted post prostate/bladder surgery	Loss of urine with activity that causes increase in intra-abdominal pressure such as coughing, sneezing, exercise.	Support to the area through the use of a vaginal tampon, urethral stents, periurethral bulking agent injections, and pessary use. Kegel and other similar exercises most helpful in younger, premenopausal patients. Pelvic floor rehabilitation with biofeedback, electrical stimulation and bladder training. Surgical intervention can be helpful in well-chosen patients.
Functional incontinence	Associated with inability to get to the toilet or lack of awareness of need to void	Usually in person with mobility issues or altered cognition. Worsened by unavailability of a helper to assist in toileting activities.	Ameliorated by having assistant who is aware of voiding cue available to help with toileting activities.
Transient incontinence	Associated with acute event such as delirium, UTI, medication use, restricted activity.	Presentation consistent with underlying process.	Treatment of underlying process, discontinuation of offending medication.

Source: Fitzgerald, M. A. (2017) <u>Nurse Practitioner Certification Examination and Practice Preparation</u>, 5th Edition, Philadelphia, PA: F.A. Davis.

10. Samantha, a healthy 32-year-old woman who is taking combined oral contraceptives, is here to review the results of her recent liquid-based Pap screening that revealed atypical squamous cells of unknown significance (ASCUS) and high-risk HPV positive. She has no history of previous abnormal cervical cytology, with her last screening obtained approximately 2 years ago. After explaining the significance of these findings, the most appropriate next step is to:

  A. Advise that she return in 6–12 months for a repeat Pap with HPV cotesting.

  B. Obtain screening tests for *N. gonorrhoeae* and *C. trachomatis* infection.

  C. Referral for colposcopy.

  D. Counsel that the usual cervical cancer screening guidelines should be followed.

11. Which of the following is demonstrated to provide the most symptom relief in treating vasomotor symptoms?

  A. Clonidine

  B. Paroxetine

  C. Conjugated estrogen

  D. Venlafaxine

12. Match the following:
  A. Hydrocele

  B. Varicocele

  C. Testicular torsion

  D. Phimosis

  E. Paraphimosis

  F. Cryptorchidism

Retracted foreskin that cannot be brought forward to cover the glans	Paraphimosis
A palpable "nest of worms" scrotal mass that is only evident in standing position	Varicocele
Collection of serous fluid that causes painless scrotal swelling, easily recognized by transillumination	Hydrocele
With this, the foreskin cannot be pulled back to expose the glans	Phimosis
Characterized by scrotal pain and loss of the cremasteric reflex	Testicular torsion
Testicle located in inguinal canal or abdomen	Cryptorchidism

Table 13-7: HIV Transmission: Risk per 10,000 Exposures*	
RAI (receptive anal intercourse)	138
Needle-sharing during injection drug use	63
Needlestick	23
IAI (insertive anal intercourse)	11
RVI (receptive vaginal intercourse)	8
IVI (insertive vaginal intercourse)	4
ROI (receptive oral intercourse)	Low
IOI (insertive oral intercourse)	Low

Source: http://www.cdc.gov/hiv/policies/law/risk.html

*With sexual activity, risk is reported without use of protection such as condom (male or female), dental dam.

Table 13-8: Summary of the Guidelines for the Use of Antiretroviral (ARV) Agents and Prevention of Opportunistic Infection in HIV-1-Infected Adults and Adolescents

Current guidelines strongly recommend initiating antiretroviral therapy (ART) for all individuals with HIV-1 infection. This includes those with early HIV-1 infection and all HIV-infected women (including pregnant women), and should be initiated regardless of CD4 T lymphocyte cell count. The goal of ART is to suppress plasma viral RNA to undetectable levels and ART can be important in preventing and managing opportunistic infections. However, in cases where ART can increase the risk of immune reconstitution inflammatory syndrome (e.g., cryptococcal meningitis), a short delay may be warranted before initiating ART.

Initiating antiretroviral therapy in treatment-naïve patients

Based on the cumulative weight of evidence, the HHS Panel recommends that:

- Antiretroviral therapy (ART) is recommended for all HIV-infected individuals to reduce the risk of disease progression.
    - The strength and evidence for this recommendation vary by pretreatment CD4 cell count: CD4 count<350 cells/mm^3 (strong recommendation); CD4 count 350–500 cells/mm^3 (strong recommendation); CD4 count>500 cells/mm^3 (moderate recommendation).
- ART also is recommended for HIV-infected individuals for the prevention of transmission of HIV.
    - The strength and evidence for this recommendation vary by transmission risks: perinatal transmission (strong recommendation); heterosexual transmission (strong recommendation); other transmission risk groups (strong recommendation)
- Patients starting ART should be willing and able to commit to treatment and understand the benefits and risks of therapy and the importance of adherence (strong recommendation). Patients may choose to postpone therapy, and providers, on a case-by-case basis, may elect to defer therapy based on clinical and/or psychosocial factors. ***Assessing and managing an antiretroviral (ARV)-experienced patient experiencing failure of antiretroviral therapy (ART) is complex. Expert advice is critical and should be sought.***

Acute and recent (early) HIV infection

- ART is recommended for all persons with HIV infection and should be offered to those with early HIV infection (moderate recommendation), although definitive data are lacking as to whether this approach will result in long-term virologic, immunologic, or clinical benefits.
- All pregnant women with early HIV infection should start ART as soon as possible to prevent perinatal transmission of HIV (strong recommendation).
- If treatment is initiated in a patient with early HIV infection, the goal is to suppress plasma HIV RNA to below detectable levels (strong recommendation).
- For patients with early HIV infection in whom therapy is initiated, testing for plasma HIV RNA levels, CD4 count, and toxicity monitoring should be performed as described for patients with chronic HIV infection (strong recommendation).
- Genotypic drug-resistance testing should be performed before initiation of ART to guide selection of the regimen (strong recommendation). If therapy is deferred, genotypic resistance testing should still be performed because the results will be useful in selecting a regimen with the greatest potential for achieving optimal virologic response when therapy is ultimately initiated (strong recommendation). If treatment is deferred, repeat testing may be considered at the time of ART initiation.
- For patients without transmitted drug-resistant virus, therapy should be initiated with a combination regimen that is recommended for patients with chronic HIV infection (strong recommendation).
- ART can be initiated before drug resistance test results.

Continued...

Table 13-8 (cont.): Summary of the Guidelines for the Use of Antiretroviral (ARV) Agents and Prevention of Opportunistic Infection in HIV-1-Infected Adults and Adolescents

ART during pregnancy

- In pregnant women, an additional goal of therapy is prevention of perinatal transmission of HIV, with a goal of maximal viral suppression to reduce the risk of transmission of HIV to the fetus and newborn (strong recommendation).
- When selecting an ARV combination regimen for a pregnant woman, clinicians should consider the known safety, efficacy, and pharmacokinetic data on use during pregnancy for each agent (strong recommendation).
- Because the risk of neural tube defects is restricted to the first 5 to 6 weeks of pregnancy and pregnancy is rarely recognized before 4 to 6 weeks, efavirenz (EFV) can be continued in pregnant women receiving an EFV-based regimen who present for antenatal care in the first trimester, provided the regimen produces virologic suppression (optional recommendation).
- When designing a regimen for a pregnant woman, clinicians should consult the most current Health and Human Services (HHS) Perinatal Guidelines (strong recommendation).

Acute opportunistic infections

- In patients with opportunistic conditions for which there is no effective therapy (e.g., cryptosporidiosis, microsporidiosis, progressive multifocal leukoencephalopathy) but for which antiretroviral therapy (ART) may improve outcomes by improving immune responses, treatment should be started as soon as possible.
- In the setting of some opportunistic infections, such as cryptococcal meningitis, for which immediate therapy may increase the risk of immune reconstitution inflammatory syndrome (IRIS), a short delay may be warranted before initiating antiretroviral treatment.
- In the setting of other opportunistic infections, such as *Pneumocystis jiroveci* pneumonia (PCP), early initiation of ART is associated with increased survival, and therapy should not be delayed (within 2 weeks of PCP diagnosis).
- In persons with active tuberculosis (TB), initiating ART during treatment for TB confers a significant survival advantage. Thus, treatment should be initiated as follows: in patients with tuberculosis and low CD4 counts (<50 cells/mm^3), ART should be started within 2 weeks; for all others, ART therapy should be initiated within 8 to 12 weeks of TB therapy initiation.
- Clinicians should refer to "Guidelines for Prevention and Treatment of Opportunistic Infections in HIV-Infected Adults and Adolescents" for more detailed discussion on when to initiate ART in the setting of a specific opportunistic infection.

Screening for HIV (U.S. Preventive Services Task Force)

- Screening is recommended in adolescents and adults ages 15–65 years, as well as younger adolescents or older adults at increased risk of infection.
- Screening is recommended for all pregnant women, including those who present in labor who are untested and whose HIV status is unknown.
- Men who have sex with men and active injection drug users are at very high risk for new HIV infection. Other persons at high risk include those who have acquired or request testing for other sexually transmitted infections. Behavioral risk factors for HIV infection include: 1) having unprotected vaginal or anal intercourse, 2) having sexual partners who are HIV-infected, bisexual, or injection drug users, and 3) exchanging sex for drugs or money.
- The conventional serum test for diagnosing HIV infection is repeated reactive immunoassay, followed by a confirmatory Western blot or immunofluorescent assay. The test is highly accurate (sensitivity and specificity >99.5%), and results are available within 1 to 2 days from most commercial laboratories.
- Rapid HIV testing may use either blood or oral fluid specimens and can provide results in 5 to 40 minutes. The sensitivity and specificity of the rapid test are also both greater than 99.5%; however, initial positive results require confirmation with conventional methods.
- Other FDA-approved tests for detection and confirmation of HIV infection include combination tests (for p24 antigen and HIV antibodies) and qualitative HIV-1 RNA.

Sources: Guidelines for the Use of Antiretroviral Agents in HIV-1-Infected Adults and
Adolescents (July 2016), available at
aidsinfo.nih.gov/contentfiles/lvguidelines/adultandadolescentgl.pdf.
Guidelines for Prevention and Treatment of Opportunistic Infections in HIV-Infected Adults
and Adolescents (August 2016), available at
http://aidsinfo.nih.gov/contentfiles/lvguidelines/adult_oi.pdf.
Screening for HIV: Clinical Summary of U.S. Preventive Services Task Force
Recommendation (April 2013), available at
http://www.uspreventiveservicestaskforce.org/Page/Topic/recommendation-
summary/human-immunodeficiency-virus-hiv-infection-screening

Table 13-9: Summary of the Guidelines for the Use of Preexposure Prophylaxis (PrEP) for HIV Prevention

Recommended Use of Daily Oral PrEP

Daily oral PrEP with fixed-dose combination of tenofovir disoproxil fumarate (TDF) 300 mg and emtricitabine (FTC) 200 mg (Truvada®) has been shown to be safe and effective in reducing the risk of HIV acquisition in adults.

- PrEP is recommended as one prevention option for adults at substantial risk of HIV acquisition, including:
  - Men who have sex with men (MSM)
  - Heterosexually active men and women
  - Injection drug users
- PrEP should be discussed with heterosexually active HIV-discordant couples as one of several options to protect the uninfected partner during conception and pregnancy so that an informed decision can be made in awareness of what is known and unknown about the benefits and risks of PrEP for mother and fetus.

Considerations for PrEP

- Data on the efficacy and safety of PrEP for adolescents is insufficient.
- Acute and chronic HIV infection must be excluded immediately before PrEP is prescribed.
- The only FDA-approved regimen for PrEP is daily TDF 300 mg co-formulated with FTC 200 mg.
  - TDF alone can be considered as an alternative regimen for injection drug users and heterosexually active adults, but not MSM.
  - The use of antiretroviral medications for PrEP, either in place or in addition to TDF/FTC, is not recommended.
  - The prescription of oral PrEP for coitally-timed or other noncontinuous daily use is not recommended.
- HIV infection should be assessed at least every 3 months while patients are taking PrEP so that it can be discontinued with an incident infection; continued use of PrEP following infection may engender resistance to one or both drugs.
- Renal function should be assessed at baseline and monitored at least every 6 months while patients are taking PrEP; PrEP should be discontinued at the first signs of developing renal failure.

Initiating PrEP

- Clinically eligible patients include those with:
  - Documented negative HIV test result before prescribing PrEP
  - No signs/symptoms of acute HIV infection
  - Normal renal function and no contraindicated medications
  - Documented hepatitis B virus infection and vaccination status
- Prescription: Daily, continuing, oral doses of TDF/FTC, ≤90-day supply.
- Follow-up services
  - At least every 3 months: HIV test, medication adherence counseling, behavioral risk reduction support, adverse effect assessment, and sexually transmitted infection (STI) symptom assessment
  - At 3 months and every 6 months thereafter: renal function
  - Every 6 months: test for bacterial STIs
  - Oral/rectal STI testing (for MSM)
  - Pregnancy intent and pregnancy test every 3 months (for heterosexual women and men)
  - Access to clean needles/syringes and drug treatment services (for injection drug users)

Source: Preexposure Prophylaxis for the Prevention of HIV Infection in the United States - 2014, available at http://www.cdc.gov/hiv/pdf/prepguidelines2014.pdf

Important additional study resources available through your Fitzgerald Health online learning portal at fhea.com/npexpert

- Resource 13-1: Male GU Examination
- Resource 13-2: Treatment Options for Relief of Menopausal Symptoms

Bonus questions for this chapter available through your Fitzgerald Health learning portal at fhea.com/npexpert.

Resources for Additional Study

Books:

Fitzgerald, M. A. (2017) Female Reproductive and Genitourinary Systems, Nurse Practitioner Certification Examination and Practice Preparation, 5th Edition, Philadelphia, PA: F.A. Davis.

Fitzgerald, M. A. (2017) Male Genitourinary System, Nurse Practitioner Certification Examination and Practice Preparation, 5th Edition, Philadelphia, PA: F.A. Davis.

Hawkins, J.W. (2011) Guidelines for Nurse Practitioners in Gynecologic Settings, 10th Edition, New York, NY: Springer Publishing.

Audio programs:

Fitzgerald, M. A. Antimicrobial Update: A Focus on Treatment Recommendations in Sexually Transmitted Infection (STI), North Andover, MA: Fitzgerald Health Education Associates.

Fitzgerald, M. A. Antimicrobial Update: A Focus on Treatment Recommendations in Urinary Tract Infections (UTI), North Andover, MA: Fitzgerald Health Education Associates.

Table 14-1: Major Depressive Episode ≥5 symptoms present in the same 2-week period SIGECAPS Mnemonic	
*S*leep	Insomnia or hypersomnia, staying asleep problematic
*I*nterest	Depressed mood (marked diurnal variation)*, loss of interest or pleasure*, irritability common in teens, children
*G*uilt	Feelings of worthlessness
*E*nergy	Fatigue
*C*oncentration	Diminished ability to think clearly or make decisions
*A*ppetite	Weight change (increase or decrease), loss of food enjoyment
*P*sychomotor	Psychomotor retardation or agitation
*S*uicide	Recurrent thoughts of death, passive without plan most common

*Must include one of these

Sources: American Psychiatric Association. (2013). Diagnostic and statistical manual of mental disorders: DSM-5. Washington, D.C: American Psychiatric Association. http://www.mdedge.com/currentpsychiatry/article/63313/mnemonics-mnutshell-32-aids-psychiatric-diagnosis

Table 14-2: Generalized Anxiety Disorder (GAD) ≥3 of the following must be reported as occurring on most days, ≥6 months WATCHERS Mnemonic
*W*orry *A*nxiety *T*ension in muscles *C*oncentration difficulty *H*yperarousal (or irritability) *E*nergy loss *R*estlessness *S*leep disturbance (typically difficulty initiating sleep)

Sources:
American Psychiatric Association. (2013). Diagnostic and statistical manual of mental disorders: DSM-5. Washington, D.C: American Psychiatric Association. http://www.mdedge.com/currentpsychiatry/article/63313/mnemonics-mnutshell-32-aids-psychiatric-diagnosis

Table 14-3: Overlapping Symptoms of Depression and GAD		
Depression	**Overlapping symptoms**	**GAD**
Depressed mood	Sleep disturbance	Palpitation
Anhedonia	Psychomotor agitation	Muscle tension
Appetite disturbance	Concentration difficulty	Sweating
Worthlessness	Irritability	Dry mouth
Suicidal ideation	Fatigue	Nausea

Table 14-4: Therapeutic Goals in Treatment of Mood Disorders

Treatment goal	Comment
Remission of symptoms for ≥4–5 months, aimed at the virtual elimination of a person's symptoms of depression or anxiety and restoration of his or her psychosocial and occupational functioning *Consider longer-term therapy if ≥2nd episode.*	*Remission is most often achieved with a combination of therapies, including pharmacologic, psychologic, and social services.* *If antidepressant therapy is discontinued, a slow taper of the medication is advised. Ongoing monitoring for relapse is needed.* The goal of continuation treatment is to prevent relapse in the vulnerable period immediately following symptomatic recovery. Remission allows the patient to return to enjoying life and making strides toward recovery. Incomplete response with partial improvement of symptoms is common in mental healthcare and is associated with a greater risk for relapse and symptom recurrence.
Electroconvulsant therapy (ECT) should be considered for patients with major depressive disorder with a high degree of symptom severity and functional impairment or for cases in which psychotic symptoms or catatonia are present.	ECT likely the treatment modality of choice for patients in whom there is an urgent need for response, such as patients who are suicidal or refusing food and nutritionally compromised.

Source: Practice Guideline for the Treatment of Patients With Major Depressive Disorder, available at http://psychiatryonline.org/guidelines

Table 14-5: Choosing a Therapeutic Agent in Mood Disorder

Clinical question	Comment	Medication characteristic
What are the most bothersome symptoms? What medication will possibly be helpful in treating these symptoms? (Note: Primary care providers write for ≥80% of all mental health medications, usually dosing too low, treating for too short a time period.)	Vegetative symptoms present (altered sleep, such as hypersomnia, low libido, altered appetite, unexplained fatigue, psychomotor retardation, altered concentration, GI disturbance)? Energized or anxious?	Selective serotonin reuptake inhibitors (SSRIs) listed from most to least energizing: Fluoxetine (Prozac®), sertraline (Zoloft®), citalopram (Celexa®), escitalopram (Lexapro®), paroxetine (Paxil®). *Best effect on lifting and smoothing mood.* Selective serotonin norepinephrine reuptake inhibitors (SNRIs): Venlafaxine (Effexor®), duloxetine (Cymbalta®), desvenlafaxine (Pristiq®), others. Occasional reports of being energizing, helpful in anxious and/or resistant depression. *Best effect on lifting and smoothing mood plus increasing focus.* Selective dopamine reuptake inhibitor (SDRI) bupropion (Wellbutrin®). Potentially activating, usually used as add-on therapy with SSRI. *Best effect on improving mood when insufficient response with SSRI or as solo agent.* Increased the risk of suicidal thinking and behavior (suicidality) in children, adolescents, and young adults age≤24 years in short-term studies of major depressive disorder (MDD) and other psychiatric disorders. Not noted in adults >24 years, reduction in risk with antidepressant use compared to placebo in adults ≥65 years. Anxiolytics: Benzodiazepines, buspirone (BuSpar®). *Potentially helpful in alleviating hypervigilance associated with anxiety, but use does not decrease worry.*
What is the given medication's profile?	Include T½, potential drug interactions, adverse effect profile, others	Rate of sexual adverse effects with SSRI, SNRI=~40%, SDRI=~20% (anorgasmia, erectile dysfunction, impaired libido most common).

Source: Practice Guideline for the Treatment of Patients With Major Depressive Disorder, available at http://psychiatryonline.org/guidelines

Table 14-6: SSRIs T½	
SSRI	**T½**
Paroxetine (Paxil®)	21 h
Sertraline (Zoloft®)	26 h
Escitalopram (Lexapro®)	27–32 h
Citalopram (Celexa®)*	33 h
Fluoxetine (Prozac®)	84 h, metabolite=7–15 days

*See FDA safety communication warning about citalopram and potential abnormal rhythms in higher doses, with maximum 40 mg/d in all, maximum 20 mg/d in adults, age≥60 years or hepatic impairment, history of prolonged QTc interval, others; full warning available at www.fda.gov/drugs/drugsafety/ucm297391.htm

Table 14-7: CYP450 Isoenzyme Inhibition by SSRIs					
	CYP isoenzymes				
	1A2	**2C9**	**2C19**	**2D6**	**3A4**
Escitalopram	0	0	0	0	0
Citalopram	+	0	0	+	0
Fluoxetine	+	++	+ to ++	+++	++
Paroxetine	+	+	+	+++	+
Sertraline	+	+	+ to ++	+	+

0=Minimal or weak inhibition; +, ++, +++ =Mild, moderate, or strong inhibition.

1. Which of the following is likely to cause cardiac dysrhythmia and seizures when taken in an intentional ingestion equivalent to a typical adult therapeutic dose?

    A. A 4-week supply of fluoxetine

    B. A 2-week supply of nortriptyline

    C. A 3-week supply of venlafaxine

    D. A 3-day supply of diazepam

2. Of the following in need of an antidepressant, who is the best candidate for fluoxetine (Prozac®) therapy?

    A. An 80-year-old woman who is taking multiple medications and who presents with depressed mood and agitation

    B. A 45-year-old man with anorgasmia who is an occasional marijuana user

    C. A 28-year-old woman who occasionally "skips a dose" of her prescribed medication and is using a progestin implant (Nexplanon®) for contraception

    D. A 44-year-old woman with decreased appetite who is on hydrochlorothiazide for the treatment of hypertension

3. You see a 45-year-old woman with major depressive disorder (MDD) who started taking standard dose sertraline one week ago. She returns today with a chief complaint of "not really feeling any better. In fact, I think I might feel worse. I have this on-and-off headache right over my eyes since I started the medication." Results of physical examination reveal the following: Well-groomed and appropriately dressed for the occasion, PERLA, fundi WNL, CN 2–12 intact, clear, fluid speech. Today, you provide the following advice, choosing two of the following responses.

   A. The sertraline dose is likely inadequate and needs to be increased.

   B. She should be switched to a SNRI such as venlafaxine.

   C. Due to her headache report, the sertraline should be immediately discontinued.

   D. A lag of a number of weeks in the onset of SSRI therapeutic effect is expected.

   E. Frontal headache is a common short-term problem with early SSRI use.

4. Ms. Yancy is a 56-year-old woman with a history of depression and has been taking citalopram for about 6 months. Four days ago, she decided to discontinue the citalopram as she states her depressive symptoms have been much improved. Today, she presents with "not feeling well," with a 2-day history of persistent frontal headache. When assessing Ms. Yancy for additional findings of antidepressant discontinuation syndrome, the NP anticipates that Ms.Yancy will report all of the following except:

   A. Nausea.

   B. Fever.

   C. Flu-like symptoms.

   D. Anxiety.

Table 14-8: Antidepressant Discontinuation Syndrome FINISH Mnemonic
Typically noted when SSRI, SNRI, TCA taken for ≥6 weeks then rapidly discontinued. Typically lasts <7 days. Avoided with medication taper over ~6 weeks. Bothersome but not life-threatening.
*F*lu-like symptoms *I*nsomnia *N*ausea *I*mbalance (dizziness, difficulty with coordination) *S*ensory disturbances (nightmares common) *H*yperarousal (anxiety/agitation), *H*eadache

PHQ-2 Depression Screening Tool

- http://www.cqaimh.org/pdf/tool_phq2.pdf

PHQ-9 Depression Screening Tool

- http://www.phqscreeners.com/sites/g/files/g10016261/f/2014
  12/PHQ-9_English.pdf

General Anxiety Disorder Screening Tool (GAD-7)

- http://www.integration.samhsa.gov/clinical-
  practice/screening-tools#anxiety

5. Which of the following provides the most accurate information on assessing for alcohol abuse in a 55-year-old man who states, "I drink 5–6 beers every night but I get to work every day."

   A. Elevated ALT/AST to ≥6 times upper limit of normal

   B. Positive response to two items on the CAGE questionnaire

   C. Modest RBC macrocytosis

   D. Elevated serum triglycerides

Table 14-9: CAGE Questionnaire
Have you ever felt you ought to *Cut* down on drinking?
Have people *Annoyed* you by criticizing your drinking?
Have you ever felt bad or *Guilty* about your drinking?
Have you ever had a drink first thing in the morning to steady your nerves or get rid of a hangover? (*Eye-opener**)
*Modify for use with other forms of substance abuse by substituting N (normal) for E (eye-opener), i.e. Do you ever use heroin in order to keep from getting sick or withdrawing? With ≥2 positive responses, questionnaire has a sensitivity of 93% and a specificity of 76%

Source: Ewing JA. Detecting Alcoholism: The CAGE Questionnaire. *JAMA*. 1984;252:1905-1907.

For additional alcohol abuse screening tools, see National Institute on Alcohol Abuse and Alcoholism at www.niaaa.nih.gov

6. Rank the following from highest alcohol content (1) to lowest (3).	
12 oz (0.36 L) beer (7.2-proof)	
6 oz (0.19 L) wine (22-proof)	
3 oz (0.09 L) liquor (80-proof)	

Table 14-10: Risk Factors for Suicide	
Psychiatric illness	Severity of psychiatric illness Recent psychiatric inpatient hospitalization Higher among alcoholics
Hopelessness	More important than depression in explaining suicidal ideation Often mediates between • Low self-esteem • Loneliness • Interpersonal losses • Suicide
History of previous suicide attempt or threat	Strongest single predictive factor Up to 50% of successful victims have made a prior attempt. • 1 of every 100 attempt survivors will die by suicide within 1 year.
Age, sex and race	Young people attempt more often Females attempt 4× more than men Men complete 3× more than women • Likely reflects lethality of method (firearm use, hanging, others) Elderly white men (>85 years) have highest suicide rate. Whites>blacks, but this gap is narrowing.
Marital status	Living alone increases the suicide risk. Lost loved one or failed relationship within one year
Occupation	Unemployed and unskilled at greater risk
Health status	Higher risk with chronic pain or terminal illness HIV alone does not seem to increase risk.
Adverse childhood experiences	The more adverse events, the higher the suicidal risk
Family history	6× greater risk with a first-degree relative who committed suicide
Antidepressants	No clear increase in suicides Increase in suicidal thought/ideation, especially in younger adults
Other	Accessibility to weapons Anniversary of significant relationship loss Rural areas greater than urban areas LGBT youth

Source: Kaplan, H., Sadock, B. (2007). Kaplan & Sadock's Synopsis of Psychiatry: Behavioral Sciences/Clinical Psychiatry, (10th Ed.). Philadelphia, PA: Lippincott Williams & Wilkins.

Important additional study resources available through your Fitzgerald Health online learning portal at fhea.com/npexpert

- Resource 14-1: Stuart and Lieberman's "15-minute-hour" method of primary care counseling
- Resource 14-2: Understanding the Risk of Opioid Addiction
- Resource 14-3: Erik Erikson's Stages of Psychosocial Development
- Resource 14-4: Family Systems Theory

Bonus questions for this chapter available through your Fitzgerald Health learning portal at fhea.com/npexpert.

Resources for Additional Study

Books:

Desai, S. (2009) <u>Clinician's Guide to Laboratory Medicine: Pocket</u>, Houston, TX: MD2B.

Ferri, F. (2014) <u>Ferri's Best Test: A Practical Guide to Clinical Laboratory Medicine and Diagnostic Imaging</u>, 3<u>rd</u> Edition, St. Louis, MO: Elsevier Health Sciences.

Fitzgerald, M. A. (2017) Psychosocial Disorders, <u>Nurse Practitioner Certification Examination and Practice Preparation</u>, 5<u>th</u> Edition, Philadelphia, PA: F. A. Davis.

Audio programs:

Fitzgerald, M. A. <u>Anxiety and Panic Disorder: The Latest Treatment Recommendations</u>, North Andover, MA: Fitzgerald Health Education Associates.

Fitzgerald, M. A. <u>Depression: The Latest Treatment Recommendations</u>, North Andover, MA: Fitzgerald Health Education Associates.

Fitzgerald, M. A. <u>Laboratory Data Interpretation: A Case Study Approach</u>, North Andover, MA: Fitzgerald Health Education Associates.

Miller, S. K. <u>Prescribing for the Relief of Symptoms Update</u>, North Andover, MA: Fitzgerald Health Education Associates.

Video programs:

Wright, W. L. <u>Expert Exam: The Primary Care Neurologic Exam</u>, North Andover, MA: Fitzgerald Health Education Associates.

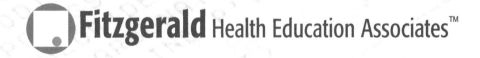

Chapter 15: Select Health Issues in the Older Adult

*Learning activities are an integral part of the course
available through your Fitzgerald Health learning portal at
fhea.com/npexpert:*

*Online component for Family and Adult-Gerontology NPs:
Common Musculoskeletal Problems*

*Special Considerations in Geriatric Prescribing: Issues of
Safety and Efficacy*

*Online component for Adult-Gerontology NPs:
Primary Care of the Adolescent*

*Foundations of Gerontology: Theories of Aging, Care of the
Frail Elder*

Table 15-1: Delirium vs. Dementia		
	Delirium	**Dementia**
Defined	A sudden state of rapid changes in brain function reflected in confusion, changes in cognition, activity, and level of consciousness	A slowly developing impairment of intellectual or cognitive function that is progressive and interferes with normal functioning
Etiology	Precipitated by an acute underlying cause, such as an acute illness	Variety of causes
Onset	Abrupt onset, over hours to days, usually a precise date, rapidly progressive change in mental status *"Mom was fine 4 days ago when I took her grocery shopping but is very confused today."*	Insidious onset that cannot be related to a precise date, gradual change in mental status, with reports of "good and bad days" *"Three years ago, we took over paying Dad's bills since he kept forgetting. This year, we realize he cannot be alone anymore."*
Memory	Impaired but variable recall	Memory loss, especially for recent events
Duration	Hours to days	Months to years
Reversible?	Usually reversible to baseline mental status when underlying illness resolves	Chronically progressive and irreversible
Sleep disturbance	Disturbed sleep-wake cycle with hour-to-hour variability, often worse as the day progresses ("sundowning")	Disturbed sleep-wake cycle but lacks hour-to-hour variability, often day-night reversal
Psychomotor	Usually a change in psychomotor activity, either hyperkinetic (25%), hypoactive (25%), or mixed (35%). No change in motor activity in approximately 15%.	No psychomotor changes until later in disease
Perceptual disturbances	Perceptual disturbances, including hallucinations	No perceptual disturbances until later in disease
Speech	Speech content incoherent, confused, with a wide variety of often inappropriately-used words, such as misnamed persons and items	In earlier stages, word searching, progressing to sparse speech content Mute in later disease
Note: Delirium and dementia often coexist. The diagnosis of delirium must be considered in the presence of a sudden-onset change in mental status in the person with dementia.		

Sources: Pierson, C. (2014) Older Patients, in Goolsby, M. J., Grubbs, L. Advanced Assessment: Interpreting findings and formulating differential diagnoses, 3rd Edition. Philadelphia, PA: F. A. Davis.

Merck Manual: Overview of Delirium and Dementia, available at www.merckmanuals.com/professional/neurologic_disorders/delirium_and_dementia/overview_of_delirium_and_dementia.html#v1036234

Delirium etiology

- Drugs
  - When any medication is added or dose is adjusted. Problematic medications include systemic anticholinergics (TCA, first-generation antihistamines, such as diphenhydramine), 1st- and 2nd-generation antipsychotics, opioids, opiates, benzodiazepines, alcohol, other
- Emotional (mood disorders, loss); Electrolyte disturbance (in particular, hyponatremia)
- Low PO_2 (hypoxemia from CAP, COPD, MI, pulmonary embolism [PE]); Lack of drugs (withdrawal from alcohol, other habituating substances)
- Infection
  - ***UTI, CAP (most common delirium etiology)***
- Retention of urine or feces; Reduced sensory input (blindness, deafness, darkness, change in surroundings)
- Ictal or postictal state
  - Alcohol withdrawal relatively common reason for isolated seizure in the older adult
- Undernutrition
  - Protein/calorie malnutrition, vitamin B_{12} or folate deficiency, dehydration, including postoperative volume disturbance
- Metabolic (poorly-controlled DM, under- or untreated hypo- or hyperthyroidism); Myocardial problems (MI, heart failure, dysrhythmia)
- Subdural hematoma
  - Can be a result of minor head trauma, due to a combination of brain atrophy and fragile blood vessels

Source: Merck Manual: Overview of Delirium and Dementia, available at www.merckmanuals.com/professional/neurologic_disorders/delirium_and_dementia/overview_of_delirium_and_dementia.html#v1036234

Delirium intervention

- Assess those at greatest risk to help avoid this condition.
- Treat underlying cause, recognizing that infection, medications, fractures are most common contributors to the development of delirium.

Table 15-2: Dementia Etiology

Dementia type	Comment
Alzheimer-type	Approximately 50–80%
Vascular (multi-infarct) dementia	Approximately 20%
Parkinson disease	5%
Miscellaneous causes	HIV, dialysis encephalopathy, neurosyphilis, normal-pressure hydrocephalus, Pick's disease, Lewy body disease, frontotemporal dementia, others
Approximately 30% of people with Alzheimer-type dementia also have vascular dementia.	

Table 15-3: Evaluation of the Person with New-onset Mental Status Change

The evaluation of the person with mental status change starts with the comprehensive health history and physical examination. Diagnostic testing should be focused in order to reveal the diagnosis of underlying etiology with potentially reversible conditions.

Definite	As directed by patient risk factors and presentation
BUN, Cr Glucose Calcium Sodium Hepatic enzymes Vitamin B_{12}/folate TSH RPR/VDRL (syphilis testing) CBC with WBC differential UA, U C & S ECG	Brain imaging (CT vs. MRI) PET scan Toxic screen CXR ESR HIV Additional studies as needed

Source: Merck Manual: Overview of Delirium and Dementia, available at www.merckmanuals.com/professional/neurologic_disorders/delirium_and_dementia/overview_of_delirium_and_dementia.html#v1036234

Notes:

Table 15-4: American Academy of Neurology Standards for Alzheimer-type Dementia (AD) Care	
Strategy	**Comment**
To slow decline in AD	Vitamin E 1,000 international units twice daily or selegiline 5 mg twice daily No added benefit to using both products The use of NSAIDs and postmenopausal hormone therapy has not been supported for this purpose.
In mild-to-moderate–stage disease, the use of the cholinesterase inhibitors is considered to be the mainstay of treatment.	Cholinesterase inhibitors (donepezil [Aricept®], rivastigmine [Exelon®], galantamine [Razadyne®]) have *clear though minor and time-limited benefits* by increasing availability of acetylcholine. At the same time, this small effect is clinically significant.
In moderate-to-severe AD, further studies of multiple interventions are needed.	Approved for use in *moderate-to-severe AD, the N-methyl-D-aspartate receptor antagonist memantine (Namenda®).* Through its effect on glutamate, helps to create an environment that allows for storage and retrieval of information. Also used in earlier disease with cholinesterase inhibitor. Donepezil (Aricept®) also approved for use in more advanced disease.
Treat agitation and depression.	Approximately 40% of individuals with dementia will also have depression. Standard antidepressant therapy is indicated, keeping in mind potential drug-drug and drug-food interactions.
Consider non–AD-related (noncognitive) reasons for behavioral issues, such as behavioral disturbances.	Evaluate for pain, infection, and other clinical conditions commonly found in the older adult population.
If environmental manipulation fails to eliminate agitation or psychosis in the person with dementia, consider treatment with psychotropic medication.	Second-generation antipsychotics such as risperidone best studied for this indication, recognizing the increased risk of stroke and cardiovascular events associated with the use of this drug class in older adults with dementia.

Source: AAN Guideline Summary for Clinicians: Detection, diagnosis and management of dementia, available at
http://tools.aan.com/professionals/practice/pdfs/dementia_guideline.pdf

For a helpful clinical tool, see AAN Dementia Encounter Kit, available at
http://www.aan.com/Guidelines/Home/ByTopic?topicId=15

1. Mrs. Little is a 78-year-old woman with recently-diagnosed Alzheimer-type dementia (AD) who is here today for an office visit with her 55-year-old daughter. According to her daughter, Mrs. Little struggles with word-finding and has difficulty following directions. She appears "not to care about what is going on around her," while other times is engaged in family activities. According to her daughter, Mrs. Little will have an angry verbal outburst that is triggered by a minor problem. Her daughter states, "This is not like my mother. Usually she is very patient." When evaluating Mrs. Little, the NP considers that irritability in a person with early-stage dementia is often indicative of a:

   A. Mood disorder.

   B. Thought disorder.

   C. Normal pressure hydrocephalus.

   D. Hyperparathyroidism.

2. Mrs. Little currently resides with her daughter's family and they voice a desire for this to continue "as long as possible and safe." When evaluating Mrs. Little's healthcare needs, choose the two options that do not apply.

   A. A home safety evaluation should be conducted and appropriate modifications carried out.

   B. If Mrs. Little has a sudden change in mental status, her healthcare provider should be contacted as soon as possible.

   C. Behavioral difficulties often arise in individuals with AD if their usual routine is disrupted.

   D. The use of a cholinesterase inhibitor will likely improve her mental status to a point that is nearly equivalent to her predementia baseline.

   E. The most common adverse effects from cholinesterase inhibitor use include nausea and diarrhea.

   F. A second-generation antipsychotic such as risperidone should be started to help minimize the angry outburst risk.

*Boxed warning: Elderly patients with dementia-related psychosis treated with antipsychotic drugs are at an increased risk of death. Analyses of 17 placebo-controlled trials (modal duration of 10 weeks), largely in patients taking atypical antipsychotic drugs, revealed a risk of death in drug-treated patients of between 1.6 to 1.7 times the risk of death in placebo-treated patients. The causes of death were varied; most of the deaths appeared to be either cardiovascular (e.g., heart failure, sudden death) or infectious (e.g., pneumonia) in nature. See http://www.fda.gov/Drugs/DrugSafety/PostmarketDrugSafetyInformationforPatientsandProviders/ucm124830.htm for additional information.

Table 15-5: Strategies to Improve Functional Performance and Reduce Problem Behaviors in Dementia

Strategy	Strength of evidence
To improve functional performance	
Behavior modification, scheduled toileting, prompted voiding to reduce urinary incontinence	Strong
Graded assistance, practice and positive reinforcement to increase functional independence	Good

Source: AAN Guideline Summary for Clinicians: Detection, Diagnosis and Management of Dementia, available at
http://tools.aan.com/professionals/practice/pdfs/dementia_guideline.pdf

Table 15-6: Medications with Significant Systemic Anticholinergic Effect: Tricyclic antidepressants (amitriptyline [Elavil®], doxepin [Sinequan®, Silenor®]), overactive bladder medications (oxybutynin [Ditropan®]), first-generation antihistamines, select antipsychotics, others
Potential adverse effects due to systemic anticholinergic effect

Dry mouth, skin	Hyperpnea
Blurred vision	Mydriasis
Urinary retention (usually w/BPH)	Flushing
Sedation	Psychosis
Agitation	Seizure
Tachycardia	Coma
	Hyperthermia

Source: 2015 Beers Criteria Update Expert Panel. American Geriatrics Society Updated Beers Criteria for Potentially Inappropriate Medication Use in Older Adults.
https://www.guideline.gov/summaries/summary/49933?f=rss&osrc=12

Or

- Dry as a bone (dry mouth)
- Red as a beet (flushing)
- Mad as a hatter (confusion)
- Hot as a hare (hyperthermia)
- Can't see (vision changes)
- Can't pee (urinary retention)
- Can't spit (dry mouth)
- Can't (something that rhymes with spit [constipation])

3. According to the recommendations found in the Beers Criteria, the use of certain medications and the other members of its class should be avoided in the older adult. Match the medication with the rationale for avoiding or using with caution in the elder.

A. Zolpidem (Ambien®)

B. Amitriptyline (Elavil®)

C. Naproxen sodium (Aleve®, Anaprox®)

D. Sertraline (Zoloft®)

Significant risk of orthostatic hypotension	Elavil
Increase in fall and fracture risk	Ambien
Potential to promote fluid retention	Naproxen
Increased risk for hyponatremia	Sertraline

For further information on medications to avoid in the older adult, see American Geriatrics Society: 2015 Beers Criteria Update Expert Panel. American Geriatrics Society Updated Beers Criteria for Potentially Inappropriate Medication Use in Older Adults. https://www.guideline.gov/summaries/summary/49933?f=rss&osrc=12

4. Match the patient presentations with the following terms:

A. "All of a sudden, I passed out and woke up on the floor."

B. "I feel lightheaded."

C. "The room is spinning."

Syncope	A
Dizziness	B
Vertigo	C

Table 15-7: Syncope			
Condition	**Definition**	**Common etiology**	**Comment**

Patient presentation, "I passed out. I don't know what happened, but I woke up on the floor."	A transient loss of consciousness characterized by a loss of postural tone, typically sudden in onset, with no warning, with spontaneous recovery
	
	Since the patient has no warning of the event and therefore makes no attempt to break the fall, patient often has injury as a result of the fall associated with a syncopal episode.
		• Neurally-mediated syncope: Example: Vasovagal syncope
		  o Causes: Fear, pain, anxiety, prolonged standing in one place, warmth, nausea, sweating, lightheadedness
		• Situational syncope:
		  o Causes: Cough, defecation, micturition, swallow
		• Cardiac outflow tract obstruction: Examples:
		  o Hypertrophic cardiomyopathy
		  o Valvular, especially high-grade aortic stenosis
		  o Aortic dissection
		  o Dysrhythmia, including ventricular tachycardia, SVT, prolonged QT interval (consider use of QT-prolonging medications, such as macrolides and fluoroquinolone antibiotics, second-generation antipsychotics, others), AV heart block with HR<30 BPM
		• Orthostatic hypotension
		  o Dehydration, including excessive diuresis
		  o Medications implicated in orthostatic syncope: TCA, alpha-blockers, calcium channel blockers, clonidine, diuretics, alcohol, PDE-5 inhibitors (erectile dysfunction medications)
			Intervention primarily involves an accurate diagnosis of the underlying condition and treating the underlying cause.

Source: Merck Manual: Syncope, available at
www.merck.com/mmpe/sec07/ch069/ch069f.html#sec07-ch069-ch069e-140

Table 15-8: Dizziness vs. Vertigo		
	Dizziness	**Vertigo**
Condition	Sense of disturbed relationship to space, but surroundings are not moving.	Surroundings are moving; sensation of motion with eyes closed.
Patient presentation	"I feel lightheaded."	"The room is spinning."
Common etiology	Multiple causes including circulatory or neurologic disorders	Usually inner-ear disturbance (i.e., small crystals within the inner ear become displaced and incorrectly stimulate nerve cells within the semicircular canals)
Common causes	Circulatory disorder (e.g., orthostatic hypotension), neurologic conditions (e.g., Parkinson's), certain medications, anxiety disorders, hypoglycemia, hyperthermia, dehydration	Inflammation of inner ear, Meniere's disease, head trauma, stroke, multiple sclerosis, tumors, certain types of migraine headaches
Intervention	Treat underlying cause	If symptomatic, treat underlying cause

Source: MedlinePlus. Dizziness and Vertigo, available at:
https://medlineplus.gov/dizzinessandvertigo.html

5. Ms. Hopkins is a 78-year-old woman with a history of hypertension, dyslipidemia, and stable angina pectoris who presents for follow-up care. She is a former smoker who quit 25 years ago with a 40 pack-year history. She denies chest pain or shortness of breath. Her current medications include a beta-adrenergic antagonist, sustained-release nitrate, angiotensin-converting enzyme inhibitor, statin, low-dose aspirin, and a thiazide diuretic. She complains of feeling a "catch or cramp" in her lower posterior legs bilaterally when she walks for extended periods. This is promptly relieved by rest. Which of the following do you anticipate finding on examination of her lower extremities?

   A. Hyperpigmentation with bilateral ankle edema

   B. Diminished bilateral pedal pulses with thinning of the skin

   C. Extensive dry skin with evidence of lichenification on the plantar aspects of both feet

   D. Diminished sensory perceptions and abnormal monofilament examination

6. An appropriate diagnostic test to perform next for Ms. Hopkins is:

   A. Venography of lower legs.

   B. Ankle-Brachial Index (ABI).

   C. ECG.

   D. Serum B-type natriuretic peptide (BNP).

Table 15-9: Peripheral Artery Disease vs. Venous Insufficiency vs. Peripheral Neuropathy

Presentation	Etiology	Diagnosis	Treatment
Peripheral artery disease (PAD)			
Leg pain and numbness during activities (intermittent claudication); persistent infections or sores on the leg and feet; pale or bluish color to skin. Some patients may be asymptomatic.	Systemic build-up of plaque in the arteries, limiting blood flow (usually observed in the legs). Smoking is the main risk factor. Other factors include age, high blood pressure, hypercholesterolemia, and elevated blood sugar.	Ankle-brachial Index (ABI) value <0.9; doppler ultrasound or MRI to assess bloodflow; treadmill test to evaluate severity of symptoms; arteriogram to identify blocked arteries	Lifestyle modifications (e.g., smoking cessation, physical activity, weight loss if overweight). Treatments to control blood pressure, cholesterol, and blood sugar. Antiplatelets (e.g., aspirin) to prevent blood clots. Cilostazol and pentoxifylline to reduce symptoms of PAD. Surgery to improve blood flow.
Venous insufficiency			
Common symptoms include burning, swelling, throbbing, cramping, aching, and heaviness in the legs; restless legs and leg fatigue; telangiectasias (spider veins).	Congenital absence of or damage to venous valves resulting in reflux through superficial veins; thrombus formation can also cause valve failure.	Physical exam of the appearance of leg veins. Duplex ultrasound can be used to assess blood flow in veins and eliminate other causes (e.g., blood clots).	Lifestyle changes (physical activity, weight loss if overweight), use of compression stockings to decrease swelling. Various techniques to remove the refluxing superficial vessels (e.g., sclerotherapy or ablation).
Peripheral neuropathy			
Gradual onset of numbness and tingling in hands and feet; burning pain; sharp electric-like pain; muscle weakness; extreme sensitivity to touch.	Damage to nerves extending to peripheral system. Diabetes is the most common cause, though others include traumatic injuries, infections, and exposure to toxins.	Nerve damage identified via nerve function test (electromyography) or nerve biopsy. Full medical history and physical to identify underlying cause of neuropathy.	Pain can be alleviated with NSAIDs (mild pain), anti-seizure and antidepressant medications, lidocaine patch, and opioids (when other treatments fail). Transcutaneous electrical nerve stimulation (TENS) can help relieve symptoms.

Source: National Heart, Lung, and Blood Institute. Peripheral Arterial Disease. Available at: http://www.nhlbi.nih.gov/health/health-topics/topics/pad/

Robert Weiss. Venous Insufficiency. Available at: http://emedicine.medscape.com/article/1085412-treatment

Table 15-10: Tap Water Temperature Safety: Primary Prevention of Burns	
Tap water temperature	**Length of time to 3rd degree burn if adult exposed to water of this temperature**
150°F (65.6°C)	2 seconds
140°F (60°C)	6 seconds
130°F (54.4°C)	30 seconds
120°F (48.9°C)	5 minutes

Note: Children and the elderly will likely burn at lower temperatures and with shorter exposure. As a result, it is recommended that hot water heaters should be set to a temperature of no more than 120°F (48.9°C). Bath and shower water should be hand-tested prior to use to ensure a safe temperature.

Source: Consumer Product Safety Commission, available at http://www.cpsc.gov//PageFiles/121522/5098.pdf

Bonus questions for this chapter available through your Fitzgerald Health learning portal at fhea.com/npexpert.

195

Table 15-11: Possible Warning Signs of Alzheimer-type Dementia vs. Typical Age-related Memory Changes		
Challenge	**Possible warning sign of Alzheimer-type dementia**	**Part of typical age-related memory changes**
Memory loss that disrupts daily life	Memory loss, especially forgetting recently learned information, forgetting important dates or events, asking for the same information over and over Reliance on memory aids, such as reminder notes, electronic devices, or family members for activities the person could at one time handle independently	*Sometimes forgetting names or appointments, but remembering this information later*
Challenges in planning or solving problems	Changes in ability to develop and follow a plan or work with numbers, trouble following a familiar recipe or keeping track of monthly bills Difficulty concentrating, taking much longer to do things than in past	*Making occasional errors when balancing a checkbook or other similar task*
Difficulty completing familiar tasks at home, at work, or at leisure	Difficulty in completing typical daily tasks, such as trouble driving to a familiar location, managing a budget, or remembering rules of a favorite game	*Occasionally needing help to perform a task, such as using the settings on a microwave or recording a television show*
Confusion with time or place	Losing track of dates, seasons, and overall passage of time Trouble understanding something if it is not happening immediately Sometimes they may forget where they are or how they got there.	*Occasionally getting the date or day of the week incorrect but correcting this later*
Trouble understanding visual images and spatial relationships	Vision problems are often an early sign. Difficulty reading, judging distance, and determining color or contrast Altered perception, such as passing a mirror and thinking someone else is in the room or not realizing that he/she is the person in the mirror	*Vision changes related to cataracts or other common age-related changes*
New problems with words in speaking or writing	Trouble following or joining a conversation, often stopping in the middle of a conversation without idea of how to continue, often repeating parts of the conversation Struggle with vocabulary, difficulty finding the right word, calling items by the wrong name, developing new ways to describe an item, such as calling French fried potatoes, "those skinny things you eat with ketchup"	*Sometimes having trouble finding the right word*
Misplacing things and losing the ability to retrace steps	Placing items in unusual places, such as shoes in the refrigerator, repeatedly misplacing items, occasionally accusing others of stealing the misplaced item This problem tends to accelerate in frequency over time.	*Misplacing items from time to time, such as a pair of glasses or the remote control, with the ability to retrace steps to locate the item*

Table 15-12: Depression vs. Pseudodementia vs. Dementia in the Older Adult			
Finding	Depression (Mental status improvement to predepression baseline with treatment)	Pseudodementia (Dementia syndrome or cognitive impairment of severe depression, mental status improvement to predepression baseline with treatment)	Dementia (Slowly progressive change in mental status)
Change in mental status	Relatively rapid	Onset fairly well demarcated	Slow mental decline
Orientation	Can usually report correct time, date, location	Can usually report correct time, date, location with encouragement and coaching	Confused, often becomes lost in a familiar location
Memory	Notices or worries about memory problem, can report nature of memory difficulty, has trouble with concentration	Takes increased effort to complete mental status exam (MSE), likely to answer "I don't know." Improved performance with coaching and encouragement.	Difficulty with short-term memory, usually does not notice memory problems
Language and motor skills	Usually slow when compared to baseline but normal	Usually slow when compared to baseline but normal	Writing, speaking, motor skills impaired

Source: Pierson, C. (2011) Older Patients, in Goolsby, M. J., Grubbs, L. <u>Advanced Assessment: Interpreting findings and formulating differential diagnoses</u>, 2nd Edition. Philadelphia, PA: F. A. Davis. Pp. 477-507

Table 15-13: Dementias: An Overview					
	Mild cognitive impairment (MCI)	**Alzheimer's dementia (AD)**	**Vascular dementia (VaD)**	**Dementia with Lewy body (DLB)**	**Frontotemporal dementias (FTDs)**
Definition and prevalence	Decline in cognition more expected for age. No change in ADLs 3–19% in those at age>65 years	AD=50–70% of all cases of dementia At age 85, 11% of men, 14% females have AD	Often co-occurs with AD=mixed dementia- likely the second most common dementia As solo cause, third most common dementia 8–15% of dementia	15–20% of late-onset dementia Patients with dementia symptoms around the same time as having symptoms of Parkinson's	Group of related disorders that cause degeneration of the frontal and temporal lobes. (e.g., Pick's dementia)
First symptoms	Memory loss	Memory loss	Often, but not always sudden; variable; apathy, falls, focal weakness, disorientation, anxiety/depression	Fluctuating presentation, visual hallucinations (may present as a psychiatric disorder), REM sleep disorder, delirium, parkinsonism, repeated and unexplained falls	Insidious onset and gradual progression. Personality changes cause more problems than cognitive problems. Apathy; poor judgment/insight, speech/language; hyperorality
Risk factors	Age, low education level, h/o depression or anxiety, lack of exercise, African ancestry, HTN, hyperlipidemia, presence of apolipoprotein E (ApoE) E4 allele	Age, female gender, AA and Hispanics > Caucasian. Down syndrome, being a mother of child with Down syndrome, genetic vulnerability (chromosomes 1, 6, 12, 14, 21) Acquired risk factors include HTN, lipoproteins, cerebrovascular disease, altered glucose metabolism, and brain trauma.	Increasing age, male gender, cardiovascular risk factors (e.g., HTN, smoking, T2DM, dyslipidemia, etc.)	More common in men ApoE E4 allele found more often in patients with DLB	Familial risk possible

Continued...

Table 15-13 (cont.): Dementias: An Overview					
	Mild cognitive impairment (MCI)	**Alzheimer's dementia (AD)**	**Vascular dementia (VaD)**	**Dementia with Lewy body (DLB)**	**Frontotemporal dementias (FTDs)**
Biological basis	Multiple possible etiologies: Alzheimer's, vascular, metabolic, medical disorder, traumatic events, depression, substance abuse With MCI, changes in temporal lobe, hippocampus with brain volume decrease	Characteristic neuritic plaques, neurofibrillary tangles, and synaptic loss throughout the cerebral cortex and limbic system	Cortical and subcortical infarcts (e.g., small-vessel disease, multi-infarcts, cerebral hypoperfusion)	Lewy bodies are dense intracellular neuronal inclusions found in the cortical, subcortical area of brain. EEG can help distinguish between DLB and AD, but not between VaD and AD or diffuse DLB.	In Pick's disease, the brain has marked frontal and temporal lobe atrophy.
Pharmacologic treatment	Acetylcholinesterase inhibitors can delay but not prevent the progression of MCI.	Mild-moderate AD: Acetylcholinesterase inhibitors Moderate-severe AD: NMDA receptor antagonists SGAs with caution	Cholinesterase inhibitors may help. Treat vascular risks (e.g., HTN, dyslipidemia, diabetes)	First-generation antipsychotic use can result in neuromuscular sensitivity (e.g. NMS). SGAs helpful with psychosis w/o adverse effects. Treat depression; anticholinesterase use can benefit memory.	Symptomatic psychiatric treatment (e.g., SSRI for depression, psychostimulant for apathy, risperidone for problem behaviors)
Non-pharmacologic treatment	Good health habits to reduce risk factors Volunteer or stay cognitively active	Reminiscence therapy, personalized music, non-confrontational and enjoyable social interactions, redirection, reassurance Support family	Physical activities, intellectually stimulating and social activity	Variable course, but generally more rapid progression than AD. Time from diagnosis to death is ~6 years.	Protect patients from his or her indiscretions
Course of illness	>50% will progress to dementia w/in 5 years. Depression doubles the risk	Average life span after diagnosis is 6–9 years. Progressive illness with impairment in function and dependence on others for care.	Shortens lifespan by 3 years.	Progresses more rapidly than AD. Mean age at diagnosis is 68 years, death at 75 years	Generally slow progression

Source: Perese, E. (2012). <u>Psychiatric Advanced Practice Nursing: A biopsychosocial foundation for practice</u>. Philadelphia, PA: F.A. Davis.

Organ System, Therapeutic Category, Drug(s)	Recommendation, Rationale, Quality of Evidence (QE), Strength of Recommendation (SR)
Anticholinergics	
First-generation antihistamines: ■ Brompheniramine ■ Carbinoxamine ■ Chlorpheniramine ■ Clemastine ■ Cyproheptadine ■ Dexbrompheniramine ■ Dexchlorpheniramine ■ Dimenhydrinate ■ Diphenhydramine (oral) ■ Doxylamine ■ Hydroxyzine ■ Meclizine ■ Promethazine ■ Triprolidine	*Avoid* Highly anticholinergic; clearance reduced with advanced age, and tolerance develops when used as hypnotic; risk of confusion, dry mouth, constipation, and other anticholinergic effects or toxicity Use of diphenhydramine in situations such as acute treatment of severe allergic reaction may be appropriate *QE = Moderate; SR = Strong*
Antiparkinsonian agents ■ Benztropine (oral) ■ Trihexyphenidyl	*Avoid* Not recommended for prevention of extrapyramidal symptoms with antipsychotics; more-effective agents available for treatment of Parkinson disease *QE = Moderate; SR = Strong*
Antispasmodics: ■ Atropine (excludes ophthalmic) ■ Belladonna alkaloids ■ Clidinium-Chlordiazepoxide ■ Dicyclomine ■ Hyoscyamine ■ Propantheline ■ Scopolamine	*Avoid* Highly anticholinergic, uncertain effectiveness *QE = Moderate; SR = Strong*
Antithrombotics	
Dipyridamole, oral short-acting (does not apply to the extended-release combination with aspirin)	*Avoid* May cause orthostatic hypotension; more effective alternatives available; IV form acceptable for use in cardiac stress testing *QE = Moderate; SR = Strong*
■ Ticlopidine	*Avoid* Safer, effective alternatives available *QE = Moderate; SR = Strong*

CNS=central nervous system; NSAIDs=nonsteroidal anti-inflammatory drugs; SIADH, syndrome of inappropriate antidiuretic hormone.

Table 1 *(continued on page 3)*

From THE AMERICAN GERIATRICS SOCIETY

A POCKET GUIDE TO THE

AGS 2015 BEERS CRITERIA

This guide has been developed as a tool to assist healthcare providers in improving medication safety in older adults. The role of this guide is to *inform* clinical decision-making, research, training, quality measures and regulations concerning the prescribing of medications for older adults to improve safety and quality of care. It is based on *The AGS 2015 Updated Beers Criteria for Potentially Inappropriate Medication Use in Older Adults.*

Originally conceived of in 1991 by the late Mark Beers, MD, a geriatrician, the Beers Criteria catalogues medications that cause side effects in the elderly due to the physiologic changes of aging. In 2011, the AGS sponsored its first update of the criteria, assembling a team of experts and using an enhanced, evidence-based methodology. In 2015, the AGS again funded the development of the Updated Criteria using an evidence-based methodology and rating each Criterion (quality of evidence and strength of evidence) using the American College of Physicians' Guideline Grading System, which is based on the GRADE scheme developed by Guyatt et al.

The full document, along with accompanying resources can be viewed in their entirety online at geriatricscareonline.org.

INTENDED USE

The goal of this guide is to improve care of older adults by reducing their exposure to Potentially Inappropriate Medications (PIMS).

■ This should be viewed as a guideline for identifying medications for which the risks of their use in older adults outweigh the benefits.

■ These criteria are not meant to be applied in a punitive manner.

■ This list is not meant to supersede clinical judgment or an individual patient's values and needs. Prescribing and managing disease conditions should be individualized and involve shared decision-making.

■ These criteria also underscore the importance of using a team approach to prescribing and the use of non-pharmacological approaches and of having economic and organizational incentives for this type of model.

■ Two companion pieces were developed for the 2015 update. The first addresses the best way for patients, providers, and health systems to use (and not use) the 2015 AGS Beers Criteria. The second is a list of alternative medications included in the current use of High-Risk Medications in the Elderly and Potentially Harmful Drug-Disease Interactions in the Elderly quality measures. Both pieces can be found on geriatricscareonline.org.

The criteria are not applicable in all circumstances (i.e. patient's receiving palliative and hospice care). If a provider is not able to find an alternative and chooses to continue to use a drug on this list in an individual patient, designation of the medication as potentially inappropriate can serve as a reminder for close monitoring so that adverse drug effects can be incorporated into the electronic health record and prevented or detected early.

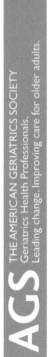

AGS THE AMERICAN GERIATRICS SOCIETY
Geriatrics Health Professionals.
Leading change. Improving care for older adults.

Table 1 Continued

Organ System, Therapeutic Category, Drug(s)	Recommendation, Rationale, QE, SR
Anti-infective	
■ Nitrofurantoin	**Avoid in individuals with creatinine clearance <30 mL/min or for long-term suppression of bacteria** Potential for pulmonary toxicity, hepatoxicity, and peripheral neuropathy, especially with long-term use; safer alternatives available QE = Low; SR = Strong
Cardiovascular	
Peripheral alpha-1 blockers ■ Doxazosin ■ Prazosin ■ Terazosin	*Avoid use as an antihypertensive* High risk of orthostatic hypotension; not recommended as routine treatment for hypertension; alternative agents have superior risk/benefit profile QE = Moderate; SR = Strong
Central alpha blockers ■ Clonidine ■ Guanabenz ■ Guanfacine ■ Methyldopa ■ Reserpine (>0.1 mg/d)	**Avoid clonidine as first-line antihypertensive. Avoid others as listed** High risk of adverse CNS effects; may cause bradycardia and orthostatic hypotension; not recommended as routine treatment for hypertension QE = Low; SR = Strong
Disopyramide	**Avoid** Disopyramide is a potent negative inotrope and therefore may induce heart failure in older adults; strongly anticholinergic; other antiarrhythmic drugs preferred QE = Low; SR = Strong
Dronedarone	**Avoid in individuals with permanent atrial fibrillation or severe or recently decompensated heart failure** Worse outcomes have been reported in patients taking dronedarone who have permanent atrial fibrillation or severe or recently decompensated heart failure QE = High; SR = Strong
Digoxin	**Avoid as first-line therapy for atrial fibrillation. Avoid as first-line therapy for heart failure. If used for atrial fibrillation or heart failure, avoid dosages >0.125 mg/d** Use in atrial fibrillation: should not be used as a first-line agent in atrial fibrillation, because more-effective alternatives exist and it may be associated with increased mortality Use in heart failure: questionable effects on risk of hospitalization and may be associated with increased mortality in older adults with heart failure; in heart failure, higher dosages not associated with additional benefit and may increase risk of toxicity Decreased renal clearance of digoxin may lead to increased risk of toxic effects; further dose reduction may be necessary in those with Stage 4 or 5 chronic kidney disease. QE = Atrial fibrillation: moderate. Heart failure: low. Dosage >0.125 mg/d: moderate; SR = Atrial fibrillation: strong. Heart failure: strong. Dosage >0.125 mg/d: strong

Table 1 (continued on page 4)

Table 1 Continued

Organ System, Therapeutic Category, Drug(s)	Recommendation, Rationale, QE, SR
■ Nifedipine, immediate release	**Avoid** Potential for hypotension; risk of precipitating myocardial ischemia QE = High; SR = Strong
Amiodarone	**Avoid amiodarone as first-line therapy for atrial fibrillation unless the patient has heart failure or substantial left ventricular hypertrophy** Amiodarone is effective for maintaining sinus rhythm but has greater toxicities than other antiarrhythmics used in atrial fibrillation; it may be reasonable first-line therapy in patients with concomitant heart failure or substantial left ventricular hypertrophy if rhythm control is preferred over rate control QE = High; SR = Strong
Central nervous system	
Antidepressants, alone or in combination ■ Amitriptyline ■ Amoxapine ■ Clomipramine ■ Desipramine ■ Doxepin >6 mg/d ■ Imipramine ■ Nortriptyline ■ Paroxetine ■ Protriptyline ■ Trimipramine	**Avoid** Highly anticholinergic, sedating, and cause orthostatic hypotension; safety profile of low-dose doxepin (≤6 mg/d) comparable with that of placebo QE = High; SR = Strong
Antipsychotics, first- (conventional) and second- (atypical) generation	**Avoid, except for schizophrenia, bipolar disorder, or short-term use as antiemetic during chemotherapy** Increased risk of cerebrovascular accident (stroke) and greater rate of cognitive decline and mortality in persons with dementia Avoid antipsychotics for behavioral problems of dementia and/or delirium unless nonpharmacological options (e.g., behavioral interventions) have failed or are not possible *and* the older adult is threatening substantial harm to self or others QE = Moderate; SR = Strong
Barbiturates ■ Amobarbital ■ Butabarbital ■ Butalbital ■ Mephobarbital ■ Pentobarbital ■ Phenobarbital ■ Secobarbital	**Avoid** High rate of physical dependence, tolerance to sleep benefits, greater risk of overdose at low dosages QE = High; SR = Strong

Table 1 (continued on page 5)

Table 1 Continued

Page 6

Organ System, Therapeutic Category, Drug(s)	Recommendation, Rationale, QE, SR
Estrogens with or without progestins	***Avoid oral and topical patch. Vaginal cream or tablets: acceptable to use low-dose intravaginal estrogen for management of dyspareunia, lower urinary tract infections, and other vaginal symptoms*** Evidence of carcinogenic potential (breast and endometrium); lack of cardioprotective effect and cognitive protection in older women. Evidence indicates that vaginal estrogens for the treatment of vaginal dryness are safe and effective; women with a history of breast cancer who do not respond to nonhormonal therapies are advised to discuss the risk and benefits of low-dose vaginal estrogen (dosages of estradiol <25 mcg twice weekly) with their health care provider *QE = Oral and patch: high. Vaginal cream or tablets: moderate.; SR = Oral and patch: strong. Topical vaginal cream or tablets: weak*
Growth hormone	***Avoid, except as hormone replacement following pituitary gland removal*** Impact on body composition is small and associated with edema, arthralgia, carpal tunnel syndrome, gynecomastia, impaired fasting glucose *QE = High; SR = Strong*
Insulin, sliding scale	***Avoid*** Higher risk of hypoglycemia without improvement in hyperglycemia management regardless of care setting: refers to sole use of short- or rapid-acting insulins to manage or avoid hyperglycemia in absence of basal or long-acting insulin; does not apply to titration of basal insulin or use of additional short- or rapid-acting insulin in conjunction with scheduled insulin (ie, correction insulin) *QE = Moderate; SR = Strong*
Megestrol	***Avoid*** Minimal effect on weight; increases risk of thrombotic events and possibly death in older adults *QE = Moderate; SR = Strong*
Sulfonylureas, long-duration: ■ Chlorpropamide ■ Glyburide	***Avoid*** Chlorpropamide: prolonged half-life in older adults; can cause prolonged hypoglycemia; causes SIADH Glyburide: higher risk of severe prolonged hypoglycemia in older adults *QE = High; SR = Strong*
Gastrointestinal	
Metoclopramide	***Avoid, unless for gastroparesis*** Can cause extrapyramidal effects, including tardive dyskinesia; risk may be greater in frail older adults *QE = Moderate; SR = Strong*
Mineral oil, given orally	***Avoid*** Potential for aspiration and adverse effects; safer alternatives available *QE = Moderate; SR = Strong*

Table 1 *(continued on page 7)*

Table 1 Continued

Page 5

Organ System, Therapeutic Category, Drug(s)	Recommendation, Rationale, QE, SR
Benzodiazepines *Short- and intermediate-acting:* ■ Alprazolam ■ Estazolam ■ Lorazepam ■ Oxazepam ■ Temazepam ■ Triazolam *Long-acting:* ■ Clorazepate ■ Chlordiazepoxide (alone or in combination with amitriptyline or clidinium) ■ Clonazepam ■ Diazepam ■ Flurazepam ■ Quazepam	***Avoid*** Older adults have increased sensitivity to benzodiazepines and decreased metabolism of long-acting agents; in general, all benzodiazepines increase risk of cognitive impairment, delirium, falls, fractures, and motor vehicle crashes in older adults May be appropriate for seizure disorders, rapid eye movement sleep disorders, benzodiazepine withdrawal, ethanol withdrawal, severe generalized anxiety disorder, and periprocedural anesthesia *QE = Moderate; SR = Strong*
Meprobamate	***Avoid*** High rate of physical dependence; very sedating *QE = Moderate; SR = Strong*
Nonbenzodiazepine, benzodiazepine receptor agonist hypnotics ■ Eszopiclone ■ Zolpidem ■ Zaleplon	***Avoid*** Benzodiazepine-receptor agonists have adverse events similar to those of benzodiazepines in older adults (e.g., delirium, falls, fractures); increased emergency room visits/hospitalizations; motor vehicle crashes; minimal improvement in sleep latency and duration *QE = Moderate; SR = Strong*
Ergoloid mesylates (dehydrogenated ergot alkaloids) Isoxsuprine	***Avoid*** Lack of efficacy *QE = High; SR = Strong*
Endocrine	
Androgens ■ Methyltestosterone ■ Testosterone	***Avoid unless indicated for confirmed hypogonadism with clinical symptoms*** Potential for cardiac problems; contraindicated in men with prostate cancer *QE = Moderate; SR = Weak*
Desiccated thyroid	***Avoid*** Concerns about cardiac effects; safer alternatives available *QE = Low; SR = Strong*

Table 1 *(continued on page 6)*

Table 1 Continued

Organ System, Therapeutic Category, Drug(s)	Recommendation, Rationale, QE, SR
Proton-pump inhibitors	**Avoid scheduled use for >8 weeks unless for high-risk patients (e.g., oral corticosteroids or chronic NSAID use), erosive esophagitis, Barrett's esophagitis, pathological hypersecretory condition, or demonstrated need for maintenance treatment (e.g., due to failure of drug discontinuation trial or H_2 blockers)** Risk of C difficile infection and bone loss and fractures *QE = High; SR = Strong*
Pain medications	
Meperidine	**Avoid, especially in those with chronic kidney disease** Not effective oral analgesic in dosages commonly used; may have higher risk of neurotoxicity, including delirium, than other opioids; safer alternatives available *QE = Moderate; SR = Strong*
Non-cyclooxygenase-selective NSAIDs, oral: ■ Aspirin >325 mg/d ■ Diclofenac ■ Diflunisal ■ Etodolac ■ Fenoprofen ■ Ibuprofen ■ Ketoprofen ■ Meclofenamate ■ Mefenamic acid ■ Meloxicam ■ Nabumetone ■ Naproxen ■ Oxaprozin ■ Piroxicam ■ Sulindac ■ Tolmetin	**Avoid chronic use, unless other alternatives are not effective and patient can take gastroprotective agent (proton-pump inhibitor or misoprostol)** Increased risk of gastrointestinal bleeding or peptic ulcer disease in high-risk groups, including those aged >75 or taking oral or parenteral corticosteroids, anticoagulants, or antiplatelet agents; use of proton-pump inhibitor or misoprostol reduces but does not eliminate risk. Upper gastrointestinal ulcers, gross bleeding, or perforation caused by NSAIDs occur in approximately 1% of patients treated for 3–6 months and in ~2–4% of patients treated for 1 year; these trends continue with longer duration of use *QE = Moderate; SR = Strong*
■ Indomethacin ■ Ketorolac, includes parenteral	**Avoid** Indomethacin is more likely than other NSAIDs to have adverse CNS effects. Of all the NSAIDs, indomethacin has the most adverse effects. Increased risk of gastrointestinal bleeding/peptic ulcer disease, and acute kidney injury in older adults *QE = Moderate; SR = Strong*
Pentazocine	**Avoid** Opioid analgesic that causes CNS adverse effects, including confusion and hallucinations, more commonly than other opioid analgesic drugs; is also a mixed agonist and antagonist; safer alternatives available *QE = Low; SR = Strong*
Skeletal muscle relaxants: ■ Carisoprodol ■ Chlorzoxazone ■ Cyclobenzaprine ■ Metaxalone ■ Methocarbamol ■ Orphenadrine	**Avoid** Most muscle relaxants poorly tolerated by older adults because some have anticholinergic adverse effects, sedation, increased risk of fractures; effectiveness at dosages tolerated by older adults questionable *QE = Moderate; SR = Strong*
Genitourinary	
Desmopressin	**Avoid for treatment of nocturia or nocturnal polyuria** High risk of hyponatremia; safer alternative treatments *QE = Moderate; SR = Strong*

TABLE 2. 2015 American Geriatrics Society Beers Criteria for Potentially Inappropriate Medication Use in Older Adults Due to Drug–Disease or Drug–Syndrome Interactions That May Exacerbate the Disease or Syndrome

Disease or Syndrome	Drug(s)	Recommendation, Rationale, Quality of Evidence (QE), Strength of Recommendation (SR)
Cardiovascular		
Heart failure	NSAIDs and COX-2 inhibitors Nondihydropyridine CCBs (diltiazem, verapamil)—avoid only for heart failure with reduced ejection fraction Thiazolidinediones (pioglitazone, rosiglitazone) Cilostazol Dronedarone (severe or recently decompensated heart failure)	**Avoid** Potential to promote fluid retention and exacerbate heart failure *QE = NSAIDs: moderate. CCBs: moderate. Thiazolidinediones: high. Cilostazol: low. Dronedarone: high; SR = Strong*
Syncope	Acetylcholinesterase inhibitors (AChEIs) Peripheral alpha-1 blockers ■ Doxazosin ■ Prazosin ■ Terazosin Tertiary TCAs ■ Chlorpromazine ■ Thioridazine ■ Olanzapine	**Avoid** Increases risk of orthostatic hypotension or bradycardia *QE = Peripheral alpha-1 blockers: high. TCAs, AChEIs, antipsychotics: moderate; SR = AChEIs, TCAs: strong. Peripheral alpha-1 blockers, antipsychotics: weak*
Central nervous system		
Chronic seizures or epilepsy	Bupropion Chlorpromazine Clozapine Maprotiline Olanzapine Thioridazine Thiothixene Tramadol	**Avoid** Lowers seizure threshold; may be acceptable in individuals with well-controlled seizures in whom alternative agents have not been effective *QE = Low; SR = Strong*
Delirium	Anticholinergics* Antipsychotics Benzodiazepines Chlorpromazine Corticosteroids[a] H_2-receptor antagonists ■ Cimetidine ■ Famotidine ■ Nizatidine ■ Ranitidine Meperidine Sedative hypnotics	**Avoid** Avoid in older adults with or at high risk of delirium because of potential of inducing or worsening delirium Avoid antipsychotics for behavioral problems of dementia and/or delirium unless nonpharmacological options (e.g., behavioral interventions) have failed or are not possible **and** the older adult is threatening substantial harm to self or others. Antipsychotics are associated with greater risk of cerebrovascular accident (stroke) and mortality in persons with dementia *QE = Moderate; SR = Strong*

Table 2 *(continued on page 9)*

Table 2 Continued

Disease or Syndrome	Drug(s)	Recommendation, Rationale, QE, SR
Dementia or cognitive impairment	Anticholinergics* Benzodiazepines H₂-receptor antagonists Nonbenzodiazepine, benzodiazepine receptor agonist hypnotics ■ Eszopiclone ■ Zolpidem ■ Zaleplon Antipsychotics, chronic and as-needed use	**Avoid** Avoid due to adverse CNS effects Avoid antipsychotics for behavioral problems of dementia and/or delirium unless nonpharmacological options (e.g., behavioral interventions) have failed or are not possible *and* the older adult is threatening substantial harm to self or others. Antipsychotics are associated with greater risk of cerebrovascular accident (stroke) and mortality in persons with dementia *QE = Moderate; SR = Strong*
History of falls or fractures	Anticonvulsants Antipsychotics Benzodiazepines Nonbenzodiazepine, benzodiazepine receptor agonist hypnotics ■ Eszopiclone ■ Zaleplon ■ Zolpidem TCAs SSRIs Opioids	**Avoid unless safer alternatives are not available; avoid anticonvulsants except for seizure and mood disorders. Opioids: avoid, excludes pain management due to recent fractures or joint replacement** May cause ataxia, impaired psychomotor function, syncope, additional falls; shorter-acting benzodiazepines are not safer than long-acting ones If one of the drugs must be used, consider reducing use of other CNS-active medications that increase risk of falls and fractures (ie, anticonvulsants, opioid-receptor agonists, antipsychotics, antidepressants, benzodiazepine-receptor agonists, other sedatives/hypnotics) and implement other strategies to reduce fall risk *QE = High. Opioids: Moderate; SR = Strong. Opioids: Strong*
Insomnia	Oral decongestants ■ Pseudoephedrine ■ Phenylephrine Stimulants ■ Amphetamine ■ Armodafinil ■ Methylphenidate ■ Modafinil Theobromines ■ Theophylline ■ Caffeine	**Avoid** CNS stimulant effects *QE = Moderate; SR = Strong*

*See Table 7 in full criteria available on www.geriatricscareonline.org.

Table 2 *(continued on page 10)*

Table 2 Continued

Disease or Syndrome	Drug(s)	Recommendation, Rationale, QE, SR
Parkinson disease	All antipsychotics (except aripiprazole, quetiapine, clozapine) Antiemetics ■ Metoclopramide ■ Prochlorperazine ■ Promethazine	**Avoid** Dopamine-receptor antagonists with potential to worsen parkinsonian symptoms Quetiapine, aripiprazole, clozapine appear to be less likely to precipitate worsening of Parkinson disease *QE = Moderate; SR = Strong*
Gastrointestinal		
History of gastric or duodenal ulcers	Aspirin (>325 mg/d) Non-COX-2 selective NSAIDs	**Avoid unless other alternatives are not effective and patient can take gastroprotective agent (ie, proton-pump inhibitor or misoprostol)** May exacerbate existing ulcers or cause new/additional ulcers *QE = Moderate; SR = Strong*
Kidney/Urinary tract		
Chronic kidney disease Stages IV or less (creatinine clearance <30 mL/min)	NSAIDs (non-COX and COX-selective, oral and parenteral)	**Avoid** May increase risk of acute kidney injury and further decline of renal function *QE = Moderate; SR = Strong*
Urinary incontinence (all types) in women	Estrogen oral and transdermal (excludes intravaginal estrogen) Peripheral Alpha-1 blockers ■ Doxazosin ■ Prazosin ■ Terazosin	**Avoid in women** Aggravation of incontinence *QE = Estrogen: High. Peripheral alpha-1 blockers: Moderate; SR = Estrogen: Strong. Peripheral alpha-1 blockers: Strong*
Lower urinary tract symptoms, benign prostatic hyperplasia	Strongly anticholinergic drugs, except antimuscarinics for urinary incontinence.*	**Avoid in men** May decrease urinary flow and cause urinary retention *QE = Moderate; SR = Strong*

*excludes inhaled and topical forms. Oral and parenteral corticosteroids may be required for conditions such as exacerbations of COPD but should be prescribed in the lowest effective dose and for the shortest possible duration.
CCB=calcium channel blocker; AChEI=acetylcholinesterase inhibitor; CNS=central nervous system; COX=cyclooxygenase; NSAIDs=nonsteroidal antiinflammatory drug; TCAs=tricyclic antidepressant

Table 2 *(continued on page 11)*

TABLE 4. 2015 American Geriatrics Society Beers Criteria for Potentially Clinically Important Non-anti-infective Drug–Drug Interactions That Should Be Avoided in Older Adults

Object Drug and Class	Interacting Drug and Class	Recommendation, Risk Rationale, Quality of Evidence (QE), Strength of Recommendation (SR)
ACEIs	Amiloride or triamterene	**Avoid routine use; reserve for patients with demonstrated hypokalemia while taking an ACEI** Increased risk of hyperkalemia *QE = Moderate; SR = Strong*
Anticholinergic	Anticholinergic	**Avoid; minimize number of anticholinergic drugs** Increased risk of cognitive decline *QE = Moderate; SR = Strong*
Antidepressants (ie, TCAs and SSRIs)	≥2 other CNS-active drugs[a]	**Avoid total of ≥3 CNS-active drugs[a]; minimize number of CNS-active drugs** Increased risk of falls *QE = Moderate; SR = Strong*
Antipsychotics	≥2 other CNS-active drugs[a]	**Avoid total of ≥3 CNS-active drugs[a]; minimize number of CNS active drugs** Increased risk of falls *QE = Moderate; SR = Strong*
Benzodiazepines and nonbenzodiazepine, benzodiazepine receptor agonist hypnotics	≥2 other CNS-active drugs[a]	**Avoid total of ≥3 CNS-active drugs[a]; minimize number of CNS active drugs** Increased risk of falls and fractures *QE = High; SR = Strong*
Corticosteroids, oral or parenteral	NSAIDs	**Avoid: if not possible, provide gastrointestinal protection** Increased risk of peptic ulcer disease or gastrointestinal bleeding *QE = Moderate; SR = Strong*
Lithium	ACEIs	**Avoid; monitor lithium concentrations** Increased risk of lithium toxicity *QE = Moderate; SR = Strong*
Lithium	Loop diuretics	**Avoid; monitor lithium concentrations** Increased risk of lithium toxicity *QE = Moderate; SR = Strong*
Opioid receptor agonist analgesics	≥2 other CNS-active drugs[a]	**Avoid total of ≥3 CNS-active drugs[a]; minimize number of CNS drugs** Increased risk of falls *QE = High; SR = Strong*
Peripheral Alpha-1 blockers	Loop diuretics	**Avoid in older women, unless conditions warrant both drugs** Increased risk of urinary incontinence in older women *QE = Moderate; SR = Strong*
Theophylline	Cimetidine	**Avoid** Increased risk of theophylline toxicity *QE = Moderate; SR = Strong*
Warfarin	Amiodarone	**Avoid when possible; monitor INR closely** Increased risk of bleeding *QE = Moderate; SR = Strong*
Warfarin	NSAIDs	**Avoid when possible; if used together, monitor for bleeding closely** Increased risk of bleeding *QE = High; SR = Strong*

[a]Central nervous system (CNS)-active drugs: antipsychotics; benzodiazepines; nonbenzodiazepine, benzodiazepine receptor agonist hypnotics; tricyclic antidepressants (TCAs); selective serotonin reuptake inhibitors (SSRIs); and opioids.

ACEI = angiotensin-converting enzyme inhibitor; NSAID=nonsteroidal antiinflammatory drug.

TABLE 3. 2015 American Geriatrics Society Beers Criteria for Potentially Inappropriate Medications to Be Used with Caution in Older Adults

Drug(s)	Recommendation, Rationale, Quality of Evidence (QE), Strength of Recommendation (SR)
Aspirin for primary prevention of cardiac events	**Use with caution in adults ≥80 years old** Lack of evidence of benefit versus risk in adults ≥80 years old *QE = Low; SR = Strong*
Dabigatran	**Use with caution in adults ≥75 years old and in patients with CrCl <30 mL/min** Increased risk of gastrointestinal bleeding compared with warfarin and reported rates with other target-specific oral anticoagulants in adults ≥75 years old; lack of evidence of efficacy and safety in individuals with CrCl <30 mL/min *QE = Moderate; SR = Strong*
Prasugrel	**Use with caution in adults aged ≥75** Increased risk of bleeding in older adults; benefit in highest-risk older adults (e.g., those with prior myocardial infarction or diabetes mellitus) may offset risk *QE = Moderate; SR = Weak*
Antipsychotics Diuretics Carbamazepine Carboplatin Cyclophosphamide Cisplatin Mirtazapine Oxcarbazepine SNRIs SSRIs TCAs Vincristine	**Use with caution** May exacerbate or cause SIADH or hyponatremia; monitor sodium level closely when starting or changing dosages in older adults *QE = Moderate; SR = Strong*
Vasodilators	**Use with caution.** May exacerbate episodes of syncope in individuals with history of syncope *QE = Moderate; SR = Weak*

CrCl= creatinine clearance; SNRIs = Serotonin-nonrepinephrine reuptake inhibitors; SSRIs = Selective serotonin reuptake inhibitors; TCA=tricyclic antidepressant.

TABLE 5. 2015 American Geriatrics Society Beers Criteria for Non-Anti-Infective Medications That Should Be Avoided or Have Their Dosage Reduced with Varying Levels of Kidney Function in Older Adults

Medication Class and Medication	Creatinine Clearance, mL/min, at Which Action Required	Recommendation, Rationale, Quality of Evidence (QE), Strength of Recommendation (SR)
Cardiovascular or hemostasis		
Amiloride	<30	***Avoid*** Increased potassium and decreased sodium *QE = Moderate; SR = Strong*
Apixaban	<25	***Avoid*** Increased risk of bleeding *QE = Moderate; SR = Strong*
Dabigatran	<30	***Avoid*** Increased risk of bleeding *QE = Moderate; SR = Strong*
Edoxaban	30–50 <30 or >95	***CrCl 30-50: Reduce dose*** ***CrCl <30 or >95: Avoid*** Increased risk of bleeding *QE = Moderate; SR = Strong*
Enoxaparin	<30	***Reduce dose*** Increased risk of bleeding *QE = Moderate; SR = Strong*
Fondaparinux	<30	***Avoid*** Increased risk of bleeding *QE = Moderate; SR = Strong*
Rivaroxaban	30–50 <30	***CrCl 30-50: Reduce dose*** ***CrCl <30: Avoid*** Increased risk of bleeding *QE = Moderate; SR = Strong*
Spironolactone	<30	***Avoid*** Increased potassium *QE = Moderate; SR = Strong*
Triamterene	<30	***Avoid*** Increased potassium and decreased sodium *QE = Moderate; SR = Strong*
Central nervous system and analgesics		
Duloxetine	<30	***Avoid*** Increased gastrointestinal adverse effects (nausea, diarrhea) *QE = Moderate; SR = Weak*
Gabapentin	<60	***Reduce dose*** CNS adverse effects *QE = Moderate; SR = Strong*

Table 5 Continued

Medication Class and Medication	Creatinine Clearance, mL/min, at Which Action Required	Recommendation, Rationale, QE, SR
Levetiracetam	≤80	***Reduce dose*** CNS adverse effects *QE = Moderate; SR = Strong*
Pregabalin	<60	***Reduce dose*** CNS adverse effects *QE = Moderate; SR = Strong*
Tramadol	<30	***Immediate release: Reduce dose*** ***Extended release: avoid*** CNS adverse effects *QE = Low; SR = Weak*
Gastrointestinal		
Cimetidine	<50	***Reduce dose*** Mental status changes *QE = Moderate; SR = Strong*
Famotidine	<50	***Reduce dose*** Mental status changes *QE = Moderate; SR = Strong*
Nizatidine	<50	***Reduce dose*** Mental status changes *QE = Moderate; SR = Strong*
Ranitidine	<50	***Reduce dose*** Mental status changes *QE = Moderate; SR = Strong*
Hyperuricemia		
Colchicine	<30	***Reduce dose; monitor for adverse effects*** Gastrointestinal, neuromuscular, bone marrow toxicity *QE = Moderate; SR = Strong*
Probenecid	<30	***Avoid*** Loss of effectiveness *QE = Moderate; SR = Strong*

CNS=central nervous system.

The primary target audience is the practicing clinician. The intentions of the criteria include 1) improving the selection of prescription drugs by clinicians and patients; 2) evaluating patterns of drug use within populations; 3) educating clinicians and patients on proper drug usage; and 4) evaluating health-outcome, quality-of-care, cost, and utilization data.

Reprinted with permission from American Geriatrics Society 2015 Beers Criteria Update Expert Panel. (2015). American Geriatrics Society 2015 updated Beers Criteria for potentially inappropriate medication use in older adults. Journal of the American Geriatrics Society. Volume 63, Issue11, pages 2227-2246, November 2015.

Table 5 *(continued on page 14)*

Resources for Additional Study

Books:

Fitzgerald, M. A. (2017) Older Adults, <u>Nurse Practitioner Certification Examination and Practice Preparation</u>, 5th Edition, Philadelphia, PA: F. A. Davis.

Audio programs:

Fitzgerald, M. A. <u>Laboratory Data Interpretation: A Case Study Approach</u>, North Andover, MA: Fitzgerald Health Education Associates.

Miller, S. K. <u>Gerontological Nurse Practitioner Certification Exam Review and Advanced Practice Update</u>, North Andover, MA: Fitzgerald Health Education Associates.

Chapter 16: Primary Care of the Well and Sick Infant, Child, and Teen

(FNP track only)

Learning activities are an integral part of the course available through your Fitzgerald Health learning portal at fhea.com/npexpert:

Online programs for Family NPs only:

Primary Care of the Woman during Pregnancy and Common Infant Dermatological Conditions

While children are not miniature adults, many adult therapeutic concepts apply to pediatrics.

- Examples: Asthma care, antimicrobial therapy

- *Pharmacodynamics knows no age.*

Most children are healthy. As a family NP and primary care provider, you help ensure the child and family remain well. When approaching your practice and examination, keep in mind your role as coach, counselor, and advocate.

For a helpful guide to pediatric well-child visits, see Bright Futures, Promoting Child Development, available at https://brightfutures.aap.org/Bright%20Futures%20Documents/BF3%20pocket%20guide_final.pdf

For help with conducting the pediatric health history and physical examination, please see Feeney, S., Fitzgerald, M.A. Pediatric Physical Assessment Cue Cards, 10th Edition, North Andover, MA: Fitzgerald Health Education Associates, Inc., available at fhea.com

1. A full-term pregnancy is one where the birth occurs between:

   A. 37 weeks and 38 weeks of gestation.

   B. 37 weeks and 38 weeks plus 6 days of gestation.

   C. 39 weeks and 40 weeks plus 6 days of gestation.

   D. 41 weeks and 41 weeks plus 6 days of gestation.

Table 16-1: Classification of Term Pregnancy EDD=40 weeks	
Early-term	37 weeks through 38 weeks plus 6 days
Full-term	39 weeks through 40 weeks plus 6 days
Late-term	41 weeks through 41 weeks plus 6 days
Post-term	42 weeks and beyond

Source: http://www.acog.org/Resources-And-Publications/Committee-Opinions/Committee-on-Obstetric-Practice/Definition-of-Term-Pregnancy

Table 16-2: Defining Times in Earlier Childhood	
Neonate	Ages 0–28 days
Infancy	First year of life
Toddler	Ages 1–2 years
Preschool	Ages 3–4 years
School-age	Ages 5–12 years

2. Which of the following do you not expect to find in the examination of a full-term healthy newborn?

    A. Holding the baby about 16–20 inches (41–51 cm) away from the caregiver's face takes advantage of the newborn's visual range.

    B. Bluish scleral tint is noted regardless of ethnicity or eye color.

    C. The newborn's eyes are quite light and glare sensitive.

    D. If an object goes towards the newborn's eye, the baby will likely react with a defensive blink reflex.

3. During a well neonate visit for Christopher, a healthy 2-week-old boy born at 41 weeks' gestation, you anticipate that the baby will have:

    A. A visual preference for the human face.

    B. Hear low-pitched voices best.

    C. Will not react to the cry of other neonates.

    D. A poorly-developed sense of smell.

4. When counseling the parents of Joshua, a healthy term newborn, about sleeping safety, the NP advises the following:

    A. Position the baby on the side with a positioning wedge or back, as he is most comfortable.

    B. Place the baby in a face-up position for sleep.

    C. Place a soft bumper in the crib to minimize the risk of injury.

    D. Even when a caregiver is in attendance, the tummy-down position is not safe in the first two months of life.

Table 16-3: Summary and Strength of Recommendations: Task Force on Sudden Infant Death Syndrome "Back to sleep, tummy to play"	
Supervised, awake "tummy time" is recommended to facilitate development and to minimize development of positional plagiocephaly. Start immediately post-birth, building up slowly to a total of 30 minutes per day until such time as child easily turns tummy-to-back, back-to-tummy without assistance.	
Level A recommendations	• Back to sleep for every sleep. • Use a firm sleep surface. • Room-sharing without bed-sharing is recommended. • Keep soft objects and loose bedding out of the crib. • Pregnant women should receive regular prenatal care. • Avoid smoke exposure during pregnancy and after birth. • Avoid alcohol and illicit drug use during pregnancy and after birth. • Breastfeeding is recommended. • Consider offering a pacifier at nap time and bedtime. • Avoid infant overheating. • Do not use home cardiorespiratory monitors as a strategy for reducing the risk of SIDS. • Expand the national campaign to reduce the risk of SIDS to include a major focus on the safe sleep environment and ways to reduce the risk of all sleep-related infant deaths, including SIDS, suffocation, and other accidental deaths; pediatricians, family physicians, and other primary care providers should actively participate in this campaign.
Level B recommendations	• Infants should be immunized in accordance with recommendations of the AAP and Centers for Disease Control and Prevention. • Avoid use of commercial devices marketed to reduce the risk of SIDS.
Level C recommendations	• Healthcare professionals, staff in newborn nurseries and NICUs, and child care providers should endorse the SIDS risk-reduction recommendations from birth. • Media and manufacturers should follow safe-sleep guidelines in their messaging and advertising. • Continue research and surveillance on the risk factors, causes, and pathophysiological mechanisms of SIDS and other sleep-related infant deaths, with the ultimate goal of eliminating these deaths entirely.

Sources: SIDS and Other Sleep-Related Infant Deaths: Expansion of Recommendations for a Safe Infant Sleeping Environment, available at pediatrics.aappublications.org/content/early/2011/10/12/peds.2011-2284

Laughlin J, Luerssen TG, Dias MS, and the Committee on Practice and Ambulatory Medicine. Prevention and Management of Positional Skull Deformities in Infants. *Pediatrics.* 2011;128;1236-41.

During breastfeeding with proper latch, no dimpling of the baby's cheeks, no clicking sound with sucking.

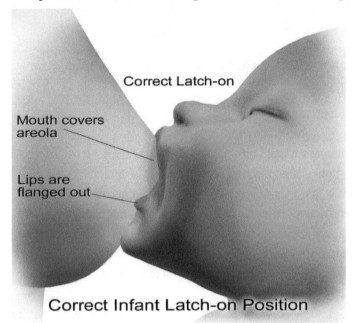

Correct Latch-on

Mouth covers areola

Lips are flanged out

Correct Infant Latch-on Position

Figure 16-12

5. In considering newborn jaundice, all of the following are correct except:

A. All forms of neonatal jaundice are usually seen first in the face and then progress caudally to the trunk and extremities.

B. Using only visual evaluation of bilirubin levels to estimate the degree of jaundice can lead to errors in clinical judgment.

C. The onset of physiologic jaundice is usually within the first 12 hours of life.

D. Encouraging feedings at minimum every 2–3 hours at the breast per day while avoiding dextrose and water feedings will help minimize the newborn's risk of hyperbilirubinemia.

For additional information on guidelines for management of jaundice in the breastfeeding infant ≥35 weeks' gestation, please visit
https://pediatrics.aappublications.org/content/124/4/1193

6. You are providing counseling for the parents and caregivers of a healthy full-term newborn who is being breastfed. The counseling should include information on all of the following except:

    A. The baby should make at least 6 wet diapers a day.

    B. Newborns often lose up to 10% of birth weight in the first week of life.

    C. A breastfed baby usually has 4 or more bowel movements per day.

    D. The baby should be back up to birth weight by age 3–4 weeks.

Table 16-4: Infant Feeding		
	Formula: Frequency and amount	**Breastfeeding: Average frequency**
Newborn	1.5–3 ounces (45–90 mL) every 2–3 hours	Every 1.5–3 hours, no more than 4 hours without feeding, minimum 8–12 feedings per day,
2 months	4–5 ounces (120–150 mL) every 2–4 hours	At least 7 to 9 times per day, usually dictated by infant
4 months	4–6 ounces (120–180 mL) every 3–4 hours	At least 6 to 8 times per day, usually dictated by infant and if supplemental feedings
6 months	6–8 ounces (180–230 mL) every 4–5 hours while awake	At least 4 to 6 times per day, usually dictated by infant and if supplemental feedings

7. You see Alexandra, born at 40.5 weeks' gestation, who is now 14 days old. According to her mother, she is a vigorous eater and is both breast- and formula-fed. On examination of the neonate, you note bilateral breast engorgement with physiologic galactorrhea on the left. You appreciate all of the following are correct concerning this condition except:

    A. Its onset is usually at approximately day 3–4 of life.

    B. That maternal hormonal influences are likely the cause.

    C. This breast engorgement will resolve without intervention within the first two months of life.

    D. Further evaluation is required to confirm this assessment.

8. A 12-day-old infant who is otherwise well presents with a 2-day history of irritation of both eyes. He was born at a local birth center and received standard newborn care including ocular chemoprophylaxis. Examination reveals bilateral lid swelling, chemosis, and mucoid discharge. The most likely cause of this condition is:

    A. Chemical irritation from neonatal chemoprophylaxis.

    B. Chlamydial (inclusion) conjunctivitis.

    C. Gonococcal conjunctivitis.

    D. Neonatal adenovirus infection.

Source: http://www.cdc.gov/conjunctivitis/newborns.html

9. You are rounding in the nursery and see the neonate of a mother who is HBsAg-positive. Your most appropriate action is to:

    A. Check the baby for HBsAb.

    B. Inform the mother that she should not breastfeed.

    C. Administer hepatitis B immunization to mother and infant.

    D. Give hepatitis B immunization and hepatitis B immune globulin to the newborn.

10. Indicate the appropriate neonatal reflex for each description.

    A. Moro reflex

    B. Palmar grasp

    C. Babinski reflex

    D. Parachute reflex

    E. Tonic neck reflex

    F. Stepping reflex

    G. Rooting reflex

Walking motion made with legs and feet when held upright and feet touching the ground. Appears for first 3–4 months, then reappears at 12–24 months.	
Turning of head and sucking when cheek is stroked. No longer seen by 6–12 months.	
Throwing out arms and legs followed by pulling them back to the body following a sudden movement or loud noise. No longer seen by 16 weeks.	
Arching of back and head raises when placed on stomach. Lasts until about 12 months.	
When stimulating the back, the trunk and hips move toward the side of the stimulus. No longer seen by 9 months.	
Grasping of an object when placed in the palm. No longer seen by 2–3 months.	
Stroking the sole of the foot elicits fanning of the toes. No longer seen by 6 months.	

11. Which of the following is the most important time to screen for hearing defects?

    A. In the first days of life

    B. During the time of most intense speech formation

    C. Before the child enters school

    D. Once antimicrobial therapy for AOM is completed

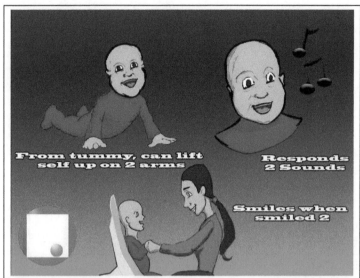

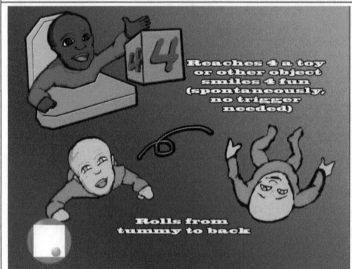

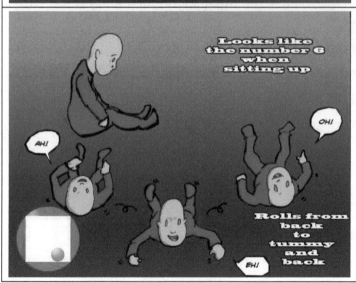

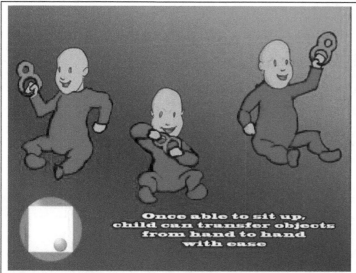

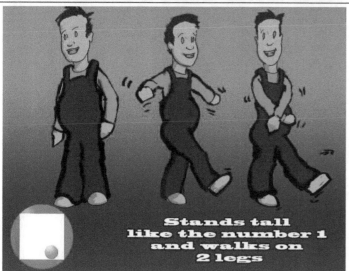

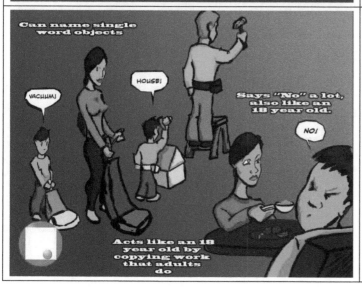

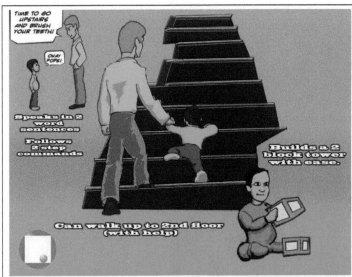

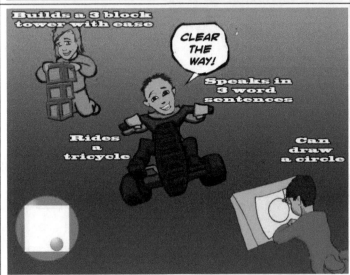

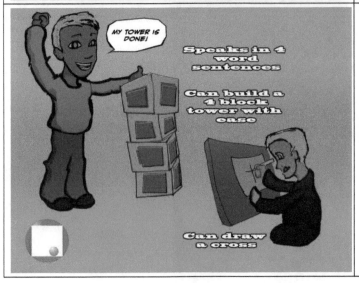

Table 16-5: Discipline	
Question	**Answer**
What is discipline?	A method of teaching children rules of conduct through providing limits and setting boundaries
Is punishment the same as discipline?	No, punishment is a part of discipline and is the consequence of not adhering to the rules.
How does "time out" work as a form of punishment?	This is a method of short-term isolation to decrease the undesirable behavior.
Where is the child placed for "time-out?"	The child sits in a special place that is safe, easily observed by parent or caregiver, uninteresting, and only used for "time out." Avoid the use of bed, bedroom, or any place where the child could be frightened.

12. In teaching a family about "time out," this method is appropriate to use beginning at about age _____.

13. The child remains in "time out" for what period of time?

_____.

Source: Communication and Discipline, available at
www.healthychildren.org/English/family-life/family-dynamics/communication-discipline/Pages/default.aspx

14. In a healthy 3½-year-old, what percentage of speech should be intelligible by people who are not in daily contact with the child?

   A. About 25%

   B. About 50%

   C. About 75%

   D. Nearly 100%

15. You see a well child who resists being placed in a supine position on the exam table, cries loudly when her parent is out of view, and has visibly erupting lower central incisors. This child is approximately what age?

   A. 6–8 weeks

   B. 3–4 months

   C. 7–8 months

   D. 2–3 years

Table 16-6: Tooth Eruption

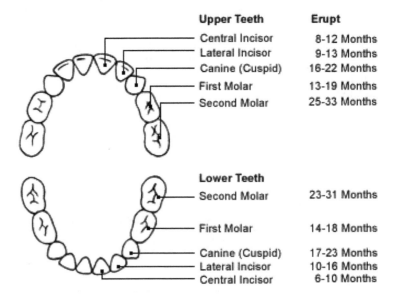

Upper Teeth	Erupt
Central Incisor	8-12 Months
Lateral Incisor	9-13 Months
Canine (Cuspid)	16-22 Months
First Molar	13-19 Months
Second Molar	25-33 Months

Lower Teeth	
Second Molar	23-31 Months
First Molar	14-18 Months
Canine (Cuspid)	17-23 Months
Lateral Incisor	10-16 Months
Central Incisor	6-10 Months

16. Which of the following is most consistent with a normal developmental exam for a thriving 6-month-old infant born at 32 weeks' gestation?

   A. Responds to own name and sits without support

   B. Reaches for toy with one hand and recognizes familiar people and objects at a distance

   C. Babbles mamama, bababa and transfers objects hand-to-hand without difficulty

   D. Vocalizes "ah" and "oh" sounds, and is able to lift head briefly when positioned on the tummy and turn it from side-to-side

For a helpful review of early childhood development with developmental "red flags," please see www.cdc.gov/ncbddd/actearly/milestones/index.html

17. Thomas is a neonate who was born at 32 weeks' gestation. The adjusted age calculation should be used to assess his development until age:

   A. 6 months.

   B. 12 months.

   C. 18 months.

   D. 24 months.

18. You examine a healthy 2-month-old boy and note that his foreskin cannot be retracted. You consider that:

    A. The foreskin should be forcibly retracted to facilitate cleaning.

    B. In most instances, the foreskin is not easily retractable until the child is about 3 years old.

    C. The risk for hypospadias or epispadias is increased in the presence of this finding.

    D. Persistent maternal hormonal influences contribute to this problem.

19. You examine a thriving 4-week-old boy who was born at 39 weeks' gestation and note a painless, tense, non-reducible, relatively symmetric scrotal enlargement that brightly and evenly transilluminates. The parents report that the scrotum "always looks like this," without change in size during the course of the day. Bilateral testes, approximately 1 cm in length, are palpable and held within the scrotum. The penis is approximately 4 cm in length. You consider these findings are most consistent with:

    A. A normal examination.

    B. Bilateral inguinal hernias.

    C. Micropenis.

    D. Noncommunicating hydrocele.

Table 16-7: Hydrocele in the Infant			
	Causes	**Presentation**	**Management**
Non-communicating hydrocele **Most common**	Sealing of abdominal cavity during gestation with residual trapped peritoneal fluid in scrotal sac	Fluid-filled scrotal sac; transilluminates, nontender; testes normal; no change in scrotal size with position change, same at bedtime and on awakening	Reassurance, no risk of herniation; no special skin care needed Usually resolves by age 2 years without intervention; referral only if size interferes with activity, comfort
Communicating hydrocele **Relatively uncommon**	Incomplete sealing of peritoneal cavity at inguinal area during gestation, leaving communication between abdominal cavity and scrotum	Fluid-filled scrotal sac; transilluminates, nontender; testes normal; however, amount of fluid in scrotum (scrotal size) varies with position of neonate; larger with dependent upright position (day) and smaller after lying flat (upon awakening)	Due to communication, an infant is at risk for herniation of abdominal contents; referral to pediatric urologist or surgeon is recommended.

Source: UpToDate®, Brenner, J.S. & Ojo, A., Causes of painless scrotal swelling in children and adolescents, available at www.uptodate.com/contents/causes-of-painless-scrotal-swelling-in-children-and-adolescents

20. Which of the following is most consistent with pyloric stenosis (upper GI obstruction [PS]) or intussusception (lower GI obstruction [I]) or both?

_____ A. Significantly more common in males.

_____ B. Sudden onset, colicky, severe, and intermittent abdominal pain.

_____ C. Accompanied by loose stools that are often described as currant jelly appearance (mixture of blood and sloughed mucous).

_____ D. Most common time for symptom onset= Approximately age 3 weeks.

_____ E. Post-fed projectile vomiting is present, with the baby eager to eat again immediately post emesis.

_____ F. Accompanied by a sausage-shaped abdominal mass.

_____ G. Olive-shaped RUQ abdominal mass occasionally noted.

_____ H. Usually occurs between ages 6–12 months.

_____ I. Ultrasonography is usually first-line diagnostic study.

Table 16-8: Pyloric Stenosis vs. Intussusception				
Condition	**Definition**	**Presentation**	**Diagnostics**	**Intervention**
Pyloric stenosis	Thickening of the pylorus muscle, preventing food from moving from the stomach to the small intestines.	Nonbilious vomiting (often projectile) or regurgitation; dehydration and malnutrition; jaundice. Condition usually presents at ~3 weeks of life.	Ultrasonography is preferred to detect thickened pyloric muscle. An enlarged pylorus ("olive") can often be palpated in the right upper quadrant of the abdomen.	Surgical correction is considered the standard of care.
Intussusception	Caused when a section of intestines invaginates into the adjoining intestinal lumen, causing bowel obstruction. If left untreated, is uniformly fatal in 2–5 days.	Vomiting, abdominal pain, rectal passage of blood and mucus, lethargy, and a palpable abdominal mass. Symptoms often preceded by an upper respiratory tract infection.	Ultrasonography to identify target and pseudokidney signs; contrast enema is the traditional and most reliable diagnostic approach; plain abdominal radiography only identifies about 60% of cases.	Non-operative approaches include hydrostatic or pneumatic enemas; surgical reduction needed if non-operative approaches are unsuccessful or if an obvious perforation is present.

Sources: Nazer H. Pediatric hypertrophic pyloric stenosis. Available at: http://emedicine.medscape.com/article/929829-overview

Blanco FC. Intussusception. Available at: http://emedicine.medscape.com/article/930708-overview

21. Pediatric immunizations: True or false?

    (T/F) MMR should not be given to a 12-month-old whose mother is pregnant.

    (T/F) A 6-month-old who is taking amoxicillin for acute otitis media (AOM) should have immunizations delayed until the antimicrobial course is completed.

    (T/F) Preterm infants are usually immunized at the schedule that corresponds with their birth or extrauterine age.

    (T/F) One of the best ways to protect infants younger than 6 months of age from influenza is to make sure members of their household and their caregivers are vaccinated against the disease.

    (T/F) The risk of autism can be reduced through the use of an early childhood vaccination schedule that minimizes the number of immunizations given at a single visit.

    (T/F) In order to avoid post-vaccine discomfort, younger children should be given a weight- and age-appropriate dose of an antipyretic, such as acetaminophen or ibuprofen, prior to receiving immunizations.

    (T/F) Children 6–11 months of age who are traveling outside the United States should receive 1 dose of MMR.

22. Which of the following vaccine(s) are recommended during pregnancy to achieve passive immunity in the newborn? (Select all that apply).

    A. Influenza

    B. Tdap

    C. Rubella

    D. Varicella

    Sources: http://www.cdc.gov/vaccines/hcp/acip-recs/vacc-specific/flu.html

    Chart of Contraindications and Precautions to Commonly Used Vaccines, available at www.cdc.gov/vaccines/recs/vac-admin/contraindications-vacc.html

23. As part of a well-child visit, you advise the parents of a well 6-month-old that a mild fever of 1–2 days in duration is most likely to occur after the baby receives:

    A. Inactivated polio virus (IPV) vaccine.

    B. *Haemophilus influenzae* type B (Hib) vaccine.

    C. Pneumococcal conjugate 13-valent vaccine (PCV13).

    D. Injectable influenza vaccine.

24. The American Academy of Pediatrics recommends screening for autism at which of the following times in early childhood?

    A. 6 and 12 months

    B. 12 and 18 months

    C. 18 and 24 months

    D. 24 and 30 months

Table 16-9: Developmental "Red Flags" in the Young Child **Persistent presence of ≥1 of these indicators warrants further evaluation.**
• **By 6 months:** No big smiles or other warm, joyful expressions
• **By 9 months:** No back-and-forth sharing of sounds, smiles, or other facial expressions
• **By 12 months:** Lack of response to name, no babbling or "baby talk," and/or no back-and-forth gestures, such as pointing, showing, reaching, or waving
• **By 16 months:** No spoken words
• **By 24 months:** No meaningful two-word phrases that don't involve imitating or repeating

Source: Modified Checklist for Autism in Toddlers (M-CHAT), available at:
http://www.firstsigns.org/downloads/m-chat.PDF, and at
www2.gsu.edu/~psydlr/Diana_L._Robins,_Ph.D._files/M-CHAT_new.pdf

Table 16-10: DSM-5 Criteria for Autism Spectrum Disorder (ASD) **(Encompasses the DSM-IV autistic disorder, childhood disintegrative disorder, and Rett's disorder)**
ASD is characterized by deficits in 2 core domains:

Persistent deficits in social communication and social interaction across multiple contexts, with notable deficits in:
  • Social-emotional reciprocity
  • Nonverbal communication behaviors
  • Developing, maintaining, and understanding relationships

Restricted, repetitive patterns of behavior, interests, or activities, ≥2 present
  • Stereotyped or repetitive motor movements, use of objects or speech
  • Insistence on sameness, inflexible adherence to routines or ritualized patterns of verbal or nonverbal behavior
  • Highly-restricted, fixated interests that are abnormal in intensity or focus
  • Hyper- or hyporeactivity to sensory input, or unusual interest in sensory aspects of environment

Severity is specified by degree of impairment on social communication and restricted, repetitive patterns of behavior.
Symptoms must be present in the early developmental period, though may not manifest until social demands exceed capacity.
Symptoms cause clinically significant impairment in social, occupational, or other important areas of functioning.

Source: American Psychiatric Association. (2013). Diagnostic and Statistical Manual of
Mental Disorders: DSM-5 (5th ed). Arlington, VA.

25. A 2½-year-old boy is brought by his mother who reports that, approximately 10 minutes ago, the child was injured when he pulled a pot of boiling water off the stove. The child is alert and crying, and age-appropriately resists the examination. Skin survey reveals approximately 18% body surface area of moist, red skin with peeling borders, largely involving the posterior thighs, buttocks, and scrotum. No other injury is noted. Identify the two most important considerations in his care.

    A. The injury should be débrided as soon as possible.

    B. The affected area should be promptly washed with an antiseptic solution.

    C. Specialty burn care should be promptly sought.

    D. Child protective services should be immediately notified.

    E. A course of oral antibiotics should be initiated.

Table 16-11: Child Maltreatment Risk Factors
Child <4 years of age
Special needs that can increase caregiver burden (disabilities, mental or physical health problems)
Parents' lack of understanding of child's needs, lack of parenting skills and knowledge of child development
Parental history of child maltreatment
Substance abuse/mental health issues in family
Parental characteristics (e.g., low education, low income)
Nonbiological, transient caregivers in the home (e.g., mother's male partner)
Family social isolation, disorganization, violence
Parenting stress, poor parent-child relationships
Community violence
Concentrated neighborhood disadvantage (e.g., residential instability, high unemployment rates)

Source:
http://www.cdc.gov/ViolencePrevention/childmaltreatment/riskprotectivefactors.html

Table 16-12: Defining Times and Tasks in Later Childhood and Adolescence

	Social Development	Psychological Development
Early adolescence 10–13 years	Concrete thinking with early moral concept struggles, progression of sexual identity development, reassessment of body image	Early work on emotional separation from parents, beginning to identify as a person other than parents' child; early strong peer identification, often early exploration of potentially harmful health behaviors including as substance use, others.
Mid-adolescence 14–17 years	Increased abstract thinking, often views self still seen as "bullet proof;" growing verbal abilities; identification of law with morality; start of fervent ideology (religious, political)	Increasing emotional separation from parents; strong peer identification, often increased health risk (smoking, alcohol, etc.); early educational and vocational plans
Late adolescence 18–21 years	Complex abstract thinking, increased impulse control; further development of personal identity; further development or rejection of religious and political ideology	Development of social autonomy, increasingly complex intimate relationships, moving towards development of vocational capability and financial independence

Sources: http://www.education.com/articles/middle-school/ and
http://www.education.com/articles/high-school/

Table 16-13: Tanner Stages:

Evaluation of Secondary Sexual Characteristics and Reproductive Capacity

Puberty occurs during, but is not synonymous with, adolescence.

Tanner stage	Male	Female
1	Pre-puberty	Pre-puberty
2	Testes enlarge; scrotal skin reddening with change in texture; sparse growth of long, slightly pigmented pubic hair at base of penis	Breast buds and papilla elevated, downy pigmented pubic hair along labia majora
3	Increase in penile length but minimal change in width, sometimes called the "pencil penis" stage; further scrotal enlargement; pubic hair darker, coarser, covers greater area; onset of growth spurt	Breast mound enlargement; darker, coarser, curling pubic hair on mons, labia majora; onset of growth spurt
4	Increase in penile length and width with development of glans; further darkening of scrotal skin; adult-type pubic hair with no spread to medial surface of thighs	Areola and papilla elevated to form a second mound above level of rest of breast; adult-type pubic hair with no spread to medial surface of thighs; menarche
5	Full adult genitalia; adult-type pubic hair with spread to medial surface of thighs, possibly abdomen	Recession of areola to mound of breast, extension of pubic hair to medial thigh

Source: Duderstadt, K. (2013) Pediatric Physical Examination, 2nd Edition, St. Louis, MO:
Elsevier Health Sciences

Tanner staging

Five stages like the five fingers

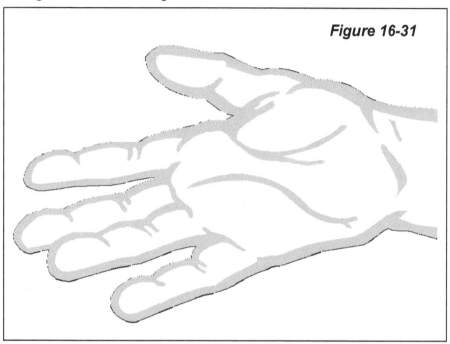

Figure 16-31

Table 16-14: Puberty: Normative vs. Alterations		
Gender	**Age range at onset of Tanner 2 changes (earliest pubertal changes)**	**Alterations in puberty: Early or late onset**
Female	7 y (thelarche only, earliest breast development) 8 y (pubarche, earliest pubic hair development)–13 y	<7–8 y: Idiopathic in majority (≥85%). Most common puberty disorder. Continuous GnRH agonist analog an option to delay progress, requires specialty evaluation for treatment. >13 y: Multiple factors: Nutrition (low weight), hormonal, genetic (Turner syndrome [XO female]), others
Male	9–14 y	<9 y: Idiopathic in <40% (CNS tumors most often implicated) >14 y: Multiple factors: Nutritional, hormonal, genetic, others

26. You see Sharon for a well-child visit. She is a 12-year-old who is at Tanner stage 2–3 and states unhappily, "I am the shortest girl in my class." When reviewing her growth chart, you notice she has been consistently between the 10th and 15th percentile for height and weight during her childhood. The rest of her examination is within normal limits. You advise that:

   A. She should have an evaluation by a pediatric endocrinology specialist.

   B. Her growth spurt will start soon.

   C. Due to her age, she is likely near her adult height.

   D. X-ray determination of bone age should be obtained.

27. Physiologic gynecomastia is usually found in which of the following?

    A. A 14-year-old male who is at Tanner stage 3

    B. A 12-year-old male who is at Tanner stage 2

    C. A 17-year-old male who is at Tanner stage 5

    D. A 10-year-old male who is at Tanner stage 1

28. You see a Tanner stage 4 14-year-old male who you suspect has Fragile X syndrome because of the notation of all of the following except:

    A. Macroorchidism.

    B. Large body habitus.

    C. History of learning differences.

    D. Hip and breast enlargement.

Table 16-15: Common Genetic Syndromes	
	Findings
Fragile X syndrome (FXS)	**In males:** Large forehead, ears, prominent jaw, tendency to avoid eye contact. Large testicles (macroorchidism) noted only after the beginning of puberty, large body habitus, learning and behavioral differences (hyperactivity, developmental disability common).
	In females: Significantly less common with fewer prominent findings, usually with less severe developmental issues
	Most common known cause of autism in either gender, occurs in all racial and ethnic groups.
	Blood testing available for carrier state (genetic risk for having a child with fragile X syndrome) or for diagnosis of the condition. Antenatal diagnosis possible.
Klinefelter syndrome, XXY male	Only males affected, with specific physical habitus: Low testicular volume, hip and breast enlargement, infertility. Mostly developmental issues, most commonly language impairment.
	Most common form of sex hormone aneuploidy (abnormal number of chromosomes within a cell) in males, some without symptoms.
	Blood testing available for carrier state (genetic risk for having a child with Klinefelter syndrome) or for diagnosis of the condition. Antenatal diagnosis possible.
Turner syndrome, XO female	Usually characterized by short stature (5 feet [152 cm] tall or under), usually evident by age 5 years; wide, webbed neck; broad, shield-shaped chest, absent menses, infertility. Often noticeable at birth, narrow, high-arched palate, retrognathia (lower jaw not prominent), low-set ears, edema of hands and feet. Females who are classified as mosaic Turner's syndrome, with chromosomal changes in some but not all cells, typically have milder features.
	High rate of spontaneous pregnancy loss in XO female fetus. Blood testing available for diagnosis of the condition. Antenatal diagnosis possible.

Sources: The National Fragile X Foundation. Fragile X Syndrome, available at https://fragilex.org/fragile-x/fragile-x-syndrome/
Turner Syndrome Society, available at http://www.turnersyndrome.org/

29. A 12-year-old boy presents with his mother for a well-child visit. What is the most helpful approach to this visit?

    A. Interview and examine the child in the absence of the mother.

    B. Interview the child with the mother, asking her to leave for the examination.

    C. Ask the child if he wishes his mother to be there for the interview and examination.

    D. Ask the mother if she wishes to be included in the interview and examination.

30. You see a 13-year-old boy with no immunizations documented. In updating this child's immunizations, which of the following should be omitted?

    A. Hepatitis B

    B. *Haemophilus influenzae* type B (Hib)

    C. Tetanus, diphtheria, acellular pertussis (Tdap)

    D. Measles, mumps, rubella (MMR)

Table 16-16: Acne Vulgaris	
Pathophysiology	**Comment**
Follicular epidermal hyperproliferation with subsequent follicle plugging, excess sebum production, presence of pathogenic *Propionibacterium acnes,* accompanying inflammation Keratolytic and antibacterial agents guide acne vulgaris therapy.	Affects 80% of all teens, with 20% having severe acne and subsequent scarring Affects areas of skin where sebaceous follicles located: Face, upper chest, and back

Table 16-17: Treatment Options in Acne Vulgaris

Key patient teaching points: All acne therapies take 6–8 weeks of use prior to significant clinical effect. Topical therapies should be used over entire skin region, not simply for spot therapy of existing lesions.

Acne medication	Mechanism of action, indications, considerations for use
Topical benzoyl peroxide cream, lotion, various concentrations (2.5% as effect as 10%, less irritating)	• *Antibacterial* • Inexpensive, available OTC. Most helpful in mild acne, usually with a keratolytic acne wash with salicylic acid 2%. Also comedolytic effects.
Topical retinoids including tretinoin gel, cream, various concentrations, other retinoid-like compounds, such as adapalene (Differin®) gel or cream, tazarotene (Tazorac®), tretinoin (Retin-A®), azelaic acid (Azelex®), lower strength OTC formulation	• *Keratolytic, significant antiinflammatory effect. Indicated in all acne types* • With initial use, mild to moderate skin irritation, improves over time. • Photosensitizing, provide advice on sunscreen use, regardless of skin tone
Topical antibiotics (clindamycin, erythromycin, dapsone [sulfa-based], others)	• *Antibacterial, antiinflammatory* • Most effective for mild acne; less effective than oral antibiotics for moderate and severe acne; often used in combination with comedolytic such as benzoyl peroxide and/or retinoid.
Oral antibiotics (doxycycline, minocycline, erythromycin, TMP/SMX, azithromycin, others)	• *Antibacterial, antiinflammatory* • Indicated for the treatment of moderate inflammatory acne, usually when topical therapy has been inadequate • Once skin is clear (usually after 3 months of continuous therapy), taper off slowly over a few months while adding topical antibiotic agents; rapid discontinuation results in return of acne to pretreatment baseline. Long-term or repeat therapy is often needed.
Combined estrogen-progestin hormonal contraceptive (females only, in pill, patch, or ring form)	• *Reduction in androgen levels, decreased sebum production*. • Best suited for females with moderate to severe acne. About 3 months of continuous use prior to significant acne improvement. With discontinuation, acne usually gradually returns to pretreatment baseline.
Isotretinoin (Accutane®) capsules, various strengths	• *Mechanism of action not well understood*. • Indicated for treatment of cystic (severe) acne that does not respond to other therapies such as oral antibiotics and topical retinoids. Usual course of treatment is 4–6 months; discontinue when nodule count is reduced by 70%; repeat course only if needed after 2 months off drug. • Careful monitoring for mood destabilization and/or suicidal thoughts is an important part of patient care during isotretinoin use, although mental health risk is low. • Prescriber and patient must be properly educated in use of drug and fully aware of adverse reactions profile, including cheilitis, conjunctivitis, hypertriglyceridemia, xerosis, photosensitivity, and potent teratogenicity. Females of childbearing age must use two types of highly-effective contraception 1 month prior to, during, and 1 month after use of isotretinoin. iPLEDGE Program is designed to prevent pregnancies in patients taking isotretinoin by using iPLEDGE prescribers and pharmacies, and signing iPLEDGE card.

Sources: Gilbert, D., Chambers, H., Eliopoulos, G., Saag, M, Pavia A. (2016) <u>The Sanford Guide to Antimicrobial Therapy</u>, 46th Edition, Sperryville, VA: Antimicrobial Therapy, Inc.

Habif, T. (2012) <u>Dermatology DDxDeck</u>, 2nd Edition, St. Louis, MO: Elsevier Health Sciences.

iPLEDGE Program, available at www.ipledgeprogram.com/default.aspx

Table 16-18: Classification and Treatment of Acne Vulgaris		
Acne type	**Description**	**Preferred treatment**
Mild	<20 comedones, or <15 inflammatory lesions, or <30 total lesions	Topical retinoid alone often helpful, consider addition of topical antibiotic and/or benzoyl peroxide
Moderate	20 to 100 comedones, or 15 to 50 inflammatory lesions, or 30 to 125 total lesions	Oral antibiotic with topical retinoid
Severe	>5 cysts, or total comedone count >100, or total inflammatory lesion count >50, or >125 total lesions	Oral antibiotic with topical retinoid. If ineffective, oral isotretinoin (Accutane®). For large, painful cysts, consider intralesional corticosteroid injection.

Source: Acne and Related Disorders: Acne Vulgaris, available at
http://www.merckmanuals.com/professional/dermatologic_disorders/acne_and_related_dis
orders/acne_vulgaris.html

---

31. Match the following.

    A. Benzoyl peroxide

    B. Isotretinoin (Accutane®)

    C. Tretinoin (Retin-A®)

    D. Combined oral contraceptive

Indicated for treatment of cystic acne	
Most cost-effective topical antibacterial in mild acne	
Used as a keratolytic in acne treatment	
Use results in reduction of androgen levels	

        32. In the USA, which of the following is the most common cause of adolescent death?

           A. Suicide

           B. Homicide

           C. Accidental injury

           D. Malignancy

33. Adolescent issues: True or false?

> (T/F) Although adolescents tend to drink alcohol less frequently than adults, they drink considerably more alcohol per occasion of drinking.

> (T/F) USPSTF recommends depression screening using a validated questionnaire in adolescents (ages 12–18 years).

> (T/F) In all states, parental notification or consent is not required for an adolescent (generally considered to be ages 14 up until 18th birthday) to receive contraceptive services, prenatal care, or evaluation and treatment for STIs or substance abuse.

> (T/F) The majority of states require either parental consent or notification for teenagers younger than 18 to have a pregnancy termination.

Sources: Underage Drinking—Highlights From the Surgeon General's Call to Action to Prevent and Reduce Underage Drinking, available at http://www.ncbi.nlm.nih.gov/books/NBK44360

http://www.drugabuse.gov/publications/principles-adolescent-substance-use-disorder-treatment-research-based-guide/introduction

U.S. Preventive Services Task Force, Major Depressive Disorder in Children and Adolescents, available at www.uspreventiveservicestaskforce.org/uspstf/uspschdepr.htm

CRAFFT questions: A brief screening test for adolescent substance abuse

- *C*ar
  - Have you ever ridden in a CAR driven by someone (including yourself) who has been high or been using drugs or alcohol?
- *R*elax
  - Do you ever use alcohol or drugs to RELAX, feel better about yourself, or fit in?
- *A*lone?
  - Do you ever use alcohol or drugs while you are by yourself (ALONE)?
- *F*orget
  - Do you ever FORGET things you did while using alcohol or drugs?
- *F*riends
  - Do your family or FRIENDS ever tell you that you should cut down on your drinking or drug use?
- *T*rouble
  - Have you ever gotten into TROUBLE while you were using alcohol or drugs?
    - ≥2 yes answers suggest a serious problem.

Source: The Center for Adolescent Substance Abuse Research (CeASAR), available at www.ceasar-boston.org/

34. James is a 15-year-old who arrives for a well-teen visit with his mother. Prior to the beginning of the visit, his mother pulls you aside and states, "I want him checked for all drugs, but he said he is not using anything and does not want to be tested." Which of the following is your most appropriate response?

　　A. "What drugs do you think James is taking?"

　　B. "I cannot force James to take a drug test."

　　C. "Let's discuss your concerns with James."

　　D. "Since you are concerned, I can order the test without James' consent."

35. The most common contraceptive method used by teens is:

    A. Male condom.

    B. Combined oral contraceptives.

    C. DMPA injection (Depo-Provera®).

    D. Withdrawal.

36. In which of the following scenarios is parental consent for care required?

    A. An 18-year-old female who is seeking a pregnancy termination

    B. A 16-year-old female requesting a prescription for oral contraceptives

    C. A 15-year-old male requesting testing for sexually transmitted infection

    D. A 17-year-old male who requests treatment for contact dermatitis

Legal rights of the adolescent patient

- All 50 states and DC entitle adolescents to consent to care for medically emancipated conditions, including:
    - Contraception
    - Pregnancy
    - Sexually transmitted infection
    - Substance abuse
        - Fewer than 20% of teens report they would get treatment for STI, family planning, or substance abuse if parent notification was required.
    - Mental health
        - 45% of teens report they would not get treatment for depression if parental notification was required.
- A policy guaranteeing confidentiality for the teenager except in life-threatening situations should be clearly stated to the parent or guardian and the adolescent at the initiation of the relationship with the healthcare provider, either verbally or in writing.

Source: Center for Children's Advocacy.
http://www.kidscounsel.org/legalresources/legalresources_teenrights/legal-rights-info-for-teens-2

http://www.advocatesforyouth.org/publications/publications-a-z/516-adolescent-access-to-confidential-health-services

The Society for Adolescent Medicine: Summary of positions on delivery of health services to adolescents

- Confidentiality is an essential component of adolescent healthcare.

- Confidentiality should be available to encourage adolescents to seek care and provide candid information.

- Healthcare providers should educate adolescents and their families about the meaning, importance, scope, and limitations of confidentiality protection.

- Communication between adolescents and their parents or caretakers should be supported; parental participation should be encouraged, but not mandated.

- To the extent possible, providers and delivery systems should review and revise as needed all procedures, such as scheduling, billing, and record keeping, to protect confidentiality.

- Providers should receive ongoing training related to state and federal consent and confidentiality laws related to adolescent healthcare and are skilled in applying these laws.

- Laws allowing minors to consent to certain types of healthcare and protect the confidentiality of their healthcare information are necessary and should be maintained.

- Research should focus on increasing the numbers of adolescents receiving high-quality, confidential healthcare.

**Available online at Society for Adolescent Medicine, available at
http://www.adolescenthealth.org/SAHM_Main/media/Advocacy/Positions/Aug-04-
Confidential_Health_Care_for_Adolescents.pdf**

Table 16-19: Recommendations for Promoting the Health and Well-Being of Lesbian, Gay, Bisexual, and Transgender Adolescents: A Position Paper of the Society for Adolescent Health and Medicine
All healthcare providers who care for adolescents should be educated to provide competent and nonjudgmental care for lesbian, gay, bisexual, or transgendered (LGBT) youth.
Healthcare providers should understand that the majority of LGBT young people are healthy and well-adjusted teenagers and young adults.
Sexual orientation and gender identity are dynamic constructs. Healthcare providers, educators, policy makers, and researchers should be cautious in assigning labels to an adolescent's sexual orientation because this often evolves over time. Providers should ask adolescents how they self-identify, and should be guided by the youth's language and self-concept.
Family connectedness and support are important protective factors against depression, drug use, and high-risk sexual behavior in LGBT adolescents. However, practitioners also should understand that not all LGBT adolescents may be ready to disclose their sexuality to their family. When LGBT teens decide to disclose their sexuality or gender identity, providers should aim to assist families with acceptance of their LGBT teenagers.
Lesbian, gay, bisexual, or transgender youth are often at increased risk of bullying and victimization by peers and adults, including teachers, coaches, and family members; and victimization is associated with an increased risk for depression and suicide. Healthcare providers should be comfortable discussing these issues with their LGBT patients and should take an active role in educating the schools and community on prevention efforts to prevent and stop victimization.
Because victimized LGBT youth are at increased risk of depression and suicidality, providers should screen for these mental health issues and intervene as appropriate.
Antidiscrimination policies should be implemented to protect LGBT youth in foster care settings. Municipalities should disseminate policy guidelines to ensure appropriate care for LGBT youth in out-of-home venues.
Lesbian, gay, bisexual, or transgender youth in juvenile detention settings are at risk of harassment and bullying from fellow detainees as well as staff. Local juvenile justice systems should adopt policies to ensure the physical and mental well-being of incarcerated youth.
For youth who are struggling with sexual orientation or gender identity, affirmative therapeutic approaches can help adolescents explore their identities in a healthy manner. Reparative "therapy," which attempts to change one's sexual orientation or gender identity, is inherently coercive and inconsistent with current standards of medical care.
Adolescent healthcare providers should be educated regarding the healthcare needs of sexually-active LGBT teenagers. Guidance for screening individuals who are sexually active with members of the same sex is described in the Centers for Disease Control's *Sexually Transmitted Disease Treatment Guidelines*.
Future research on all of these aspects of LGBT health is needed to direct provider interventions, education, and community policy.

Source: http://www.jahonline.org/article/S1054-139X(13)00057-8/abstract

37. You are seeing 17-year-old Cynthia. As part of the visit, you consider her risk factors for type 2 diabetes mellitus would likely include all of the following except:

  A. Obesity.

  B. Pacific Islander ancestry.

  C. Family history of type 1 diabetes mellitus.

  D. Personal history of polycystic ovary syndrome (PCOS).

Table 16-20: Type 2 Diabetes Mellitus (T2DM) in Children: When to Consider Testing

| Overweight or obese (BMI>85th percentile for age and sex, weight-for-height >85th percentile, or weight >120% of ideal for height)

Plus ≥2 risk factors | Additional risk factors for T2DM in children include:
• Family history of T2DM in first- or second-degree relative
• Race/ethnicity (Native American, African American, Latino, Asian American, Pacific Islander)
• Signs of, or conditions associated with, insulin resistance, including acanthosis nigricans, hypertension, dyslipidemia, polycystic ovary syndrome, small for gestational age at birth in the child's history
• Maternal history of DM or gestational DM | Initiate testing (A1C, FBS, 2-h oral GTT) at age 10 years or at onset of puberty (Tanner stage 2), if puberty occurs earlier

Frequency: Every 3 years |

Source: American Diabetes Association Standards of Medical Care in Diabetes—2014, available at http://care.diabetesjournals.org/content/37/Supplement_1/S14.full.pdf+html

38. Sam is a 15-year-old with a BMI=40 kg/m^2 who presents with a lipid profile that reveals low HDL, elevated triglycerides, and an acceptable A1C. Which of the following is the recommended treatment option?

    A. Oral niacin

    B. Oral fibrate therapy

    C. Weight loss

    D. Oral statin therapy

Table 16-21: Lipid Screening and Cardiovascular Health in Childhood

The population approach to a healthful diet should be recommended to all children older than 2 years, according to Dietary Guidelines for Americans. This approach includes the use of low-fat dairy products. For children between 12 months and 2 years of age for whom overweight or obesity is a concern or who have a family history of obesity, dyslipidemia, or CVD, the use of reduced-fat milk would be appropriate.
The individual approach for children and adolescents at higher risk for CVD and with a high concentration of LDL cholesterol (LDL-C) includes recommended changes in diet with nutritional counseling and other lifestyle interventions, such as increased physical activity.
The most current recommendation is to screen children and adolescents with a positive family history of dyslipidemia or premature (≤55 years of age for men and ≤65 years of age for women) CVD or dyslipidemia. It is also recommended that pediatric patients for whom family history is not known or those with other CVD risk factors, such as overweight (BMI≥85th percentile, <95th percentile), obesity (BMI≥95th percentile), hypertension (blood pressure≥95th percentile), cigarette smoking, or diabetes mellitus, be screened with a fasting lipid profile.
For these children, the first screening should take place after 2 years of age but no later than 10 years of age. Screening before 2 years of age is not recommended.
A fasting lipid profile is the recommended approach to screening, because there is no currently available noninvasive method to assess atherosclerotic CVD in children. This screening should occur in the context of well-child and health maintenance visits. If values are within the reference range on initial screening, the patient should be retested in 3 to 5 years.
For pediatric patients who are overweight or obese and have a high triglyceride concentration or low HDL cholesterol concentration, weight management is the primary treatment, which includes improvement of diet with nutritional counseling and increased physical activity to produce improved energy balance.
For patients 8 years and older with an LDL-C concentration of ≥190 mg/dL (or ≥160 mg/dL with a family history of early heart disease or ≥2 additional risk factors present or ≥130 mg/dL if diabetes mellitus is present), pharmacologic intervention should be considered. The initial goal is to lower LDL-C concentration to <160 mg/dL. However, targets as low as 130 mg/dL or even 110 mg/dL may be warranted when there is a strong family history of CVD, especially with other risk factors, including obesity, diabetes mellitus, metabolic syndrome, and other higher-risk situations.

Source: Lipid Screening and Cardiovascular Health in Childhood, available at http://pediatrics.aappublications.org/content/122/1/198.full

39. Tina is an otherwise well 15-year-old who presents with her mother. They report that Tina has had a one-day history of "sore throat and swollen glands" as well as a low-grade fever and rash. Examination reveals a diffuse maculopapular rash, mildly tender posterior cervical and postauricular lymphadenopathy, and pharyngeal erythema without exudate. The remainder of her history and review of systems is unremarkable. Per her mother's report, Tina has not received any immunizations since age 6 months. The most likely diagnosis is:

    A. Scarlet fever.

    B. Roseola.

    C. Rubella.

    D. Rubeola.

40. Jannetta is a 16-year-old who presents with a 3-day history of pharyngitis and fatigue. Findings include exudative pharyngitis, minimally tender anterior and posterior cervical lymphadenopathy, and right and left upper quadrant abdominal tenderness. Per Jannetta's record, she is up-to-date with all recommended vaccinations. This is most consistent with:

    A. *S. pyogenes* pharyngitis.

    B. Infectious mononucleosis.

    C. Hodgkin disease.

    D. Gonococcal pharyngitis.

41. Jared is a 17-year-old with no known medication allergy who has suspected infectious mononucleosis. He is febrile and complains of acute otalgia on the left for the past three days. Physical examination reveals a left tympanic membrane that is red and bulging. When considering therapy for Jared, which of the following should not be prescribed?

    A. Acetaminophen

    B. Ibuprofen

    C. Amoxicillin

    D. Azithromycin

Table 16-22: Differential Diagnosis of Acute Febrile Rash-producing Illness

Condition with causative agent	Presentation	Comments
Scarlet fever Agent: *S. pyogenes* (group A beta-hemolytic streptococci)	Sandpaper-like rash with exudative pharyngitis, fever, headache, tender, localized anterior cervical lymphadenopathy. Rash usually erupts on day 2 of pharyngitis and often peels a few days later.	Presence of rash does not imply a more severe or serious disease or greater risk of contagion. Treatment: Identical to streptococcal pharyngitis, penicillin (PO or IM) or oral amoxicillin as first-line therapy, oral macrolide (azithro-, clarithro-, erythromycin) only in PCN allergy due to issues of bacterial resistance.
Roseola Agent: Human herpesvirus-6 (HHV-6)	Discrete rosy-pink macular or maculopapular rash lasting hours to 3 days that follows a 3- to 7-day period of fever, often quite high	90% of cases seen in children <2 years Febrile seizures in 10% of children affected. Supportive treatment
Rubella Agent: Rubella virus	Mild symptoms; fever, sore throat, malaise, nasal discharge, diffuse maculopapular rash lasting about 3 days Posterior cervical and postauricular lymphadenopathy beginning 5–10 days prior to onset and present during rash Arthralgia in about 25% (most common in women)	Incubation period about 14–21 days with disease transmissible for ~1 week prior to onset of rash to ~2 weeks after rash appears. Generally a mild, self-limiting illness. Greatest risk is effect of virus on the unborn child, especially with first-trimester exposure (~80% rate congenital rubella syndrome). ***Vaccine-preventable disease*** Notifiable disease, usually to the state and/or public health authorities*, laboratory confirmation by presence of serum rubella IgM.
Measles Agent: Rubeola virus	Usually acute presentation with fever, nasal discharge, cough, generalized lymphadenopathy, conjunctivitis (copious clear discharge), photophobia, Koplik spots (appearing ~2 days prior to onset of rash as white spots with blue rings held within red spots in oral mucosa) Pharyngitis is usually mild without exudate. Maculopapular rash onset 3–4 days after onset of symptoms, may coalesce to generalized erythema.	Incubation period ~10–14 days with disease transmissible for ~1 week prior to onset of rash to ~2–3 weeks after rash appears. CNS and respiratory tract complications common. Permanent neurologic impairment or death possible. Supportive treatment as well as intervention for complications ***Vaccine-preventable disease*** Notifiable disease, usually to the state and/or public health authorities*, laboratory confirmation by presence of serum rubeola IgM.
Infectious mononucleosis (IM) Agent: Epstein-Barr virus (human herpesvirus 4)	Maculopapular rash in ~20%, rare petechial rash Fever, "shaggy" purple-white exudative pharyngitis, malaise, marked diffuse lymphadenopathy, hepatic and splenic tenderness with occasional enlargement Diagnostic testing: Heterophil antibody test (Monospot®), leukopenia with lymphocytosis and atypical lymphocytes	Incubation period 20–50 days >90% will develop a rash if given amoxicillin or ampicillin during the illness. Potential for respiratory distress when enlarged tonsils and lymphoid tissue impinges on the upper airway; corticosteroids may be helpful. Splenomegaly most often occurs between days 6 and 21 after onset of illness. Avoid contact sports for ≥1 month due to risk of splenic rupture.

Source: Fitzgerald, M. A., (2017) Pediatrics, <u>Nurse Practitioner Certification Examination and Practice Preparation</u>, 5th Edition, Philadelphia, PA: F. A. Davis.
*A notifiable disease is one for which regular, frequent, and timely information regarding individual cases is considered necessary for the prevention and control of the disease. Reference on diseases considered to be notifiable, usually to the state and/or public health authorities is available at website http://www.cdc.gov/mmwr/mmwr_nd/
http://www.cdc.gov/mmwr/PDF/wk/mm6153.pdf
Also check with state public health department to receive direction on notification.

Table 16-22 (cont.): Differential Diagnosis of Acute Febrile Rash-producing Illness

Condition with causative agent	Presentation	Comments
Hand, foot, and mouth disease Agent: Coxsackie virus A16	Fever, malaise, sore mouth, anorexia; 1–2 days later, lesions; also can cause conjunctivitis, pharyngitis Duration of illness: 2–7 days	Transmission via oral-fecal or droplet Highly contagious with incubation period of 2–6 weeks Supportive treatment, analgesia important
Fifth's disease Agent: Human parvovirus B19	3–4 days of mild, flu-like illness, followed by 7–10 days of red rash that begins on face with "slapped-cheek" appearance, spreads to trunk and extremities. Rash onset corresponds with disease immunity with patient. Viremic and contagious prior to but not after onset of rash.	Droplet transmission; leukopenia common Risk of hydrops fetalis with resulting pregnancy loss when contracted by woman during pregnancy Supportive treatment
Kawasaki disease Agent: Unknown	For acute-phase illness (usually lasts about 11 days), fever with T≥104°F (40°C) lasting ≥5 days, polymorphic exanthem on trunk, flexor regions, and perineum, erythema of the oral cavity ("strawberry tongue") with extensively chapped lips, bilateral conjunctivitis, usually without eye discharge, cervical lymphadenopathy, edema and erythema of the hands and feet with peeling skin (late finding, usually 1–2 weeks after onset of fever), no other illness accountable for the findings	Usually in children ages 1–8 years Treatment with IV immunoglobulin and PO aspirin during the acute phase is associated with a reduction in rate of coronary abnormalities, such as coronary artery dilation and coronary aneurysm. Requires expert consultation and treatment advice about accurate diagnosis, aspirin use and ongoing monitoring warranted, usually at a tertiary pediatric medical center.

Source: Fitzgerald, M. A. (2017) Pediatrics, <u>Nurse Practitioner Certification Examination and Practice Preparation</u>, 5th Edition, Philadelphia, PA: F. A. Davis.

42. Timmy is a 4-year-old boy who presents with his Mom today for a sick visit. For the past 8 days, he has had intermittent fever as high as 104.5°F (40.3°C) and has complained of a sore throat and increased throat pain with swallowing, but without difficulty taking fluids. He has little appetite, but his mother denies nausea, vomiting, diarrhea, or constipation. On examination, you note he is alert, appears ill without acute distress, and has extensive cervical lymphadenopathy, injected conjunctiva, oral erythema, and a peeling rash on his hands. You consider a diagnosis of:

A. Infectious mononucleosis.

B. Scarlet fever.

C. Hand, foot, and mouth disease.

D. Kawasaki disease.

Table 16-23: Anemia in Childhood

Most common type of anemia	Etiology	Comment
Iron deficiency anemia (IDA) Hemogram= • Microcytic • Hypochromic • Elevated RDW	Most common in children ages 12–30 months Major contributors: Depletion of birth iron stores (usually lasts until ~6 months of age), initiation of lower-iron diet in later infancy, early toddler stage	Most calories in first year of life should be from breast milk with iron supplementation starting at ages 4–6 months, depending on amount of iron-fortified formula intake or iron-enriched formula In child ≥12 months, most potent risk factor for IDA=Cow's milk intake in excess of 16 oz (0.47 L) per day In child <9 months, most potent risk factors for IDA=Maternal iron depletion, prematurity

Table 16-24: Diagnosis and Prevention of Iron Deficiency and Iron Deficiency Anemia in Infants and Young Children (0–3 Years)

Preterm infants receiving breast milk should receive 2 mg/kg/d of elemental iron through supplements or foods starting by age 1 month through 12 months.
Among preterm infants receiving infant formula, iron supplements could be required, depending on multiple factors influencing iron status.
Term infants taking more than one-half of feedings as human milk should receive 1 mg/kg/d of supplemental iron starting at age 4 months until the introduction of complementary foods (fortified cereals, legumes, red meats, dark green vegetables, vitamin C-containing foods [to enhance iron absorption]).
Term formula-fed infants receive enough iron from formula with the introduction of iron-containing complementary foods after ages 4 to 6 months.
Toddlers can receive adequate iron through heme sources of iron (red meat), nonheme sources (legumes, cereal), and vitamin C-containing foods to promote iron absorption.
Toddlers who do not ingest adequate iron-containing food can receive iron supplements.
In treating an infant, child, or adult with established iron deficiency anemia (IDA), supplemental iron should be continued for about 2 months after correction of the anemia and its etiologic cause in order to replenish body stores of iron.
• Ongoing evaluation for iron deficiency is an important part of providing primary care for the young child. All children should be screened for IDA through hemoglobin measurement at age 1 year. – With Hb<10 g/dL, further testing to confirm iron deficiency, such as ferritin – With milder anemia (Hb=10–11 g/dL), an alternative evaluation plan includes treating with iron for 1 month. A rise in Hb≥1 g/dL after a month of iron therapy helps to confirm iron deficiency, particularly if additional clinical assessment helps to support the diagnosis.

Source: Clinical report—diagnosis and prevention of iron deficiency and iron-deficiency anemia in infants and young children (0–3 years of age), available at http://pediatrics.aappublications.org/content/early/2010/10/05/peds.2010-2576.full.pdf+html

43. Identify the two children that are at greatest risk for iron deficiency anemia?

   A. 3-month-old who takes about 24 oz (0.71 L) of iron-fortified formula per day

   B. 11-month-old, breastfed about 7 times a day, taking iron-fortified cereal, fruit, and vegetables three times per day

   C. 16-month-old who drinks about 1 qt (0.95 L) whole milk per day and a few solids

   D. 4-year-old who eats small amounts of meat, fruit, and cheese

   E. 6-month-old who was born at 30 weeks' gestation and is exclusively breastfed without additional supplements

44. Jackson is a 13-month-old who is in for a well-child visit. Height and weight are at approximately 40th percentile and he is on target developmentally. His diet consists of approximately 18 oz (0.53 L) of whole cow's milk per day and a variety of vegetables, fruits, lean meats, and grains. You advise that Jackson:

   A. Is eating a well-balanced diet and no nutritional supplements are needed.

   B. Should receive iron supplement equivalent to 1 mg/kg/d.

   C. Receive vitamin D 400 IU as a daily oral supplement.

   D. Should be taking in more calcium via increased cow's milk intake to ≥28 fl oz (0.83 L) per day.

Table 16-25: Micronutrient Requirements for Children		
Nutrient	**Age and daily requirement**	**Comment**
Calcium	Toddler (1–3 years)=500 mg Preschool, younger school age (4–8 years)=800 mg Older children to teens (9–18 years)=1300 mg	1 cup (0.24 L) milk, yogurt=Approximately 250 mg calcium 1 cup (0.24 L) collards, frozen, boiled=357 mg calcium 1 cup (0.24 L) black-eyed peas, boiled=211 mg calcium 3 oz (1/4 block, 85.05 g) calcium-set tofu=163 mg calcium 1 cup (0.24 L) cottage cheese, 1% milk fat=138 mg calcium 1 cup (0.24 L) soy milk=93 mg calcium 1 oz (24 nuts/28.35 g) almonds=70 mg calcium
Vitamin D	400 IU daily	Difficult to achieve this level with food or with sun exposure that most children experience 1 L of infant formula or vitamin D-fortified cow's milk contains at least 400 IU vitamin D. All non-breastfed infants ingesting <1,000 mL/day of vitamin D-fortified formula or milk should receive a vitamin D supplement of 400 IU/day. AAP recommends that exclusively and partially breastfed infants receive supplements of 400 IU/day of vitamin D shortly after birth and continue to receive these supplements until they are weaned and then consume ≥1,000 mL/day of vitamin D-fortified formula or whole milk. Sun exposure's contribution to vitamin D status is dependent on latitude of residence, skin tone, use of sunscreen, amount of clothing covering the skin, and a number of other factors.

Source: Abrams SA. Dietary Guidelines for Calcium and Vitamin D: A New Era. *Pediatrics.* 2011;127;566.

45. You are seeing an 8-year-old healthy boy who is brought in by his mother who states, "He is in trouble in school and failing two classes. His teacher thinks he is too hyper and will not sit still and wants him to be evaluated. I do not understand this. He is fine at home." When considering the diagnosis of attention deficit/hyperactivity disorder in this child, you understand that:

A. In the majority of children diagnosed with ADHD, the symptoms and behaviors will resolve by early adulthood.

B. Psychostimulant use in the child with ADHD can lead to substance abuse disorders in adolescence.

C. To confirm the diagnosis of ADHD, assessment of the child's behavior at home and school should be conducted using standardized scales.

D. When psychostimulants are prescribed with the diagnosis of ADHD, concomitant behavioral therapy is usually not needed.

Notes:

Table 16-26: Attention Deficit/Hyperactivity Disorder (ADHD)
3 Subtypes: Inattentive, hyperactive/impulsive, and combined
(children up to age 17 years)

Key diagnostic components:

- Symptoms must be present before age 12 years.
- Impairment must be present in at least 2 settings (i.e., home and school).
- Must have evidence of functional interference: Socially, academically or in extracurricular activities.

Inattention: Five or more of the following must occur <u>often</u>:

- Fails to give close attention to details or makes careless mistakes in schoolwork, work, or other activities
- Difficulty sustaining attention in tasks or play activities
- Does not seem to listen when spoken to directly
- Does not follow through on instructions and fails to finish school work, chores or duties
- Difficulty organizing tasks and activities
- Avoids, dislikes or is reluctant to engage in tasks that require sustained mental effort
- Loses things necessary for tasks
- Easily distracted by extraneous stimuli
- Forgetful in daily activities

Hyperactivity-impulsivity: Five or more of the following must occur <u>often</u>:

- Fidgets with hands or feet or squirms in seat
- Leaves seat in classroom or in other situations in which remaining seated is expected
- Runs about or climbs excessively in situations when inappropriate
  - Can be subjective feelings of restlessness in adults or adolescents
- Difficulty playing or engaging in leisure activities quietly
- Acts "on the go" or acts as if "driven by a motor"
- Talks excessively
- Blurts out answers before questions have been completed
- Difficulty waiting turn
- Interrupts or intrudes on others

Source: American Psychiatric Association. (2013). Diagnostic and statistical manual of mental disorders: DSM-5 (5th ed). Arlington, VA.

Table 16-27: Differential Diagnosis of Stridor in Children: Caused by upper airway obstruction – Getting air in more of a problem than getting air out. Characteristic sound heard on inspiration

Condition	Features	Intervention
Croup (laryngotracheobronchitis)	Viral, allergic in origin, most common ages 6 months to 5 years	Supportive treatment, perhaps systemic corticosteroid therapy
Foreign body	Acute onset from mechanical obstruction, most common in toddlers	Removal, referral to appropriate care setting such as ED
Congenital obstruction	Present from birth	Surgical repair usually indicated
Peritonsillar abscess	Usually bacterial, most often in older child or adult, usually presents with "hot potato" voice, difficulty swallowing, trismus, contralateral uvula deviation	Attention to airway maintenance, referral to appropriate care setting such as ED, prompt ENT consult, antimicrobial therapy, usually inpatient admission, and perhaps surgical intervention
Acute epiglottitis	Bacterial origin (most often *H. influenzae* type B, potentially preventable with Hib vaccine), most often in children ages 2–7 years. Abrupt onset of high-grade fever, sore throat, dysphagia, and drooling	Attention to airway maintenance, referral to appropriate care setting such as ED, prompt ENT consult, antimicrobial therapy, usually inpatient admission

Source: Stridor, available at emedicine.medscape.com/article/995267-overview

Table 16-28: Differential Diagnosis of Wheeze in Children: Caused by lower airway obstruction – Getting air out more of a problem than getting air in. Characteristic sound heard initially on expiration

Condition	Features	Intervention
Acute bronchiolitis	Often called the "disease of the happy wheezer," with a mildly ill child, 3 mo–3 y (most age<1 y), viral etiology, most often from respiratory syncytial virus (RSV), less commonly from influenza or adenovirus, short-term acute illness with wheezing often persisting ~3 wk. Most serious in early infancy (<3 mos) and preterm infants. Nearly all episodes occur between November and April.	Supportive, little evidence that inhaled bronchodilators (albuterol, epinephrine) or inhaled or systemic corticosteroids are helpful. Palivizumab (Synagis®) often used to prevent RSV infection in premature infants (first RSV season for infants born at <29 weeks' gestation; infants with chronic lung disease, congenital heart disease, or immune deficiency syndromes).
Acute bronchitis	Viral etiology, short-term, self-limiting	Supportive, often inhaled $beta_2$-agonist, oral antiinflammatory treatment
Asthma	Allergic, inflammatory etiology, symptoms recurrent, persistent without treatment	Per NIH Guidelines

Sources: Evidence-based care guideline for management of first time episode bronchiolitis in infants less than 1 year of age, http://www.guideline.gov/content.aspx?id=49259&search=evidence-based+care+guideline+for+management+of+first+time+episode+bronchiolitis+in+infants+less+than+1+year+of+age; The American Academy of Pediatrics: Diagnosis and Management of Bronchiolitis: Subcommittee on Diagnosis and Management of Bronchiolitis, http://pediatrics.aappublications.org/content/118/4/1774; VA/DoD clinical practice guideline for management of asthma in children and adults, available at http://www.healthquality.va.gov/guidelines/CD/asthma/

Table 16-29: Classifying Asthma Severity and Initiating Treatment in Children 0 to 4 Years of Age

Components of Severity		Intermittent	Persistent		
			Mild	Moderate	Severe
Impairment	Symptoms	≤2 days/week	>2 days/week but not daily	Daily	Throughout the day
	Nighttime awakenings	0	1–2×/month	3–4×/month	>1×/week
	SABA use for symptom control (not prevention of EIB)	≤2 days/week	>2 days/week but not daily	Daily	Several times per day
	Interference with normal activity	None	Minor limitation	Some limitation	Extremely limited
Risk	Exacerbations requiring oral systemic corticosteroids	0–1/year (see note)	≥2 exacerbations in 6 mos requiring oral systemic corticosteroids, or ≥4 wheezing episodes/1 year lasting >1 day & risk factors for persistent asthma		
		Consider severity and interval since last exacerbation Frequency and severity may fluctuate over time Exacerbations of any severity may occur in patients in any severity category			
Recommended Step for Initiating Treatment		Step 1	Step 2	Step 3	Step 4
				and consider short course of oral systemic corticosteroids	
		In 2 to 6 weeks, depending on severity, evaluate level of asthma control that is achieved. If no clear benefit is observed in 4 to 6 weeks, consider adjusting therapy or alternative diagnoses			

Table 16-30: Stepwise Approach for Managing Asthma in Children Age 0 to 4 Years

Intermittent Asthma	Persistent Asthma: Daily Medication
	Consult with asthma specialist if Step 3 care or higher is required. Consider consultation at Step 2.

Step 6

Preferred:

High-dose ICS + either LABA or Montelukast

and

Oral Systemic Corticosteroids

Step 5

Preferred:

High-dose ICS + either LABA or Montelukast

Step 4

Preferred:

Medium-dose ICS + either LABA or Montelukast

Step 3

Preferred:

Medium-dose ICS

Step 2

Preferred:

Low-dose ICS

Alternative:

Montelukast

Step 1

Preferred:

SABA PRN

Step Up if Needed

(first check adherence, inhaler technique, & environmental control)

Assess Control

Step Down if Possible

(& asthma is well controlled at least 3 months)

Patient Education and Environmental Control at Each Step

Quick-Relief Medication for All Patients

- SABA as needed for symptoms. Intensity of treatment depends on severity of symptoms
- With viral respiratory infection: SABA q 4-6 hours up to 24 hours (longer with healthcare provider input)
- Consider short course of oral systemic corticosteroids if exacerbation is severe or patient has history of previous severe exacerbations
- Caution: Frequent use of SABA may indicate the need to step up treatment. See text for recommendations on initiating daily long-term-control therapy

www.nhlbi.nih.gov/guidelines/asthma/asthgdln.pdf.

Table 16-31: Classifying Asthma Severity and Initiating Treatment in Children 5 to 11 Years of Age

Components of Severity		Intermittent	Persistent		
			Mild	**Moderate**	**Severe**
Impairment	Symptoms	≤2 days/week	>2 days/week but not daily	Daily	Throughout the day
	Nighttime awakenings	≤2x/month	1–2×/month	3–4×/month	>1×/week
	SABA use for symptom control (not prevention of EIB)	≤2 days/week	>2 days/week but not daily	Daily	Several times per day
	Interference with normal activity	None	Minor limitation	Some limitation	Extremely limited
	Lung Function	Normal FEV_1 between exacerbations FEV_1>80% FEV_1/FVC>85%	FEV_1≥80% predicted FEV_1/FVC>80%	FEV_1=60–80% predicted FEV_1/FVC=75–80%	FEV_1<60% predicted FEV_1/FVC<75%
Risk	Exacerbations requiring oral systemic corticosteroids	0–1/year	≥2/year		
		Consider severity and interval since last exacerbation Frequency and severity may fluctuate over time for patients in any severity category Relative annual risk of exacerbations may be related to FEV_1			
Recommended Step for Initiating Treatment		Step 1	Step 2	Step 3, medium-dose ICS option	Step 3, medium-dose ICS option, or Step 4
				This & consider short course of oral systemic corticosteroids to relieve inflammation currently present	
		In 2 to 6 weeks, evaluate level of asthma control that is achieved and adjust therapy accordingly			

Table 16-32: Stepwise Approach for Managing Asthma in Children Age 5 to 11 Years

Intermittent Asthma	Persistent Asthma: Daily Medication
	Consult w/ asthma specialist if Step 4 care or higher is required. Consider consultation at Step 3.

Step 1
Preferred:
SABA PRN

Step 2
Preferred:
Low-dose ICS
Alternative:
LTM
or
Theophylline

Step 3
Preferred:
Low-dose ICS
+
either LABA, LTM or Theophylline
or
Medium-dose ICS

Step 4
Preferred:
Medium-dose ICS + LABA
Alternative:
Medium-dose ICS + either LTM or Theophylline

Step 5
Preferred:
High-dose ICS + LABA
Alternative:
High-dose ICS + either LTM or Theophylline

Step 6
Preferred:
High-dose ICS + LABA + Oral Systemic Corticosteroid
Alternative:
High-dose ICS + either LTM or Theophylline + Oral Systemic Corticosteroid

Step Up if Needed
(first, check adherence, inhaler technique, environmental control, and comorbid conditions)

Assess Control

Step Down if Possible
(and asthma is well-controlled at least 3 months)

Each Step: Patient education, environmental control, and management of comorbidities
Steps 2-4: Consider subcutaneous allergen immunotherapy for patients who have allergic asthma
Quick-Relief Medication for All Patients
- *SABA as needed for symptoms. Intensity of treatment depends on severity of symptoms: Up to 3 treatments at 20-minute intervals as needed. Short course of oral systemic corticosteroids may be needed*
- *Caution: Increasing of use of SABA or use >2 days a week for symptom relief (not prevention of EIB) indicates inadequate control and the need to step up treatment*
www.nhlbi.nih.gov/guidelines/asthma/asthgdln.pdf.

Table 16-33: Estimated Comparative Daily Dosages for ICS in Children Ages 0 to 4 Years

Drug	Low Daily Dose	Medium Daily Dose	High Daily Dose
Budesonide inhalation suspension for nebulization (child dose)	0.25–0.5 mg	0.5–1 mg	>1 mg
Fluticasone HFA MDI: 44, 110, or 220 mcg/puff	176 mcg	176–352 mcg	352 mcg

Source: http://www.nhlbi.nih.gov/guidelines/asthma/asthgdln.pdf

Table 16-34: Estimated Comparative Daily Dosages for ICS in Children Ages 5 to 11 Years

Drug	Low Daily Dose	Medium Daily Dose	High Daily Dose
Beclomethasone HFA 40 or 80 mcg/puff	80–160 mcg	>160–320 mcg	>320 mcg
Budesonide DPI 90, 180 mcg/inhalation	200–400 mcg	>400–800 mcg	>800 mcg
Budesonide inhalation suspension for nebulization (child dose)	0.5 mg	1 mg	2 mg
Fluticasone HFA MDI: 44, 110, or 220 mcg/puff	88–176 mcg	>176–352 mcg	>352 mcg
Fluticasone DPI: 50, 100, or 250 mcg/inhalation	100–200 mcg	200–400 mcg	>400 mcg

46. Adam, a 7-year-old boy with a prior diagnosis of moderate persistent asthma, presents with his parents for a well-child visit. He is new to your practice and has not had a healthcare visit in the past year. Adam's mom mentions that he took a "pill to control his breathing, but we ran out. Right now, he uses the albuterol pump once or twice a day. This keeps his cough under pretty good control. The inhaler works quickly most of the time." You advise the following:

    A. Add a twice-a-day long-acting beta$_2$-agonist as needed to ensure Adam has better cough control.

    B. An inhaled corticosteroid should be added to Adam's treatment regimen.

    C. A leukotriene modifier is an acceptable first-line controller medication for Adam.

    D. No additional medication is needed, as Adam has adequate symptom control with the current albuterol dose and frequency.

Table 16-35: Causative Organisms in Acute Bacterial Otitis Media

Overall pathogens in AOM=No pathogen (4%), virus (70%), bacteria plus virus (66%)

Organism	Comment
S. pneumoniae (Gram-positive diplococci) (49%) **Treatment target in AOM**	Consider drug-resistant *S. pneumoniae* risk (present in many children) Mechanism of resistance: Alters binding sites within bacterial cells Low rate (~10–20%) of spontaneous resolution without antimicrobial therapy
H. influenzae (Gram-negative bacillus) (29%)	Resistance via beta-lactamase production Moderate rate (~50%) of spontaneous resolution without antimicrobial therapy
M. catarrhalis (Gram-negative cocci) (28%)	Resistance via beta-lactamase production Nearly all spontaneously resolve without antimicrobial therapy

Source: Otitis Media, Acute Empiric Therapy, available at Gilbert, D., Chambers, H., Eliopoulos, G., Saag, M., Pavia, A. (2016) <u>The Sanford Guide to Antimicrobial Therapy</u> (46th ed.). Sperryville, VA: Antimicrobial Therapy, Inc.

Table 16-36: Diagnosis and Management of AOM in Children

Diagnosis of AOM in children	• Moderate or severe bulging of TM *OR* new onset of otorrhea not related to otitis externa (OE) with otalgia • Mild bulging of TM *AND* recent (≤48 hrs) onset of ear pain (in nonverbal child – tugging, holding, rubbing) *OR* intense TM erythema with otalgia
Management of AOM should include assessment for pain and, if present, the clinician should recommend treatment for pain management.	• Analgesics: Acetaminophen or ibuprofen is recommended • Topical anesthetic agent in form of otic drops can provide short-term (approximately 30 minutes) pain relief
Watchful waiting, consisting of analgesia without antimicrobial therapy, is an acceptable treatment option in AOM.	In the otherwise well child, rationale for not immediately initiating antibiotic therapy: • Low risk for adverse outcome without antimicrobial therapy • High rate of spontaneous AOM resolution without antimicrobial therapy • Watchful waiting is only appropriate for the child ≥6 months with non-severe illness based on joint decision-making with parents/caregivers for unilateral AOM. • If watchful waiting is used, follow-up must be ensured with ability to start antibiotic therapy within 48–72 hours if child fails to improve or worsens.
Nonsevere vs. severe illness	Nonsevere illness: • Mild otalgia for <48 hours *Or* • Fever <39°C (102.2°F) in the past 24 hours Severe illness: • Moderate to severe otalgia *Or* • Otalgia for >48 hours *Or* • Fever ≥39°C (102.2°F)

Continued...

Table 16-36 (cont.): Diagnosis and Management of AOM in Children

Treatment options: Initial treatment	Antibiotic therapy at time of AOM diagnosis in the following: • Non-severe or severe illness, whether unilateral or bilateral AOM, in children younger than 6 months • Severe illness with unilateral or bilateral AOM in children ≥6 months • Non-severe illness with bilateral AOM in young children (6–23 months) Either prescribe antibiotic therapy OR offer observation with close follow-up • AOM in children ≥6 months with non-severe illness based on joint decision-making with parents/caregivers for unilateral AOM • If observation is used, follow-up must be ensured with ability to start antibiotic therapy within 48–72 hours if child fails to improve or worsens

Source: Lieberthal AS, Carroll AE, Chonmaitree T, et al. The Diagnosis and Management of
Acute Otitis Media. *Pediatrics*. 2013;131:e964-99.

Table 16-37: Recommended AOM Treatment Options

Length of therapy unless otherwise specified: <2 years=10 days, 2–6 years=7 days, ≥6 years=5–7 days

	Recommended	With PCN allergy
First-line treatment	Amoxicillin (80–90 mg/kg/d PO in 2 divided doses) OR Amoxicillin-clavulanate (90 mg/kg/d PO of amoxicillin, with 6.4 mg/kg/d of clavulanate in 2 divided doses)	Cefdinir (14 mg/kg/d PO in 1 or 2 doses) OR Cefuroxime (30 mg/kg/d PO in 2 divided doses) OR Cefpodoxime (10 mg/kg/d PO in 2 divided doses) OR Ceftriaxone (50 mg IM or IV/day for 1 or 3 d)
Antibiotic treatment after 48–72 h with failure of initial antibiotic treatment	Amoxicillin-clavulanate (90 mg/kg/d PO of amoxicillin, with 6.4 mg/kg/d of clavulanate in 2 divided doses) OR Ceftriaxone (50 mg IM/IV for 3 d)	Ceftriaxone × 3 d (as above) OR Clindamycin (30–40 mg/kg/d PO in 3 divided doses) with or without a third-generation cephalosporin Consider tympanocentesis, referral to specialist

Source: Lieberthal AS, Carroll AE, Chonmaitree T, et al. The Diagnosis and Management of
Acute Otitis Media. *Pediatrics*. 2013;131:e964-99.

For additional information on prescribing cephalosporins in the presence of penicillin
allergy, please see: Fitzgerald Health Education Associates, Newsletter Article Q&A with Dr.
Fitzgerald: How Would you Prescribe Cephalosporins to Patients with Penicillin Allergies?
by Margaret A. Fitzgerald, available at
http://fhea.com/main/content/Newsletter/fheanews_volume12_issue8.pdf

Table 16-38: Otitis Media w/Effusion (OME) in Children	
Defined	Fluid in the middle ear without signs or symptoms of ear infection Formerly known as serous otitis
First-line intervention	Watchful waiting in the majority, 75–90% resolve within 3 months without specific treatment. Antimicrobial therapy not indicated, nor is therapy with oral antihistamines or decongestants.
Evaluation in OME	Consider audiologic evaluation if OME persists for at least 3 months, if concerns are noted for hearing, speech or language, by parents, teachers, or healthcare providers, or 3 months after a prior audiologic evaluation in a child being observed with OME.
Select intervention in at-risk children	With persistent effusion accompanied by language delay and/or suspected or documented hearing loss, surgical intervention should be considered. Tympanostomy tubes and/or adenoidectomy reduced time with OME and improved hearing in the short-term but were associated with expected risk. With documented speech delay, refer for speech therapy. Persistent OME is the most common cause of temporary speech delay in early childhood.

Source: American Academy of Pediatrics. Surgical treatments for OME: A systematic review, available at http://pediatrics.aappublications.org/content/133/2/296.abstract?sid=e5efb610-dfa5-4b4b-be90-4df0b353ac30

47. Taylor is a 2½-year-old otherwise well child who presents today for a sick visit. According to his father, Taylor has vomited approximately 10 times in the past 18 hours, with the last episode about 4 hours ago. He has retained sips of water during the last hour. He also developed watery stools approximately 8 hours ago with 4 episodes in total. The last stooling episode was about 1 hour ago. Fever is reported to be elevated to 38.4°C (101.2°F) on a number of occasions during the past day. Taylor is developmentally on target, and has been at 70th percentile for height, 90th percentile for weight for the past 18 months. He is up-to-date with recommended immunizations. On assessment, he is lying in his father's arms, is alert and nods his head when asked if he is thirsty. His lips are dry and slightly cracked and there is a small amount of saliva in the oral cavity. His heart rate is 110 BPM and capillary refill is <2 seconds. Dad tells you Taylor's diaper was dry when he awoke 4 hours ago but due to watery stools, he is unsure if Taylor has voided this morning. Currently, Taylor is wearing a diaper that is slightly wet in the front. Based on these findings, you consider that Taylor appears to be:

A. Mildly dehydrated.

B. Moderately dehydrated.

C. Severely dehydrated.

D. Adequately hydrated.

Table 16-39: Assessment Criteria for Hydration Status			
Parameter	Mild 3–5%	Moderate 6–9%	Severe >10%
Turgor	Normal	Recoil<2 sec	Recoil>2 sec, tenting
Fontanels	Normal	Slightly depressed	Depressed
Mucous membranes	Slightly dry lips, thick saliva	Dry lips and oral mucosa	Very dry lips, oral mucosa
Eyes	Normal, tears present	Slightly sunken, tears decreased	Deeply sunken, tears absent
Capillary refill	Normal (<1.5 seconds)	Delayed (1.5–3 sec)	Delayed (>3 sec)
Mental status	Normal	Normal, fatigued, restless, irritable	Apathetic, lethargic, unconscious
Urine output	Slightly decreased	Decreased	Minimal
Thirst	Normal to slightly increased	Moderately increased	Very thirsty or too lethargic to assess

Source: CDC Guidelines for the Management of Acute Diarrhea After a Disaster, available at http://www.cdc.gov/disasters/disease/diarrheaguidelines.html

48. You provide the following information to Taylor's father.

   A. Taylor can go home now on rehydration therapy with an appropriate oral rehydration solution and clear liquids.

   B. Taylor should be started on rehydration therapy with an appropriate oral rehydration solution in the office now with a goal of demonstrating ability to tolerate oral fluids.

   C. Given Taylor's hydration status, he should be hospitalized for parenteral fluid replacement.

   D. Taylor is able to go home on a diet of dry toast, mashed bananas, applesauce and white rice along with sips of clear liquids.

49. A father presents his 2-year-old daughter with suspected gastroenteritis. She has had two episodes of vomiting and several episodes of diarrhea beginning 24 hours ago. Her last diarrheal episode was 2 hours ago and her diaper is wet. She has been able to consume small amounts of fluid but shows signs of mild dehydration. An appropriate treatment option to prevent further dehydration is a single oral dose of:

   A. An antidiarrheal agent (e.g., kaolin-pectin).

   B. An antimotility agent (e.g., loperamide).

   C. A 5-HT$_3$ antagonist (e.g., ondansetron).

   D. Antiparasitic antimicrobial (e.g. metronidazole).

Table 16-40: Rehydration Therapy:		
For mild to moderate dehydration, oral rehydration therapy (ORT) with oral rehydration solution (ORS) is as effective as parenteral therapy, easier to administer, and more cost-effective. With vomiting, consider premedication with 5-HT3 receptor antagonist such as ondansetron to minimize risk of further upper GI fluid loss.		
Degree of dehydration	Rehydration therapy	Replacement of ongoing losses
Minimal to none	Not applicable; sips of fluid frequently as tolerated to maintain circulating volume and hydration status	<10 kg: 60–120 mL oral rehydration solution (ORS) for each loss; >10 kg: 120–240 mL for each loss
Mild to moderate	ORT with ORS, 50–100 mL/kg over 3–4 hours, often best tolerated in frequent, small volumes, preferably supplied in the office or urgent care setting to demonstrate ability to tolerate oral therapy.	Same as above
Severe	Lactated Ringers solution (LR) preferred over normal saline (NS) IVF but used if LR not available; boluses 20 mL/kg until improvement (perfusion, LOC) then 100 mL/kg over 4 hours	Same as above If unable to drink, give through NG tube or give D5W1/4 NS with K$^+$ 20 mEq IV

Source: CDC. Guidelines for the Management of Acute Diarrhea After a Disaster, available at http://www.cdc.gov/disasters/disease/diarrheaguidelines.html

Table 16-41: Evaluation of the Acutely Ill Younger Child (≥1 month–3 years) *The febrile neonate (<28 days of age) is usually treated with empiric parenteral antimicrobial therapy and admitted to the hospital for evaluation of neonatal sepsis.*	
Reassuring findings in an ill young child	**Worrisome findings in an ill young child (toxic appearance)**
Warm, dry, appropriately colored to fingertips	Pale or cyanotic skin
Brisk capillary refill (≤2 sec)	Poor capillary refill
Regards parental face, clings to parent, consolable, age-appropriately resists examination, lusty cry, especially during examination Smiling, interactive as appropriate in relationship to degree of illness	Lethargic, does not age-appropriately resist examination, weak or no cry, especially with examination, or inconsolably irritable
Respiratory rate <50% above ULN for age	Tachypnea with respiratory rate ≥50% ULN for age
Heart rate WNL, adjusted for fever	Tachycardia, even with adjustment for fever
Tolerating oral fluids without vomiting, adequately wet diapers	Unable to take or tolerate oral fluids, vomiting, dry mucous membranes, no evidence of recent (within 4 h) urinary output

Often absent in the seriously ill young child: Hypotension, cool skin, and/or nuchal rigidity

Source: Gould, J. M., Fever in the infant and toddler, available at http://emedicine.medscape.com/article/1834870-overview

50. True or false?

(T/F) The degree of temperature reduction in response to antipyretic therapy is not predictive of presence or absence of bacteremia.

(T/F) Response to antipyretic medication does not change the likelihood of a child's having a serious bacterial infection and should not be used for clinical decision-making.

(T/F) The absence of tachypnea is the most useful clinical finding for ruling out pneumonia in children.

51. You are seeing Benjamin, an 18-month-old, who presents with his mother for a sick visit. His last well-child visit was at age 5 months, when he was up-to-date for recommended immunizations. Mom states that Benjamin has not been seen by another healthcare provider nor received vaccines since his last visit at your practice. He now presents with a 2-day history of crankiness and fever. Benjamin has had a poor appetite for the past 2 days but has not vomited and has been taking small amount of fluids. His last wet diaper was approximately 2 hours ago. Exam reveals T=39.6°C (103.4°F), P=150 BPM, RR=45/min. Additional findings include slightly dry mucous membranes, capillary refill of <2 seconds, oropharyngeal redness, bilateral, red, immobile TMs, and a clear chest. The child has a high-pitched cry, is difficult to console, and does not regard his mother's face. Your next best action is to:

A. Start the child on high-dose PO amoxicillin and analgesic otic drops.

B. Give Benjamin an age- and weight-appropriate dose of an antipyretic with plans to reassess after 1 hour.

C. Initiate an evaluation for sepsis and consider for inpatient admission.

D. Administer IM ceftriaxone and arrange for revisit tomorrow.

Table 16-42: Sepsis Workup Regardless of Age	
Sepsis: Presence of pathogenic organisms or their toxins in the blood and tissues with a resulting systemic inflammatory response	
Consider obtaining serum sepsis markers (lactate, procalcitonin, others) to help stratify the sickest children.	
Test	**Possible findings**
CBC with WBC differential	Bacterial or viral shift
Blood culture	Bacteremia (presence of bacteria in the blood) usually sustained in sepsis
Urinalysis (UA) and urine culture and sensitivity via transurethral catheter or suprapubic tap	In UTI, pyelonephritis- WBC, bacteria, urine culture positive for the offending organisms
LP for CSF analysis and culture	Pleocytosis (WBC in CSF) and other findings consistent with bacterial or viral meningitis
Chest x-ray (CXR)	To assist in diagnosis of pneumonia
Stool culture, fecal WBC count, if diarrhea present	To assist in the diagnosis of shigella or other forms of infectious diarrhea

Source: Graneto, J. W. Emergent Management of Pediatric Patients with Fever, available at http://emedicine.medscape.com/article/801598-overview#a1

Notes:

Additional Study Material and Clinical Guidelines

Table 16-43: Empiric Therapy for Pediatric Community-acquired Pneumonia (CAP) in the Outpatient Setting in Children Ages 3 Months to 17 Years
Duration of therapy=7–14 days with exception of azithromycin

	Presumed bacterial pneumonia	Presumed atypical pneumonia	Presumed influenza pneumonia
<5 years old (preschool)	Amoxicillin, oral (90 mg/kg/d in 2 doses) Alternative: Oral amoxicillin-clavulanate (amoxicillin component, 90 mg/kg/d in 2 doses)	Azithromycin oral (10 mg/kg on day 1, followed by 5 mg/kg/d on days 2–5) Alternatives: Oral clarithromycin (15 mg/kg/d in 2 doses for 7–14 days) or oral erythromycin (40 mg/kg/d in 4 doses)	Oseltamivir
≥5 years old	Oral amoxicillin (90 mg/kg/d in 2 doses to a maximum of 4 g/d); for children with presumed bacterial CAP who do not have clinical, laboratory, or radiographic evidence that distinguishes bacterial CAP from atypical CAP, a macrolide can be added to a beta-lactam antibiotic for empiric therapy Alternative: Oral amoxicillin-clavulanate (amoxicillin component, 90 mg/kg/d in 2 doses to a maximum dose of 4000 mg/d, e.g., one 2000 mg tablet twice daily)	Oral azithromycin (10 mg/kg on day 1, followed by 5 mg/kg/d on days 2–5 to a maximum of 500 mg on day 1, followed by 250 mg on days 2–5) Alternatives: Oral clarithromycin (15 mg/kg/d in 2 doses to a maximum of 1 g/d); erythromycin, doxycycline for children >7 years old	Oseltamivir or zanamivir (for children ≥7 years) Alternatives: Peramivir, oseltamivir, and zanamivir (all IV) are under clinical investigation in children IV zanamivir available for compassionate use.

For children with a history of possible nonserious allergic reactions to amoxicillin, treatment is not well defined and should be individualized. Options include a trial of amoxicillin under clinical observation; a trial of an oral cephalosporin that has substantial activity against *S. pneumoniae*, such as cefpodoxime, cefprozil, or cefuroxime, provided under clinical supervision. Additional options for the penicillin-allergic child include levofloxacin, linezolid, clindamycin, a macrolide; close clinical follow-up and full knowledge of the use of all of these medications in children is needed.

Source: The Management of Community-Acquired Pneumonia in Infants and Children Older Than 3 Months of Age: Clinical Practice Guidelines by the Pediatric Infectious Diseases Society and the Infectious Diseases Society of America, available at www.idsociety.org/uploadedFiles/IDSA/Guidelines-Patient_Care/PDF_Library/2011%20CAP%20in%20Children.pdf

Table 16-44: Antimicrobials for Oral Treatment of Urinary Tract Infection (UTI) in Febrile Infants and Children Ages 2 to 24 Months, Length of Therapy=7–14 days

Antimicrobial	Daily dosage
Amoxicillin	20–40 mg/kg/d in 3 doses
Trimethoprim/sulfamethoxazole (TMP/SMX; Bactrim®)	6–12 mg TMP, 30–60 mg SMX per kg per day in 2 doses
Cephalosporin:	
Cefixime	8 mg/kg/d in 2 doses
Cefpodoxime	10 mg/kg/d in 2 doses
Cefprozil	30 mg/kg/d in 2 doses
Cephalexin	50–100 mg/kg/d in 4 doses
Loracarbef	15–30 mg/kg/d in 2 doses

Source: Urinary Tract Infection: Clinical Practice Guideline for the Diagnosis and Management of the Initial UTI in Febrile Infants and Children 2 to 24 Months, available at pediatrics.aappublications.org/content/early/2011/08/24/peds.2011-1330

Table 16-45: Diagnosis and Management of Acute Bacterial Rhinosinusitis (ABRS) in Children	
Exclusions: Neonates and children <1 year of age, children with subacute and chronic sinusitis, anatomic abnormalities of the sinuses, immunodeficiencies, cystic fibrosis, and/or primary ciliary dyskinesia	

Differentiate between acute upper respiratory infection (URI) and ABRS diagnostic criteria	• Uncomplicated viral URI course
	   o Nasal symptoms and/or cough, nasal discharge progresses from clear to purulent to clear without antibiotics, usually within 10 days
	   o Fever early in the illness associated with constitutional symptoms, such as headaches and myalgias that resolve in 24–48 hours as the respiratory symptoms worsen
	• When ABRS should be considered only in the setting of ≥1 of the following:
	   o Worsening URI course, such as double sickening, defined as acute worsening of respiratory symptoms or new fever at day 6–7 of URI
	   o Persistence of URI-like symptoms without improvement after 7–10 days, including nasal discharge, daytime cough, bad breath, fatigue, headache, decreased appetite
	   o Acute onset: T>102.2°F (39°C), purulent nasal discharge, ill appearance for 3–4 days

Treatment options	Acute URI with
	• Persistent illness (nasal discharge of any quality) or daytime cough for >10 days without improvement
	   o Option: Antibiotic treatment or 3 days' observation
	• Worsening course or new onset of nasal discharge, daytime cough, or fever after initial improvement
	   o Option: Antibiotic treatment
	• Severe onset/concurrent fever (102.2°F [39°C]) and purulent nasal discharge >3 consecutive days
	   o Option: Antibiotic treatment

Radiographic recommendations	• Imaging is not necessary in children with uncomplicated ABRS to differentiate viral from bacterial sinusitis. • Contrast CT of paranasal sinuses and/or MRI with contrast should be obtained whenever a child is suspected of having orbital or CNS complications.
Likely pathogens	• *S. pneumoniae* = 30% o Decreased secondary to pneumococcal vaccine • Non-typeable *H. influenzae* = 30% • *M. catarrhalis* = 10% • Sterile (no pathogen isolated, likely viral) = 25%

Source: Clinical Practice Guideline for the Diagnosis and Management of Acute Bacterial Sinusitis in Children Aged 1 to 18 Years. *Pediatrics.* 2013;132:e262-e280.

Table 16-46: ABRS Antimicrobial Choices in Children
Duration of therapy=10−14 days (differs from 5−10-day therapy recommended for adults)

Initial treatment	No improvement in 72 hours	Worse at 72 hours
Observation	Additional observation OR antibiotic therapy	Amoxicillin 80–90 mg/kg/d PO with or without clavulanate
Amoxicillin* 80–90 mg/kg/d PO	Additional observation OR HD amoxicillin-clavulanate PO	HD amoxicillin-clavulanate PO
HD amoxicillin-clavulanate PO	Continue HD amoxicillin-clavulanate or change to clindamycin AND cefixime OR linezolid AND cefixime OR levofloxacin (all PO)	Clindamycin AND cefixime OR linezolid AND cefixime OR levofloxacin (all PO)

*In the case of PCN allergy, both non-type I reaction (delayed or late, >72 hours) and type I (immediate, severe reaction) can safely be treated with cefdinir, cefuroxime, or cefpodoxime. Consider allergy testing for PCN and cephalosporin in both cases prior to initiation of treatment. p.e270

Source: Clinical Practice Guideline for the Diagnosis and Management of Acute Bacterial Sinusitis in Children Aged 1 to 18 Years. *Pediatrics.* 2013;132:e262-e280.

Performing Preventive Services: A Bright Futures Handbook, available at

- http://brightfutures.aap.org/continuing_education.html

Important additional study resources available through your Fitzgerald Health online learning portal at fhea.com/npexpert

- Resource 16-1: Anticipated Early Childhood Development Milestones
- Resource 16-2: Language Milestones
- Resource 16-3: Alterations in Childhood Growth
- Resource 16-4: Plumbism: Risk Factors, Assessment and Intervention (Children<15 Years old)
- Resource 16-5: Assessing Asthma Control and Adjusting Therapy in Children 0−4 Years of Age and Assessing Asthma Control and Adjusting Therapy in Children 5−11 Years of Age
- Resource 16-6: Down Syndrome (DS) Features in the Newborn
- Resource 16-7: Car Safety Seat Use: The Latest American Academy of Pediatrics Recommendations

Bonus questions for this chapter available through your Fitzgerald Health learning portal at fhea.com/npexpert.

Resources for Additional Study

Books:

Fitzgerald, M. A., (2017) Pediatrics, Nurse Practitioner Certification Examination and Practice Preparation, 5th Edition, Philadelphia, PA: F. A. Davis.

Audio programs:

Fitzgerald, M. A. Bacterial Pharyngitis, Conjunctivitis, Acute Otitis Media: A Focus on the Latest Treatment Recommendations, North Andover, MA: Fitzgerald Health Education Associates.

Miller, S.K. Prescribing for the Relief of Symptoms Update, North Andover, MA: Fitzgerald Health Education Associates.

Yates, C. M. Acute Asthma Exacerbations and Acute Uncomplicated Bronchitis: An Evidence-based Approach to Management, North Andover, MA: Fitzgerald Health Education Associates.

Yates, C. M. Asthma Update: An Evidence-based Approach to Management Throughout the Lifespan, North Andover, MA: Fitzgerald Health Education Associates.

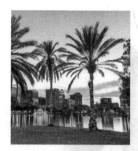
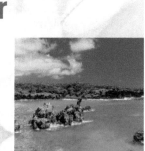
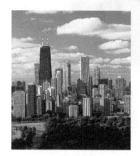
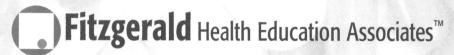

Additional Study Resources Available at <u>fhea.com</u>

Exam Prep

Fitzgerald, M.A. (2017) <u>Nurse Practitioner Certification Examination and Practice Preparation</u>, 5th Edition, Philadelphia, PA: F. A. Davis.

Kennedy-Malone, L. (2014) <u>Advanced Practice Nursing in the Care of Older Adults</u>, Philadelphia, PA: F. A. Davis.

Rhoads, J. (2014) <u>Clinical Consult to Psychiatric Nursing for Advanced Practice</u>, New York, NY: Springer Publishing.

Sefcik, D. (2012) <u>How to Study for Standardized Tests</u>, Sudbury, MA: Jones & Bartlett Publishers.

Winland-Brown, J. (2013) <u>Adult-Gerontology and Family Nurse Practitioner Certification Examination: Review Questions and Strategies</u>, 4th Edition, Philadelphia, PA: F. A. Davis.

Fitzgerald Test Bank

Fitzgerald, M.A. <u>Comprehensive 350-Question Prep Test for Adult-Gerontology NP Certifications</u>, North Andover, MA: Fitzgerald Health Education Associates.

Fitzgerald, M.A. <u>Comprehensive 350-Question Prep Test for Family NP Certification</u>, North Andover, MA: Fitzgerald Health Education Associates.

Pritham, U.A. <u>Essential 150-Question Prep Test for Women's Health Certification</u>, North Andover, MA: Fitzgerald Health Education Associates.

Quick-Look References for Practice and Exam Prep

Barankin, B. (2006) <u>Derm Notes: Dermatology Clinical Pocket Guide</u>, Philadelphia, PA: F. A. Davis.

Desai, S. (2009) <u>Clinician's Guide to Laboratory Medicine: Pocket</u>, Houston, TX: MD2B.

Feeney, S., Fitzgerald, M.A. (2017) <u>Pediatric Physical Assessment Cue Cards</u>, 10th Edition, North Andover, MA: Fitzgerald Health Education Associates.

Ferri, F. (2005) <u>Ferri's Fast Facts</u>, St. Louis, MO: Elsevier Health Sciences.

Ferri, F. (2014) <u>Ferri's Practical Guide: Fast Facts for Patient Care</u>, 9th Edition, St. Louis, MO: Elsevier Health Sciences.

Habif, T. (2012) <u>Dermatology DDxDeck</u>, 2nd Edition, St. Louis, MO: Elsevier Health Sciences.

Jones, K. B. (2015) <u>ECG Notes: Interpretation and Management Guide</u>, 3rd Edition, Philadelphia, PA: F.A. Davis.

Jones, K.B. (2016) <u>Pocket Anatomy and Physiology</u>, 3rd Edition, Philadelphia, PA: F.A. Davis.

McCaffrey, R. (2014) <u>NP Notes: Nurse Practitioner's Clinical Pocket Guide</u>, 2nd Edition, Philadelphia, PA: F. A. Davis.

McDevitt, L., Tombasco, M. (2016) <u>Orthopedic Physical Assessment Cue Cards</u>, North Andover, MA: Fitzgerald Health Education Associates

Pedersen, D. (2010) <u>Pocket Psych Drugs: Point-of-Care Clinical Guide</u>, Philadelphia, PA: F. A. Davis.

Sommers, M. (2012) <u>Pocket Diseases</u>, Philadelphia, PA: F. A. Davis.

Weston, W. (2016) <u>Pediatric Dermatology DDxDeck</u>, 2nd Edition, St. Louis, MO: Elsevier Health Sciences.

Wright, W. L. (2015) <u>Adult Physical Assessment Cue Cards</u>, 8th Edition, North Andover, MA: Fitzgerald Health Education Associates.

References

Anderson, B. C. (2006) <u>Office Orthopedics for Primary Care: Diagnosis</u>, St. Louis, MO: Elsevier Health Sciences.

Anderson, B. C. (2006) <u>Office Orthopedics for Primary Care: Treatment</u>, 3rd Edition, St. Louis, MO: Elsevier Health Sciences.

Campo, T., et al. (2015) <u>Essential Procedures for Practitioners in Emergency, Urgent, and Primary Care Settings</u>, 2nd Edition, New York, NY: Springer Publishing.

Cash, J. (2014) <u>Family Practice Guidelines</u>, 3rd Edition, New York, NY: Springer Publishing.

Dains, J. (2015) <u>Advanced Health Assessment and Clinical Diagnosis in Primary Care</u>, 5th Edition, St. Louis, MO: Elsevier Health Sciences.

Duderstadt, K. (2013) <u>Pediatric Physical Examination — An Illustrated Handbook</u>, 2nd Edition, St. Louis, MO: Elsevier Health Sciences.

Ferri, F. (2014) <u>Ferri's Best Test: A Practical Guide to Clinical Laboratory Medicine and Diagnostic Imaging</u>, 3rd Edition, St. Louis, MO: Elsevier Health Sciences.

Goolsby, M. J. (2014) <u>Advanced Assessment: Interpreting Findings and Formulating Differential Diagnoses</u>, 3rd Edition, Philadelphia, PA: F. A. Davis.

Knechtel, M. (2013) <u>EKGs for the Nurse Practitioner and Physician Assistant</u>, New York, NY: Springer Publishing.

McCance, K. (2014) <u>Pathophysiology: The Biologic Basis for Disease in Adults and Children</u>, 7th Edition, St. Louis, MO: Elsevier Health Sciences.

Mettler, F. (2013) <u>Essentials of Radiology</u>, 3rd Edition, St. Louis, MO: Elsevier Health Sciences.

Singer, A.J. (2010) <u>Skin and Soft Tissue Injuries and Infections: A Practical Evidence Based Guide</u>, Ashland, OH: PMPH-USA Ltd.

Online Skills Programs

Blumm, R. <u>Suturing Skills: The Art of Wound Repair</u>, North Andover, MA: Fitzgerald Health Education Associates.

Campo, T. M. <u>Abdominal & Pelvic Pain Evaluation: From Differential Diagnosis to Diagnostic Imaging</u>, North Andover, MA: Fitzgerald Health Education Associates.

Campo, T. M. <u>Chest Pain Evaluation: From Differential Diagnosis to Diagnostic Imaging</u>, North Andover, MA: Fitzgerald Health Education Associates.

Campo, T. M. <u>Chest X-ray Interpretation: A Systematic Approach</u>, North Andover, MA: Fitzgerald Health Education Associates.

Campo, T. M. <u>Dental Examinations: Identifying Common Disorders</u>, North Andover, MA: Fitzgerald Health Education Associates.

Campo, T. M. <u>Ophthalmology Examinations: Identifying Common Disorders</u>, North Andover, MA: Fitzgerald Health Education Associates.

Campo, T. M. <u>Radiology Diagnostic Fundamentals: When & What to Order</u>, North Andover, MA: Fitzgerald Health Education Associates.

Fitzgerald, M.A. <u>Honing Your Cardiac Exam: A Focus on Heart Sounds and Murmurs</u>, North Andover, MA: Fitzgerald Health Education Associates.

Additional Study Resources Available at <u>fhea.com</u>

Miller, S.K. <u>12-Lead ECG Interpretation: A Primary Care Perspective</u>, North Andover, MA: Fitzgerald Health Education Associates.

Miller, S.K. <u>Cardiac Rhythms: The Clinician's Approach to Accurate Interpretation</u>, North Andover, MA: Fitzgerald Health Education Associates.

Miller, S. K. <u>Beyond the Basics in 12-Lead ECG Interpretation</u>, North Andover, MA: Fitzgerald Health Education Associates.

Also available on CD-ROM

DVD Programs (most available as online programs)

Blasen, L. S. <u>Common Dermatologic Procedures</u>, North Andover, MA: Fitzgerald Health Education Associates.

Blasen, L. S. <u>Common Office Procedures</u>, North Andover, MA: Fitzgerald Health Education Associates.

Fitzgerald, M. A. <u>Expert Exam: Abdomen</u>, North Andover, MA: Fitzgerald Health Education Associates.

Kaminsky, D. <u>Demystifying Pulmonary Function Testing</u>, North Andover, MA: Fitzgerald Health Education Associates.

McDevitt, L. <u>Expert Exam: Cervical, Thoracic and Lumbar Spine</u>, North Andover, MA: Fitzgerald Health Education Associates.

McDevitt, L., Tombasco, M. <u>Expert Exam: ENT Skills for Primary and Acute Care Practitioners</u>, North Andover, MA: Fitzgerald Health Education Associates.

McDevitt, L. <u>Expert Exam: Practical Orthopedics - Shoulder</u>, North Andover, MA: Fitzgerald Health Education Associates.

Tombasco, M., Wright, W. L. <u>Expert Exam: Conducting a Pre-sports Physical Examination</u>, North Andover, MA: Fitzgerald Health Education Associates.

Tombasco, M. <u>Expert Exam: Practical Orthopedics - Knee</u>, North Andover, MA: Fitzgerald Health Education Associates.

Wright, W. L. <u>Expert Exam: Physical Examination of the Adult</u>, North Andover, MA: Fitzgerald Health Education Associates.

Wright, W. L. <u>Expert Exam: The Primary Care Neurologic Exam</u>, North Andover, MA: Fitzgerald Health Education Associates.

Continuing Education at fhea.com

- Pharmacology Update
- Acquiring Expert Skills
- Online seminars

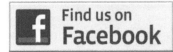

www.facebook.com/fitzgeraldhealth

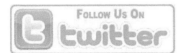

@npcert

Learn to Prescribe with Confidence through Fitzgerald Pharmacology Packages

NP students & new NPs will gain knowledge needed to prepare for certification and practice.
Available pharmacology packages:

- **Family NP Pharmacology**

- **Adult-Gerontology NP Pharmacology**

- **Gerontological Pharmacology**

For more information
or to purchase these products,
visit FHEA.com

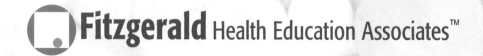

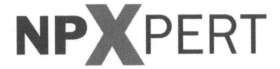

Online Course Resources

and

Review of Questions

for

All Modes of the
*Nurse Practitioner Certification
Exam Review & Advanced
Practice Update*

Fitzgerald Health course material expands and enhances the classroom learning experience. The online material is not supplemental but rather an <u>integral part of the course</u> and <u>important to your success on the exam</u>. Be sure to take advantage of the online portions of this course in order to maximize your results on the exam and preparation for practice. Printable handouts are available through your online learning portal for these lectures.

MAKE SURE YOU HAVE COMPLETED ALL PARTS OF THE COURSE.

Family nurse practitioner track (11.4 hours total)

- AANPCP vs. ANCC: A Comparison of the Examinations
- Common Infant Dermatological Conditions
- Disorders Revealed by the Cardiac Exam: A Focus on Heart Sounds and Murmurs
- Common Musculoskeletal Problems
- Principles of Family Planning
- Primary Care of the Woman during Pregnancy
- Special Considerations in Geriatric Prescribing: Issues of Safety and Efficacy
- Professional Issues

Adult-Gerontology nurse practitioner track (11.7 hours total)

- AANPCP vs. ANCC: A Comparison of the Examinations
- Disorders Revealed by the Cardiac Exam: A Focus on Heart Sounds and Murmurs
- Common Musculoskeletal Problems
- Special Considerations in Geriatric Prescribing: Issues of Safety and Efficacy
- Foundations of Gerontology: Theories of Aging, Care of the Frail Elder
- Principles of Family Planning
- Primary Care of the Adolescent
- Professional Issues

Review of course questions *PLUS* bonus questions

- Authorized users have access to an online review of course questions and bonus questions. Offered chapter-by-chapter is a review of the course questions. Following the course questions are the *bonus* questions for the chapter. <u>You will have 2 attempts for this online exam and 6 months of access to complete this portion of the program</u>. Upon completion, you may review your incorrect responses.

Take the practice exam online

- Authorized users have access to an online practice exam of 150 questions. Be sure to allow enough time to take the exam in one sitting. <u>You will have 2 attempts for this online exam and 6 months of access to complete this portion of the program</u>. Upon completion, you may review your incorrect responses.

For instructions to access the online course materials, please visit:

https://fhea.com/Access_Online_Learning.aspx